Blood & Circulatory Disorders Sourcebook

Basic Information about Disorders Such As Anemia, Hemorrhage, Shock, Embolism, and Thrombosis, along with Facts Concerning Rh Factor, Blood Banks, Blood Donation Programs, and Transfusions

Edited by Linda M. Ross. 600 pages. 1998. 0-7808-0203-9. $75.

Burns Sourcebook

Basic Information about Heat, Chemical, Electrical, and Sun Burns, along with Facts about Burn Treatment and Recovery, and Reports on Current Research Initiatives

Edited by Allan R. Cook. 600 pages. 1998. 0-7808-0204-7. $75.

Cancer Sourcebook

Basic Information on Cancer Types, Symptoms, Diagnostic Methods, and Treatments, Including Statistics on Cancer Occurrences Worldwide and the Risks Associated with Known Carcinogens and Activities

Edited by Frank E. Bair. 932 pages. 1990. 1-55888-888-8. $75.

"This publication's nontechnical nature and very comprehensive format make it useful for both the general public and undergraduate students."
— *Choice, Oct '90*

"This compact collection of reliable information, written in a positive, hopeful tone, is an invaluable tool for helping patients and patients' families and friends to take the first steps in coping with the many difficulties of cancer." — *Medical Reference Services Quarterly, Winter '91*

"An important resource for the general reader trying to understand the complexities of cancer."
— *American Reference Books Annual, '91*

Cancer Sourcebook for Women

Basic Information about Specific Forms of Cancer That Affect Women, Featuring Facts about Breast Cancer, Cervical Cancer, Ovarian Cancer, Cancer of the Uterus and Uterine Sarcoma, Cancer of the Vagina, and Cancer of the Vulva; Statistical and Demographic Data; Treatments, Self-Help Management Suggestions, and Current Research Initiatives

Edited by Allan R. Cook and Peter D. Dresser. 524 pages. 1996. 0-7808-0076-1. $75.

"This timely book is highly recommended for consumer health and patient education collections in all libraries." — *Library Journal, Apr '96*

"The availability under one cover of all these pertinent publications, grouped under cohesive headings, makes this certainly a most useful sourcebook."
— *Choice, Jun '96*

"Laudably, the book portrays the feelings of the cancer victim, as well as her mate . . . .both benefit from the gold mine of information nestled between the two covers of this book. It is hard to conceive of any library that would not want it as part of its collection. Recommended."
— *Academic Library Book Review, Summer '96*

". . . written in easily understandable, non-technical language. Recommended for public libraries or hospital and academic libraries that collect patient education or consumer health materials."
— *Medical Reference Services Quarterly, Spring '97*

New Cancer Sourcebook

Basic Information about Major Forms and Stages of Cancer, Featuring Facts about Primary and Secondary Tumors of the Respiratory, Nervous, Lymphatic, Circulatory, Skeletal, and Gastrointestinal Systems, and Specific Organs; Statistical and Demographic Data, Treatment Options, and Strategies for Coping

Edited by Allan R. Cook. 1,313 pages. 1996. 0-7808-0041-9. $75.

"This book is an excellent resource. The dialogue is simple, direct, and comprehensive."
— *Doody's Health Sciences Book Review, Nov '96*

"The amount of factual and useful information is extensive. The writing is very clear, geared to general readers. Recommended for all levels."
— *Choice, Jan '97*

Cardiovascular Diseases & Disorders Sourcebook

Basic Information about Cardiovascular Diseases and Disorders, Featuring Facts about the Cardiovascular System, Demographic and Statistical Data, Descriptions of Pharmacological and Surgical Interventions, Lifestyle Modifications, and a Special Section Focusing on Heart Disorders in Children

Edited by Karen Bellenir and Peter D. Dresser. 683 pages. 1995. 0-7808-0032-X. $75.

". . . comprehensive format provides an extensive overview on this subject." — *Choice, Jun '96*

"Easily understood, complete, up-to-date resource. This well executed public health tool will make valuable information available to those that need it most, patients and their families. The typeface, sturdy nonreflective paper, and library binding add a feel of quality found wanting in other publications. Highly recommended for academic and general libraries."
— *Academic Library Book Review, Summer '96*

Continues next page

Communication Disorders Sourcebook

Basic Information about Deafness and Hearing Loss, Speech and Language Disorders, Voice Disorders, Balance and Vestibular Disorders, and Disorders of Smell, Taste, and Touch

Edited by Linda M. Ross. 533 pages. 1996. 0-7808-0077-X. $75.

"This is skillfully edited and is a welcome resource for the layperson. It should be found in every public and medical library."
— *Doody's Health Sciences Book Review, May '96*

Congenital Disorders Sourcebook

Basic Information about Disorders Acquired during Gestation, Including Spina Bifida, Hydrocephalus, Cerebral Palsy, Heart Defects, Craniofacial Abnormalities, Fetal Alcohol Syndrome, and More, along with Current Treatment Options and Statistical Data

Edited by Karen Bellenir. 607 pages. 1997. 0-7808-0205-5. $75.

Consumer Issues in Health Care Sourcebook

Basic Information about Consumer Health Concerns, Including an Explanation of Physician Specialties, How to Choose a Doctor, How to Prepare for a Hospital Visit, Ways to Avoid Fraudulent "Miracle" Cures, How to Use Medications Safely, What to Look for when Choosing a Nursing Home, and End-of-Life Planning

Edited by Wendy Wilcox. 600 pages. 1998. 0-7808-0221-7. $75.

Contagious & Non-Contagious Infectious Diseases Sourcebook

Basic Information about Contagious Diseases like Measles, Polio, Hepatitis B, and Infectious Mononucleosis, and Non-Contagious Infectious Diseases like Tetanus and Toxic Shock Syndrome, and Diseases Occurring as Secondary Infections Such As Shingles and Reye Syndrome, along with Vaccination, Prevention, and Treatment Information, and a Section Describing Emerging Infectious Disease Threats

Edited by Karen Bellenir and Peter D. Dresser. 566 pages. 1996. 0-7808-0075-3. $75.

Diabetes Sourcebook

Basic Information about Insulin-Dependent and Noninsulin-Dependent Diabetes Mellitus, Gestational Diabetes, and Diabetic Complications, Symptoms, Treatment, and Research Results, Including Statistics on Prevalence, Morbidity, and Mortality, along with Source Listings for Further Help and Information

Edited by Karen Bellenir and Peter D. Dresser. 827 pages. 1994. 1-55888-751-2. $75.

"Very informative and understandable for the layperson without being simplistic. It provides a comprehensive overview for laypersons who want a general understanding of the disease or who want to focus on various aspects of the disease."
— *Bulletin of the MLA, Jan '96*

Diet & Nutrition Sourcebook

Basic Information about Nutrition, Including the Dietary Guidelines for Americans, the Food Guide Pyramid, and Their Applications in Daily Diet, Nutritional Advice for Specific Age Groups, Current Nutritional Issues and Controversies, the New Food Label and How to Use It to Promote Healthy Eating, and Recent Developments in Nutritional Research

Edited by Dan R. Harris. 662 pages. 1996. 0-7808-0084-2. $75.

"It is so refreshing to find a reliable and factual reference book. Recommended to aspiring professionals, librarians, and others seeking and giving reliable dietary advice. An excellent compilation."
— *Choice, Feb '97*

"Recommended for public and medical libraries that receive general information requests on nutrition. It is readable and will appeal to those interested in learning more about healthy dietary practices."
— *Medical Reference Services Quarterly, Fall '97*

Ear, Nose & Throat Disorders Sourcebook

Basic Information about Disorders of the Ears, Nose, Sinus Cavities, Tonsils, Adenoids, Pharynx, and Larynx, along with Statistical and Demographic Data and Reports on Current Research Initiatives

Edited by Linda M. Ross. 600 pages. 1998. 0-7808-0206-3. $75.

Endocrine & Metabolic Diseases & Disorders Sourcebook

Basic Information for the Layperson about Disorders Such As Graves' Disease, Goiter, Cushing's Syndrome, and Hormonal Imbalances, along with Reports on Current Research Initiatives

Edited by Linda M. Ross. 600 pages. 1998. 0-7808-0207-1. $75.

Continues on back end sheets

Endocrine
and Metabolic
DISORDERS
SOURCEBOOK

Health Reference Series

Volume Thirty-six

Endocrine and Metabolic
DISORDERS SOURCEBOOK

*Basic Information for the Layperson about
Pancreatic and Insulin-Related Disorders such as
Pancreatitis, Diabetes, and Hypoglycemia;
Adrenal Gland Disorders such as Cushing's
Syndrome, Addison's Disease, and Congenital
Adrenal Hyperplasia; Pituitary Gland Disorders
such as Growth Hormone Deficiency, Acromegaly,
and Pituitary Tumors; Thyroid Disorders such as
Hypothyroidism, Graves' Disease, Hashimoto's
Disease, and Goiter; Hyperparathyroidism; and
Other Diseases and Syndromes of Hormone
Imbalance or Metabolic Dysfunction Along with
Reports on Current Research Initiatives*

Edited by
Linda M. Shin

Omnigraphics, Inc.

Penobscot Building / Detroit, MI 48226

Bibliographic Note

Because this page cannot legibly accommodate all the copyright notices, the Bibliographic Note portion of the Preface constitutes an extension of the copyright notice.

Edited by Linda M. Shin

Peter D. Dresser, Managing Editor, *Health Reference Series*
Karen Bellenir, Series Editor, *Health Reference Series*

Omnigraphics, Inc.

Matthew P. Barbour, *Manager, Production and Fulfillment*
Laurie Lanzen Harris, *Vice President, Editorial Director*
Peter E. Ruffner, *Vice President, Administration*
James A. Sellgren, *Vice President, Operations and Finance*
Jane J. Steele, *Marketing Consultant*

Frederick G. Ruffner, Jr., Publisher

©1999, Omnigraphics, Inc.

Library of Congress Cataloging-in-Publication Data

Endocrine & metabolic disorders sourcrebook : basic information for the layperson about pancreatic and insulin-related disorders such as pancreatis, diabetes, and hypoglycemia . . . / edited by Linda M. Shin.
   p. cm. -- (Health reference series ; v. 36)
  Includes bibliographical references and index.
  ISBN 0-7808-0207-1 (alk. paper)
   1. Endocrine glands--Diseases--Popular works. 2. Metabolism--Disorders--Popular works. I. Shin, Linda M. II. Series.
  RA648.E418   1998   98-6657
  616.4--dc21   CIP

∞

This book is printed on acid-free paper meeting the ANSI Z39.48 Standard. The infinity symbol that appears above indicates that the paper in this book meets that standard.

Printed in the United States

Table of Contents

Part III: Adrenal Gland Disorders

Part IV: Pituitary and Growth Disorders

Part V: Thyroid and Parathyroid Disorders

Part VI: Other Disorders of Endocrine and Metabolic Functioning

Preface

The glands of the endocrine system are responsible for secreting the hormones necessary for normal human growth, development, and metabolism. Their balance must be precise. Too much, not enough, or improperly timed hormonal secretions can lead to serious health consequences. Yet, according to one estimate, approximately 10% of the people in many developed nations can expect to experience some form of endocrine disorder. These arise from diverse causes including tumors, dietary factors, and genetics.

Until a problem develops, many people may be unfamiliar with the endocrine system or be unaware of its role in maintaining health. As a result, early symptoms of disorder are frequently overlooked or misdiagnosed. For example, the Thyroid Foundation of America estimates that half of the people who suffer from an underactive thyroid do not know it and have never been treated.

This *Sourcebook* contains information about the glands of the endocrine system, its components, the hormones it regulates, and the metabolic consequences of various disorders. Readers will learn to recognize symptoms, understand diagnostic tests, and become acquainted with various treatment options.

How to Use This Book

This book is divided into parts and chapters. Parts focus on broad areas of interest. Chapters are devoted to single topics within a part.

Part I: Introduction to the Endocrine System and Human Metabolism provides an overview of the endocrine system, explains its various glands, and gives background information on normal hormonal functioning. A directory of organizations for endocrine and metabolic diseases, along with web site information when available, is also included.

Part II: Pancreatic and Diabetic Disorders begins with background information on the role of the pancreas, a gland responsible for the production of insulin, glucagon, and somatostatin. Individual chapters present information about diseases that affect the pancreas or that occur as a result of improper regulation or use of the pancreatic hormones. The role of insulin and metabolic control in diabetic disorders is presented. Readers with additional questions about specific diabetes treatments and complications will find more information in *Diabetes Sourcebook*, Volume 3 of Omnigraphics' *Health Reference Series*.

Part III: Adrenal Gland Disorders provides information about Cushing's Syndrome, Addison's Disease, and Congenital Adrenal Hyperplasia, disorders resulting from impaired regulation of cortisol, a hormone produced by the adrenal gland.

Part IV: Pituitary and Growth Disorders offers information about disorders that results from pituitary tumors and imbalances of the major pituitary hormones, such as growth hormone and prolactin

Part V: Thyroid and Parathyroid Disorders explains the role played by the thyroid gland in controlling the body's metabolism and the function of the parathyroid glands in regulating calcium in the blood, bones, and urine. Individual chapters address topics such as goiter, hyperthyroidism, hypothyroidism, thyroiditis, and hyperparathyroidism.

Part VI: Other Disorders of Endocrine and Metabolic Functioning presents information about enzyme deficiencies and other syndromes and diseases that result from, or impact, hormonal and metabolic processes. Readers seeking further details about inborn errors of metabolism will find additional information in *Genetic Disorders Sourcebook*, Volume 13 of Omnigraphics' *Health Reference Series*.

Bibliographic Note

This volume contains documents and excerpts from publications issued by the following government agencies: National Center for

Research Resources (NCRR), National Cancer Institute (NCI), National Heart, Lung, and Blood Institute (NHLBI), National Institute of Child Health and Human Development (NICHD), National Institute of Diabetes and Digestive and Kidney Diseases (NIDDK), Office of Medical Applications of Research (OMAR), and the U.S. Department of Health and Human Services (DHHS).

In addition, this volume contains copyrighted documents from the following organizations: Harvard Medical School, Human Growth Foundation, National Adrenal Diseases Foundation, National Graves' Disease Foundation, Pituitary Tumor Network Association, the Thyroid Foundation of America, the Thyroid Society for Education and Research, and the University of Texas Health Science Center.

Copyrighted articles from the following journals are included: *Diabetes Care, Diabetes Forecast, JAMA (Journal of the American Medical Association), Mayo Clinic Health Letter, New England Journal of Medicine, Sports Medicine,* and *Thyroid Signpost*; along with excerpts from the following books: *The Endocrine System* (Chelsea House Publishers), *How Hormones Work* (Franklin Watts), *Physician's Guide to Rare Diseases* (Dowden Publishing Company, Inc.).

All copyrighted material is reprinted with permission. Document numbers where applicable and specific source citations are provided on the first page of each chapter. Every effort has been made to secure all necessary rights to reprint the copyrighted material. If any omissions have been made, contact Omnigraphics to make corrections for future editions.

Acknowledgements

Many people and organizations helped make this book a reality. Special thanks go to the Human Growth Foundation, National Adrenal Diseases Foundation, National Graves' Disease Foundation, Pituitary Tumor Network Association, The Thyroid Foundation of America, The Thyroid Society for Education and Research, and the University of Texas Health Science Center. In addition, thanks go to Margaret Mary Missar for obtaining many of the documents included in this volume.

Note from the Editor

This book is part of Omnigraphics' *Health Reference Series*. The series provides basic information about a broad range of medical concerns. It is not intended to serve as a tool for diagnosing illness, in prescribing treatments, or as a substitute for the physician/patient relationship. All persons concerned about medical symptoms or the possibility of disease are encouraged to seek professional care from an appropriate health care provider.

Part One

Introduction to the Endocrine System and Human Metabolism

Chapter 1

An Overview of the Endocrine System

Endocrinology is the branch of medical science that explores the structure of the endocrine glands and the hormones they secrete. Although some observations of this bodily system date back to ancient times, most research on the endocrine system did not occur until the modern era.

In the 3rd century B.C., the ancient Greek philosopher and scientist Aristotle observed the varying effects of castration on calves and bulls, and long before, in the ancient civilizations of Egypt and China, human behavioral changes resulting from removal of the testes were common knowledge. (Castration was practiced in both these civilizations to produce a servile class of men called eunuchs.) It was not really until the 17th century, however, that scientists gained empirical knowledge of the system of glands and their hormonal functions.

Three Centuries of Discovery

One of the first important steps regarding physiological exploration occurred in 17th-century England, when the scientist Thomas Wharton disproved the commonly held belief that the brain was a gland that secreted mucus. Wharton was also the first to recognize the difference between the ductless and ductile glands, which differentiates the endocrine and exocrine systems.

Excerpted from *The Endocrine System*, ©1990 Chelsea House Publishers, New York, New York. All rights reserved; reprinted with permission.

The 17th century also saw the first observations concerning the existence of hormones. In the 1690s, Fredrik Ruysch, a well-respected Dutch scientist, claimed that the thyroid gland "poured important substances into the blood stream." Thirty years earlier, Theophile Bordeu, a Frenchman regarded by many as the founder of endocrinology, had declared that some parts of the body gave off "emanations" that had dramatic effects on other parts of the body.

Toward the end of the 18th century, doctors began to associate a swollen neck, staring, or "bug" eyes, a racing pulse, and uncontrollable muscle tremors with a swollen thyroid gland. Some patients had such distended glands that it appeared as if huge disfiguring growths were attempting to burst from the front of their necks. This enlargement is called a toxic-goiter, which is now known to be caused by excess production of the thyroid hormone.

The earliest information about the endocrine system was first obtained from the study of patients with diseased glands. In 1849, British scientist Thomas Addison reported on 11 patients who exhibited the symptoms of anemia: their blood lacked sufficient hemoglobin, (the compound in red blood cells that carries oxygen to all the cells of the body); they frequently felt faint or lethargic; they had weak hearts; and their skin was a sickly, gray color. They died soon after he examined them. Addison performed autopsies on all of these patients and discovered that every one of them had diseased adrenal glands. Addison named the disease "melasma suprarenale," but it was later changed to Addison's disease. (President John F. Kennedy suffered from this disorder, but his doctors were able to control its effects.)

The same year Addison made his discoveries, A. A. Berthold, a German doctor, released the results of his experiments with six young male chickens, providing the first experimental proof of the existence and functioning of hormones. Berthold had castrated four of the chickens. Two of these were left to develop without their testes. He transplanted the testes of two other chickens back into their bodies, but in a distant location from where the testes had originated. The two chickens who were not castrated grew into normal roosters, sprouting the combs, wattles, and feathers of adult male birds. In contrast, the two chickens who developed without their testes never developed adult male characteristics; their combs atrophied or shrunk. This provided the first documented proof of a hormonal deficiency.

What is equally interesting, however, is that the two birds who had their testes removed and then relocated also developed into normal, sexually mature roosters. This offered evidence that hormones travel freely through the bloodstream and that where they originate is not crucial to how they function, as long as they are directly connected to the circulatory system.

Over the last hundred years medical researchers have greatly advanced this early exploration of the endocrine system. What follows is an overview of how this system functions.

How The System Works

Whereas the respiratory system supplies oxygen to the blood, and the cardiovascular system controls the circulation of blood throughout the body, the endocrine system regulates the flow of hormones in the bloodstream. These hormones play a central role in making humans what they are; they determine rate of growth and maturation and directly influence intelligence, physical agility, and sexual drives.

Production and Secretion of Hormones

The endocrine system, along with the nervous system, controls the production and secretion of hormones. Scientists once believed that the endocrine system functioned independently of the nervous system, but they now recognize the interdependence of these two regulatory systems.

The endocrine and nervous systems both regulate bodily activities, but they do so in fundamentally different ways. Endocrine glands send chemical messengers through the bloodstream, whereas the nervous system depends on electrical rather than chemical signals and sends them along a network of specialized cells called neurons. There are exceptions to these rules, however: Some neurons secrete chemicals called neurohormones, which function much like normal hormones, and some endocrine glands secrete hormones that directly influence the activity of the nervous system. Therefore, despite the basic distinction between the functioning of the two systems, they remain intertwined to a great degree.

Working in conjunction, then, the endocrine system and the nervous system provide continual information, or feedback, about the amount of hormones that are circulating through the bloodstream. If the level of any hormone in the blood is too low, the systems will signal the appropriate gland. If the hormone level is too high, another set of signals will shut down glandular production. This is known as negative feedback control. It gets this name because it works on the principle of reversing any excess or deficit that exists. It is through negative feedback that most hormone levels are regulated, much like water in a tank: When the tank is low, the fill mechanism will automatically allow water to enter. Once the tank is full, the fill mechanism shuts off the supply of water.

A few hormones, however, operate on a positive feedback principle. In this case, the presence of one hormone stimulates the production and secretion of another. The menstrual cycle in females provides an excellent example. Each month one of the ovaries produces an egg. As the egg grows, the ovary releases the hormone estrogen into the bloodstream. The rise in estrogen triggers the pituitary gland to release an additional sex hormone called LH, which stands for luteinizing hormone. In turn, LH stimulates the ovary to release the mature egg into the nearby oviduct. This final process, called ovulation, is the result of a chain reaction that began with a chemical message from the endocrine system.

Hormonal Reception

How do hormones know where to go to find appropriate target cells? Actually, they do not. They are simply carried along in the bloodstream, where they will eventually come into contact with cells that are programmed to respond to their presence. It is up to these target cells to react as the hormones pass by. They do this through a mechanism called a receptor. Essentially a large protein molecule, a receptor is continually on the lookout for a specific type of chemical, in this case a specific hormone; when one passes by, the receptor recognizes it, attracts it, and captures it. Because hormones are normally produced in minute quantities, receptors must be extremely sensitive and efficient. This sensitivity is the most crucial factor for the expression of hormonal activity. If receptor sites break down, hormones will not be able to affect target cells. This results in conditions similar to those caused by the lack of adequate hormone production.

Most hormones—insulin, for example—are too large to enter a target cell. They attach themselves to an external receptor and use it to transmit a message to the cell's interior. Some hormones, such as testosterone, a male sex hormone, are small enough to penetrate the cell's surface. They stimulate internal receptors and travel into the nucleus. Here, they activate specific genes that carry out the hormone's function.

Then the action begins. The target cells respond. The exact nature of their response depends on the type of cell. Muscle cells may increase or decrease contraction. Epithelial cells, which are found in skin surfaces and in the walls of many internal organs, alter the rate at which liquids are allowed to pass through them. Gland cells function as a group to secrete more or less of the chemicals they produce. This allows the body to constantly adjust levels of salt and water in its tissues as well as to regulate the amount of sugar in the blood and the amount of salt in sweat. All of these constant changes help the body maintain a vital chemical balance.

After the hormone has contacted its receptor cell, the continued existence of the hormone is no longer required, and the hormone is either excreted from the circulatory system by the kidneys or degraded by enzymes within the blood, liver, kidney, lungs, or target tissues. If it were not, its biological effect would continue indefinitely as long as the hormone survived.

Endocrinologists can determine hormone levels by studying not only how quickly the glands produce hormones but also how quickly hormones are destroyed. They do this by measuring how long it takes half a dose of a hormone to leave the circulatory system. This period of time, known as a half-life, is a means of predicting the rate at which hormones are eliminated from the body. (The total elimination of a substance is not a useful gauge because it is dramatically influenced by its starting concentration.) This measurement is known as the metabolic clearance rate. It measures the elimination of hormone molecules by both the liver and kidneys. It also takes into account the hormones that target cells ingest and destroy. The metabolic clearance rate can play a significant role in determining the frequency of drug administration.

In brief, hormonal communication can be measured in seven overall stages: It begins with signals from the nervous system or endocrine system that stimulate hormonal production. This is followed by the second and third stages, which involve secretion and delivery to target cells. During the fourth stage the cell receptors recognize the hormone, and in stage five, target cells respond. Once a hormone has performed its function, it enters stage six and is destroyed or degraded. Signaling the elimination of hormone cells is the final stage of communication.

Malfunction

About 10% of the population of most developed nations will experience some form of endocrine disorder. Most endocrine system disorders involve a glandular problem, such as a tumor, which results in either overproduction (hyperfunction) or underproduction (hypofunction) of hormones. In the case of the thyroid gland, hyperthyroidism and hypothyroidism can cause gland enlargement or additional tumors. Toxic goiters provide a very visual symptom of hyperthyroidism, or excess hormone production by the thyroid gland. Simple goiters result from hypothyroidism, a condition that is primarily caused by a lack of iodine in the diet and occurs very rarely today because iodine is now a common ingredient in table salt.

In addition to the overproduction or underproduction of hormones, endocrine system disorders may involve an enhancement or diminishment in the sensitivity of target cells; genetic defects that may cause abnormalities in hormone synthesis; and tumors, cysts, or infections of endocrine glands.

Treatment for the underproduction, or hypofunction, of hormones generally involves simply administering the missing hormones directly into the bloodstream, though in some cases a different hormone or a totally separate chemical may be substituted. Treatment for the overproduction, or hyperfunction, of hormones may take a variety of approaches. If a tumor is causing a gland to hyperfunction, the tumor will usually be removed. In other cases, drugs are prescribed that can block the production of specific hormones.

Chapter 2

How Hormones Work

Hormones have an amazing number of powerful effects upon the body. Depending upon the state of the endocrine system, a person can become thin or fat, acquire many different sex-specific features, have a rapid or slow metabolism, feel pain or be insensitive to it, and grow to the height of a giant or only to that of a dwarf. Because these effects are so varied, each action of a hormone undoubtedly is somewhat unique for each type of cell affected or for each part of the body. In spite of this, many details of how hormones produce some of these amazing effects are now becoming known.

Many hormones are protein hormones, made up of long chains of simple molecules called amino acids. These hormones include insulin, glucagon, parathyroid hormone, calcitonin, IGFs, and all of the pituitary hormones. The remaining hormones—sex hormones and hormones of the adrenal cortex—are steroid hormones that are chemically quite different. These hormones are slightly different forms of the cholesterol molecule and fall into the same category of substances as fats or oils (lipids). These two types of hormones each have characteristic mechanisms of changing cell function.

Protein Hormones

Most protein hormones are long chains of amino acids typically between 50 to 100 amino acids long. The exact sequence of amino acids for each hormone has been worked out within the last five to ten years. This amino acid sequence, different for each protein hormone, causes a completed protein chain to fold up to form a tiny object with a three-dimensional shape specific for that particular sequence of amino acids. Exactly how the differing chemical properties of varying sequences of amino acids interact to cause this specific three-dimensional shape is still a basic and unsolved problem in biology.

What is known at this point is that each protein hormone takes on its own particular shape after being manufactured and secreted by an endocrine cell. Because of this, a hormone can attach to other protein molecules, called receptor proteins, that are present on the surface of target cells. All the powerful effects of protein hormones can come about without the hormone ever entering a cell: protein hormones need only to lightly stick to the surface of a cell to have their effects.

Receptor proteins for hormones float in the thin film of oil (lipid) that forms a watertight barrier around each cell in the body. This film of lipid is called the cell membrane. It is not unusual for a single cell to have 10,000 to 100,000 hormone receptor proteins scattered about on its cell membrane. Each receptor protein can bind (attach to) a hormone because it has a shape that is complementary to the hormone; that is, the hormone and the receptor fit together like two pieces of a jigsaw puzzle.

Once a hormone binds to its cell receptor, one or more intracellular substances, called second messengers, are formed to carry out the instructions the hormone is giving to the cell.

When a protein hormone binds to its receptor, the receptor reacts by changing its shape. This allows it to interact with other proteins that float around on the surface of a cell. One of these is called a G protein, after its ability to bind a small molecule called GTP (guanosine triphosphate). G proteins have very important effects upon the function of a cell. When a hormone receptor binds a protein hormone, it alters its shape and attaches to a G protein.

The G protein responds by splitting into two parts. One of the parts remains attached to the hormone receptor, while the other part floats away and attaches to yet another protein.

This third protein is an enzyme called adenylate cyclase, which responds to the G protein fragment by transforming a molecule called ATP (adenosine triphosphate) into a small molecule called cyclic AMP (cAMP). It is this small molecule that acts as a powerful second messenger in the cell. Since thousands of molecules of cAMP can be generated each time a hormone binds to a receptor, only tiny amounts of hormone can have a greatly amplified effect upon a cell. This amplifying property of this whole series of events is probably why such a complicated mechanism was evolved in the first place. The final result is that a protein hormone can cause drastic changes in proteins that control cell shape and cell metabolism.

Although these steps look complicated, they actually require a very short time to take place. As a matter of fact, within two to five minutes after injecting a hormone into the bloodstream, dramatic hormonal effects upon cell function can be detected. Conversely, if a hormone detaches from a receptor, its effects disappear within an equally short time.

While many hormones use this pathway to affect cells, some hormones have slightly different modes of action. For example, some hormone-activated G proteins don't cause the release of cAMP, but instead cause the production of small lipid molecules that themselves act as second messengers.

Steroid Hormones

Steroid hormones have a structure that is very different from that of protein hormones, and act upon cells in an equally different way. Steroids like adrenal cortical hormones and sex hormones are made from molecules of cholesterol. Various smaller molecules are added to this cholesterol to produce specific types of steroid hormones. Since cholesterol (and steroid hormones) are lipid like molecules, they dissolve in oils rather than in water and have different chemical properties than protein hormones. As a matter of fact, many steroid hormones can be injected into an animal only by dissolving them in oils like peanut oil or other vegetable oils.

Since they are so poorly soluble in water, steroid hormones are transported throughout the bloodstream by "carrier" proteins that loosely attach to them. Once a steroid hormone arrives at a cell, it appears to have the ability to pass right through the cell membrane and enter the cytoplasm, perhaps by associating with other proteins that are not well understood yet. Unlike protein hormones, steroid hormones must enter a cell and be transported to the cell nucleus to affect cell function. This is another key difference between steroid and protein hormones.

Once inside the cell, steroids also bind to receptor proteins, with the difference that these receptor proteins are found floating within the cell nucleus. When a steroid receptor protein binds to a hormone, it also changes its shape. Thus, the first step in changing cell function taken by both steroid hormones and protein hormones is to bind to a receptor protein and thereby change the shape of that protein.

When a steroid receptor protein changes its shape, it is then able to bind to DNA, the genetic material in chromosomes that dictates the functions of each of our cells. Loops of DNA belonging to a single chromosome attach to a "rope" of proteins connected to the nuclear membrane. These proteins, called nuclear matrix proteins, are thought to form the "core" of each chromosome and may help steroid hormone receptors attach to DNA.

When steroid receptors bind to DNA, they attach to specific sites on the DNA and "stick up" from it like flags. This causes other nuclear proteins to settle down on the DNA nearby and start "reading" the message on a nearby gene. This message may, for example, tell the cell to start accumulating fat, as in estrogen-stimulated fat cells beneath the skin of a woman.

All of these steps, unlike the ones activated by protein hormones, are time-consuming. As a matter of fact, changes in cell function take as long as four to six hours to develop after injection of a steroid hormone. This disadvantage is offset by the fact that steroid-induced changes in function are likely to persist far longer than effects of protein hormones.

Thyroid Hormone

The way thyroxine acts upon cells long was regarded as something of a mystery. Thyroxine is too small a molecule to act like a protein and does not bind to receptors on cell surfaces. On the other hand, it is chemically unlike steroids, so for a long while it was hard to decide how it influences cells. Now, however, it has become clear that thyroxine attaches to proteins that are very like steroid receptors, with the difference that they bind thyroxine and not steroids. Thyroxine, then, also appears to mainly influence cells via an action upon DNA.

Hormones and Cancer

It has long been known that some of the features of cancer cells resemble features of cells exposed to hormones. For example, cells in tumors grow and multiply rapidly, crowding out normal cells and robbing the rest of the body of nutrients. Cells exposed to hormones also can grow rapidly, although they don't have the wild, uncontrolled growth of tumors. Also, some organs that are sensitive to steroid hormones, such as the breasts, the prostate gland, and the testes, tend to become cancerous more frequently and have tumors that may require steroid hormones to grow. We now know that these shared properties of cancerous and hormone-induced growth are not simply coincidences.

Research over the last ten years has identified genes in the DNA that appear to cause cells to become cancerous. These genes have been given abbreviated names by molecular biologists: src, for example, is found in sarcoma-type tumors, whereas other cancer-causing genes like ras, raf, erb, myc, fos, and jun were identified in other types of cancer. These genes apparently cause the production of proteins that regulate cell growth in a variety of ways. Some of these genes are also activated by hormones to increase cell growth. Insulin and IGFs, for example, apparently cause certain muscle cells to grow by activating the myc gene. Other cancer-causing genes apparently produce hormone receptor proteins that are permanently activated even if no hormone is present, leading to uncontrolled cell growth. Still other cancer producing genes, like erb, resemble steroid hormone receptors and bind to DNA to cause uncontrolled cell growth. While an understanding of these relationships between cancerous and hormone-induced changes in cell function is still in the early stages, there is much reason for optimism that the molecular mechanisms underlying these changes will become known reasonably soon.

Chapter 3

Ovaries and Testes

Like the other endocrine glands, which usually go unnoticed unless they malfunction, the testes in men and the ovaries in women play a crucial role. Their pervasive influence is particularly evident during the teenage years, when sex hormones surge and sexual maturation takes place. At no other time, except perhaps in the first few years of life (and most of us do not remember much of that), do our bodies undergo such dramatic and rapid changes. Sex hormones affect much more than physical appearance, and their control extends even beyond the physiological processes of sexual maturation and reproduction. They also hold sway over emotions and attitudes by opening up a whole spectrum of desire.

In the Beginning

Sexual development begins at the instant of conception. The fertilized egg carries within it every piece of genetic information it will ever need to produce every type of cell for a lifetime. Thus, from the very beginning, it is determined whether an embryo will mature into a male or female. Sex organs begin to show up very early in fetal development. Testicles begin to emerge in about the seventh week, and ovaries start to form in the 16th week. Sex hormone levels in the developing fetus are high. These hormones directly influence the fetal development of the sex glands.

Some medical experts believe that these early hormones affect the developing brain and contribute to behavioral differences between men and women. There are others, though, experts or not, who argue vehemently against this. These people believe that social factors, not biological ones, are solely responsible for the differences between how men and women act.

Once a baby is born, its sex hormone production drastically reduces. No one is sure what function sex hormones serve in children. Although the testes and ovaries of children are capable of manufacturing and secreting hormones, the pituitary gland has not yet provided the activating signals.

Gonads and Ovaries

The male gonads, or testes, have a unique location. They lie suspended between the thighs in a sac called the scrotum. The testes are situated outside the body because they need a lower temperature to produce viable sperm. These two egg-shaped organs are about two inches long and together weigh less than an ounce. They have two main components. The seminiferous tubules are long, narrow, curling tubes in which sperm cells are formed. These tubes are tightly packed into the testes and compose about 95% of the glands. The little spaces between the tubes hold Leydig's cells. These cells produce nearly all of the androgens, including testosterone, the major androgen hormone secreted by the testes.

Ovaries are the female gonads. One sits on each side of the uterus and is attached to it by ligaments. They are oval-shaped and measure about an inch and a half in length. Ovaries vary in weight in different stages of a female's life but weigh the most during the years that she is fertile. The ovaries produce the hormones estrogen, progesterone, and relaxin. At birth, the ovaries of a female already contain all of the egg-forming cells, or follicles, she will ever produce. It is thought that females begin with a supply of 2 million of these follicles. Only one is used each month in the development of a mature egg.

Like the hormones of the adrenal cortex, hormones of the sex glands are steroids. Although they share a similar carbohydrate origin, they are crucially different in final form and function. Each gland contains particular enzymes that account for the synthesis of specific steroids. The manufacture and secretion of the gonads is under the control of the hypothalamus and the pituitary.

16

Puberty

Have you ever complimented a mother on her darling baby girl only to learn it was a boy? Or perhaps you called her son a girl. Do not worry; it happens to all of us. Aside from genitals, physical differences in the bodies and faces of young boys and girls are not all that different. In fact, if it were not for hairstyles and outfits, the confusion would probably continue until puberty.

As was mentioned earlier, not everyone begins puberty at the same age. In the United States, girls begin puberty somewhere between the ages of 8 and 14. Boys start about two years later than girls, usually in their early teens. There seems to be neither a set pattern nor a standard pace at which the many physical changes of puberty occur.

One boy may shoot up to a height of 5 feet 7 inches in his early teens, whereas his friend hardly grows at all until suddenly at age 17, when he spurts up to become a 6-foot man. One boy will grow a heavy beard early on, and another will not need to shave until he is in college. In the same way, one girl may begin menstruating when she is 10 years old, whereas another will not start until she is 16; yet a third girl will develop breasts in grade school, causing her best friend to worry about her own as-yet undeveloped ones. Each child has his or her own individual way of transforming into a man or woman.

It takes approximately seven years to pass from childhood into adulthood. Although puberty seems to last forever for those who are going through it, enormous bodily changes occur in a remarkably brief span of time. Puberty is characterized by a rapid increase in growth, the development of secondary sex characteristics, and the maturation of reproductive organs.

At no other time does such rapid growth occur, aside from the earliest infant years. The pituitary is stimulated to increase the production of growth hormone. Once this occurs, most children grow about 25% taller in just 4 years. No wonder many teenagers feel suddenly gawky and awkward. Their bodies have become incredible growing machines.

Secondary Sex Characteristics

In addition, the pituitary, under the direction of the hypothalamus, releases hormones that strike up activity in the gonads. The production and release of sex hormones, which were suppressed during childhood, now surge. Physical changes start occurring from head to toe. This is often both a very exciting and a very confusing time. Suddenly, secondary sex characteristics become apparent. These are physical attributes that separate men from women but are not directly involved in reproduction.

In girls, breast development tends to be the first sign. Generally, the nipples and the areolae, the dark areas that surround them, begin to grow. This is followed by the arrival of soft pubic hair and underarm hair. Weight increases as hips and thighs become more rounded. As development progresses, breasts increase in size, and pubic hair becomes darker and coarser.

In boys, the first sign of the onset of puberty is most often an increase in the size of the testicles. This is caused by an enlargement of the seminiferous tubules. Soon after, the penis also begins to enlarge. Facial hair, pubic hair, and underarm hair begin to sprout. The larynx, or voice box, grows larger, causing the voice to deepen. This change in the voice can happen gradually or very suddenly. The shoulders and chest enlarge, muscles develop, and weight increases.

Testosterone

Testosterone has a tremendous influence on a boy's transformation into a man. This hormone is responsible for both the growth and differentiation of the male genitals. It also stimulates the growth of bodily hair and the production of sperm. (Testosterone is also present in women, but in much smaller amounts.) And the list goes on. The level of a man's testosterone plays an essential role in the texture of his skin and hair, the speed at which he metabolizes food, how deep a voice he will have, whether he will lose his hair or not, and even how massive his muscles and bones will become.

The Potential for Abuse

It is this tissue-building, or anabolic, effect of testosterone that has spurred an illegal market in steroids. If you watched the television coverage of the 1988 Summer Olympics in Seoul, South Korea, you are sure to remember Ben Johnson's incredible performance. Running the 100-meter race, Johnson got off to a blazing start and left the competition far behind. He ran the race in 9.79 seconds, setting a new world record and winning a gold medal.

Three days after the race, however, the Olympic Committee stripped Johnson of the prize. Blood tests showed that the Canadian runner had been taking anabolic steroids. These are synthetic hormones that were developed to duplicate the effects of testosterone.

Although medical experts disagree as to whether steroids can improve athletic ability, they all agree that taking an abnormal amount of them can have harmful effects that may last a lifetime. In large quantities, over a long period of time, anabolic steroids can be very dangerous. In young men, they can speed up the maturation process. This can result in stunted growth or early baldness. Young girls who take steroids run the risk of developing masculine traits that will not disappear, even when they stop taking the drugs.

As it does with many other hormones, a negative feedback system regulates the secretion of testosterone to prevent its overproduction or underproduction. Athletes taking large doses of steroids are seriously challenging their bodies' ability to maintain a proper balance of testosterone. This can eventually lead to heart disease or kidney and liver damage and may even increase the risk of liver cancer. When massive amounts of anabolic steroids are present in the body, the pituitary may shut down testosterone production. In the male, this can cause the testes to shrink and breasts to develop.

Testosterone and Sexuality

Testosterone is responsible for igniting sexual desire in both men and women. So far, estrogen and progesterone, although very important to sexual reproduction, have not shown any relationship to desire. Men who have lost interest in sex frequently show an abnormally low testosterone level. Injections of this hormone can restore their sex drive. This works for both men and women. Generally though, testosterone levels remain relatively constant throughout a man's life from puberty until about age 40. After that, the levels gradually decline over the next 40 years until the sex drive and fertility are decreased by about 20%.

Although hormonal levels greatly influence the sexual behavior of both men and women, any discussion of human sexuality must consider not only hormonal influences but also the important part thoughts and feelings play concerning one's sexual drive. Moreover, no matter how much work is done studying the factors that determine a person's sex drive, human sexuality remains, to a degree, a mysterious and fluctuating aspect of life.

The Reproductive Cycle

Unlike testosterone, which is controlled by a negative feedback system, the release of estrogen and progesterone is cyclical. One period, known as the menstrual cycle, normally extends over 28 days. In pubescent girls, menstruation may begin months or even years before regular ovulation begins. Adolescent girls may begin by producing sufficient hormones to build up and shed the uterine lining each month but not enough to produce a mature egg.

Once sexual maturation is complete, however, the menstrual cycle follows a specific pattern, beginning with the release of FSH from the pituitary. This stimulates the development of an egg in one of the ovaries. As the egg grows, the follicle secretes estrogen. This prevents the pituitary from releasing additional FSH, so no other eggs begin to mature. Estrogen also causes the uterus to prepare to receive a fertilized egg by building up a lining. As estrogen levels rise, the pituitary secretes LH, which in turn causes the ovary to release the egg into the oviduct. Once the egg is on its own, the leftover body that held the egg—the corpus luteum—begins producing progesterone. This hormone stops the pituitary from releasing either FSH or LH.

If the egg is not fertilized, the corpus luteum gives up and stops producing progesterone. This will generally happen a couple of days after the egg is released. As the level of progesterone declines, the thick lining of the uterus breaks up and causes the bleeding known as menstrual flow. At the same time, the pituitary, which is no longer suppressed, begins to produce FSH again. This starts the cycle once more.

The surges and falls in hormonal levels during the course of a menstrual cycle affect women in many different ways. The sudden rise of progesterone can cause women to feel particularly tense, depressed, or nervous. Many women also retain fluids and feel irritable and bloated several days before their period begins. In recent years, the term premenstrual syndrome (PMS) has been created to cover any or all of these symptoms. For most women, PMS is only an occasional or mild event. More than once, though, an extreme case of PMS has been used as a defense during the trial of a woman accused of murder. It is obviously important that women should contact their doctor if they suffer violent mood swings caused by alterations in hormone levels.

Controlling the Cycle

If the delicate hormonal balance that controls the woman's menstrual cycle is altered, conception can be very difficult, if not impossible. This is the basis upon which birth control pills work. Most of these contain a combination of estrogen and progesterone. They raise the level of hormones in the blood. The body treats this as a pregnancy and instructs the pituitary to shut off production of FSH and LH. This prevents the development and release of a mature egg. When the pills are discontinued for a few days each month, menstruation begins. Women who go off birth control pills are often surprised that they may skip their period for many months. Their body has become so accustomed to the excessively high hormone levels that their feedback system no longer works. It can take as long as half a year for the signals to return to normal.

Many women (and men) wonder why a birth control pill for males has not yet been developed. It may be, but progress is very slow. For women, only one event a month has to be controlled—the production and delivery of a mature egg. For men, who can produce more than a million sperm a day, the development of a birth control pill becomes far more complex.

Hormones and Pregnancy

When a woman becomes pregnant, her body begins producing and secreting more sex hormones than at any other time in her life. Cells of the embryo release a hormone that keeps the corpus luteum intact for the first three months. The corpus luteum enlarges and produces greater and greater amounts of both progesterone and estrogen. The progesterone helps the embryo receive nourishment from the uterus and prevents uterine contractions. It also helps prepare the breasts to produce milk. The estrogen causes the uterus and breasts to enlarge. By the end of the third month, the corpus luteum degenerates, and the placenta becomes an endocrine gland, supplying the fetus with the necessary quantities of estrogen and progesterone for its ongoing development.

By the end of the ninth month, the level of estrogen is so high that it counters the effect of progesterone on the uterus. At this point the body is preparing for labor. Contractions will be encouraged rather than prevented. Once labor begins, the mother's hypothalamus stimulates the posterior pituitary to release oxytocin. This hormone causes uterine contractions. At the same time, the mother's ovaries secrete relaxin. This hormone helps to dilate the cervix and the birth canal in preparation for the baby's delivery.

Infertility

Ten to fifteen percent of all couples are unable to conceive. This is often caused by a hormonal problem. Deficient sperm production or delivery accounts for 40% of the cases. A medical evaluation will usually determine where the problems stem from. The pituitary, ovaries, testes, and adrenal and thyroid glands should all be examined and their hormonal production tested in evaluating fertility problems.

Menopause

Although it may seem that the female body produces an enormous quantity of hormones throughout life, the opposite is true. Women produce no more than a teaspoonful of estrogen, for example, from the time puberty begins through the end of their reproductive years. The ending of fertility, like the beginning, is a process than can take several years. Most women experience it in three stages.

During the first stage, known as premenopause, the ovaries begin to produce fewer hormones. Menstrual flow often changes. For some women it lessens, while for others it becomes heavier. During menopause, the second stage, women stop having periods. Ovarian function has ceased or is very minimal. By the time a woman has gone through one year without having a period, she is said to be in stage three, or postmenopause.

Some women begin stage one in their forties, whereas others continue to have periods through their fifties. It is very unusual, however, for a woman to enter her sixties without having gone through all three stages.

Many women go through the process without experiencing any discomforting physical symptoms. For those who do, hot flashes are the most common source of complaints. These are very sudden and temporary rushes of heat that begin in the chest and spread upward. No one is quite sure what causes hot flashes, but they are known to originate in the hypothalamus. Another problem is painful intercourse. When estrogen secretion is curtailed, the tissue lining in the vagina thins, and vaginal secretions lessen. Fortunately, there are many creams available to alleviate this problem. In addition, estrogen replacement therapy in combination with progesterone is now being administered to many women. Test results to date show this combination to be an effective and safe treatment for many of the symptoms of menopause and postmenopause. There is no proven psychological advantage to hormone replacement therapy, aside from women's improved mental outlook when hot flashes have been eliminated and vaginal atrophy prevented. Physicians are therefore reluctant to prescribe hormone therapy for the depression that may accompany menopause. Relaxation techniques, counseling, or antidepressant drugs are much more commonly used.

Chapter 4

Directory of Organizations for Endocrine and Metabolic Diseases

American Association of Diabetes Educators (AADE)
444 N. Michigan Avenue, Suite 1240
Chicago, IL 60611
(312) 644-2233 or (800) 338-3633
(800) Teamup4 (Diabetes Educator Access Line)
http://www.aadenet.org

AADE is a multidisciplinary organization, with state and regional chapters, for health professionals involved in diabetes patient education. The organization sponsors a certification program for diabetes educators and provides grants, scholarships, and awards for educational research and teaching activities. AADE's annual meeting features continuing education programs on diabetes treatment and education. The organization also established a Diabetes Educator Access Line to help people with diabetes locate diabetes education services in their areas.

Publications: AADE publishes a bimonthly journal, *The Diabetes Educator*; curriculum guides; consensus statements; self-study

Information in this chapter was compiled from National Institute on Diabetes and Digestive and Kidney Diseases (NIDDK) Web Page; www.niddk.nih.gov/EndoOrg/endoorg.html February 1997; National Diabetes Information Clearinghouse, NIDDK, NIH, June 1995; and *Pituitary Patient Resource Guide*, First Annual North American Edition, ©1995 Pituitary Tumor Network Association, 16350 Ventura Blvd., Suite 231, Encino, CA 91436, (805) 499-9973; reprinted with permission. Web site information was added in 1998.

programs; and other print and non-print resources for diabetes educators.

American Diabetes Association (ADA)
ADA National Service Center
1660 Duke Street
Alexandria, VA 22314
(703) 549-1500 or (800) 232-3472
http://www.diabetes.org

ADA is both a professional association and a private, nonprofit, voluntary organization with state and local affiliates and chapters. It serves people with diabetes and their families and friends, as well as health professionals and research scientists involved in diabetes-related activities. The organization funds diabetes research and education activities; sponsors educational programs, including an annual meeting, postgraduate courses, consensus meetings, and special symposia; administers a recognition program for diabetes outpatient education; develops professional guidelines for diabetes care; and advocates for diabetes issues in the legislative and public health arenas. Local ADA affiliates often sponsor educational programs and support groups for persons with diabetes and their families.

Publications: ADA publishes monthly and quarterly magazines for patients, including *Diabetes Forecast*; professional journals focusing on basic and clinical research, including *Diabetes, Diabetes Care, Diabetes Spectrum,* and *Diabetes Reviews*; other publications, including cookbooks, meal planning guides, pamphlets, brochures, and books for patients; and clinical manuals, nutritional guides, audiovisuals, statistical reports, and curriculum guides for professionals.

American Porphyria Foundation
P.O. Box 22712
Houston, TX 77227
(713) 266-9617
Desiree Lyon, Executive Director
http://www.enterprise.net/apf/index.html

Purpose: Provides financial support for researchers in porphyria; improves the diagnosis and treatment of porphyria through educational programs; serves as a network for porphyria patients. Also sponsors support groups, political action, seminars and fund-raising projects.

24

Publications: General brochure; Diet and Nutrition in Porphyria; Porphyria Cutanea Tarda; (AIP) Acute Intermittent Porphyria; (EEP) Erythropoietic Protoporphyria; The Prophyrias—An Overview; Hematin; and Newsletter. These brochures are all available with membership. Bulk orders are available upon request.

American Thyroid Association
Montefiore Medical Center
111 East 210th Street
Room 311
Bronx, NY 10467
(718) 882-6047
Diane Miller, Administrator
http://www.thyroid.org

Purpose: A professional organization of physicians and scientists dedicated to scientific research on the thyroid. The association refers the public to member physicians in their geographic area on request.

Publications: Newsletter (quarterly); information pamphlets.

Association for Glycogen Storage Disease
P.O. Box 896
Durant, IA 52747
(319) 785-6038
Hollie Swain, President

Purpose: Acts as a forum for the discussion of glycogen storage disease (GSD), its treatment, and the problems faced by parents raising children with GSD. Disseminates medical information; fosters communication between the families of GSD patients and health care professionals. Helps obtain equipment necessary for home care of GSD patients.

Disorder: GSD is a hereditary condition characterized by a lack of or deficiency in any of the enzymes used by the body to break down glycogen. Glycogen storage diseases include: von Gierke's disease, Pompe's disease, McArdle's disease, Forbes' disease, and Andersen's disease.

Publications: *The Ray* (periodic newsletter); Parent Handbook and other brochures.

Association for Neuro-Metabolic Disorders
5223 Brookfield Lane
Sylvania, OH 43560
(419) 885-1497
Cheryl Volk, Parent Representative

Purpose: A member organization of families with children who have metabolic disorders that affect the brain. The organization provides support through personal awareness, family understanding and participation, and professional health care intervention.

Disorder: Neuro-metabolic disorders include many different, often inherited, diseases such as maple syrup urine disease, galactosemia, and biotinidase deficiency. These diseases affect body chemistry, but the organ damaged is the brain.

Publications: Newsletter (3 times a year).

Australian Pituitary Foundation
P.O. Box 126
Yagoona 2199
NSW Australia
Phone: (61-2) 630-7209
Fax: (61-2) 790-4055

Brain Tumor Foundation of Canada
111 Waterloo Street
Suite 600
London, Ontario N6B 2M4, Canada
Phone: (519) 642-7755
Fax: (519) 642-7192

Publication: *Brain Tumor Patient Resource Handbook* (Both Adult and Pediatric Versions). For more information, please call.

Cushing's Support and Research Foundation, Inc.
65 East India Row 22B
Boston, MA 02110
(617) 723-3824
(617) 723-3674
Louise L. Pace, Founder and President
http://world.std.com/~csrf/index.html

Purpose: Provides information and support for patients along with expert medical advice from physicians. Facilitates correspondence between members and maintains a referral listing of hospitals, endocrinologists and surgeons.

Cystic Fibrosis Foundation
6931 Arlington Road
Bethesda, MD 20814
(301) 951-4422
1-800-FIGHT CF
Robert Beall, President
http://www.cff.org

Purpose: Supports medical research, professional education, and a nationwide network of care centers to benefit patients with cystic fibrosis (CF). Supports services for young adults with CF.

Publications: Information brochures.

Diabetes Insipidus and Related Disorders Network
Route 2, Box 198
Creston, IA 50801
Beth Perry
http://members.aol.com/ruudh/diapage1.htm

Purpose: Informal network

Publication: Newsletter.

Diabetes Research and Education Foundation
P.O. Box 6168
Bridgewater, NJ 08807-9998
(908) 658-9322 (Tuesday-Thursday only)
http://www.celos.psu.edu/clinics/dr&edf.htm

The foundation, funded by Hoechst-Roussel Pharmaceuticals Inc., offers grants in the form of "seed money" to support novel initiatives in diabetes research and education. The foundation's Board of Trustees includes specialists in diabetes research, clinical practice, pharmacy, and patient education.

Publication: Annual Report.

Diabetes Research and Training Centers (DRTCs)

The National Institute of Diabetes and Digestive and Kidney Diseases supports six DRTCs. These centers offer continuing education, seminars, and workshops on diabetes management for health care professionals; an array of tested evaluation and assessment instruments; professional expertise in developing and implementing diabetes programs in a variety of settings; and patient referral. DRTCs are located at major medical centers affiliated with universities.

Publications: Individual centers produce a variety of educational materials, including audiovisuals for health care professionals. For additional information about DRTC materials and programs, contact individual centers listed below.

Einstein/Montefiore DRTC
1300 Morris Park Avenue
Belfer 1308
Bronx, NY 10461
(718) 430-2646

Indiana University DRTC
Regenstrief Institute, 5th Floor
1001 West 10th Street
Indianapolis, IN 46202
(317) 630-6375

Michigan DRTC
G1205 Towsley Center, Box 0201
University of Michigan Medical Centers
Ann Arbor, MI 48109-0201
(313) 763-1426

University of Chicago DRTC
Center for Research in Medical Education and Health Care
5841 S. Maryland Avenue, MC 6091
Chicago, IL 60637
(312) 753-1310

Vanderbilt University DRTC
Vanderbilt Medical Center
305 Medical Arts Building
Nashville, TN 37232-2230
(615) 322-4257 or 322-6001 (answering service)

Washington University DRTC
Diabetes Education Center
4444 Forest Park
St. Louis, MO 63108
(314) 286-1900

Division of Diabetes Translation, Centers for Disease Control and Prevention (CDC)
National Center for Chronic Disease Prevention and
Health Promotion
TISB Mail Stop K-13
4770 Buford Highway, NE
Atlanta, GA 30341-3724
(404) 488-5080

An agency of the Public Health Service, Department of Health and Human Services, CDC develops public health approaches to reduce the burden of diabetes in the United States. The agency supports diabetes control programs in 26 states and 1 territory; carries out state and national surveillance activities to assess diabetes prevalence, impact, and possible contributing factors; develops consensus guidelines for clinical and public health practice; supports community-based preventive programs for minority populations and the elderly; and coordinates Federal activities concerned with translating research findings into clinical practice, including issues related to cost and reimbursement practices, disability, and quality of life.

Publications: CDC distributes a practice manual for primary care practitioners and a companion guide for patients, surveillance reports, and guidelines on patient education, educational reimbursement, and maternal and child health. State programs have produced patient and professional publications.

The Endocrine Society
9650 Rockville Pike
Bethesda, MD 20814-3998
http://www.endo-society.org

Publication: *The Journal of Clinical Endocrinology & Metabolism*

The Health Resource, Inc.
564 Locust Street
Conway, AR 72032
Phone: (501) 329-5272
Fax: (501) 329-9489
http://thehealthresource.com

Patient Services: Receive an individualized, comprehensive research report on your specific medical condition so you can survey your treatment options—both conventional and alternative. Call for additional information.

H.E.L.P., The Institute for Body Chemistry
P.O. Box 1338
Bryn Mawr, PA 19010
(610) 525-1225
Edward A. Krimmel and Patricia T. Krimmel Co-Directors

Purpose: Promotes medical/scientific research concerning the relationship between food chemistry and body chemistry specifically related to hypoglycemia. Disseminates information on body chemistry.

Hemochromatosis Research Foundation
P.O. Box 8569
Albany, NY 12208
(518) 489-0972
Margaret A. Krikker, M.D., President

Purpose: Seeks to increase public and professional awareness of hereditary hemochromatosis (HH) and the hazards of supplemental iron. Encourages routine use of screening tests by physicians. Assists public, patients, families, and physicians with HH diagnosis, treatment, and genetic counseling and in forming regional support networks. Provides telephone referral service to patients requesting names of physicians and research centers concerned with HH.

Disorder: Hereditary hemochromatosis is a disorder of iron metabolism in which dietary iron absorption exceeds body needs. If not diagnosed and treated, the accumulating iron may result in one or more complications such as liver enlargement, heart irregularities and failure, diabetes and other hormonal deficiencies, and arthritis.

Publications: *Hemochromatosis Awareness* (quarterly newsletter); information booklets and videotapes.

Human Growth Foundation
7777 Leesburg Pike
Suite 202 South
Falls Church, VA 22043
(703) 883-1773
1-800-451-6434
Kimberly Frye, Executive Director
http://www.genetic.org/hgf

Purpose: A member organization of families of children with physical growth problems and interested persons united to help medical science better understand the process of growth. Distributes funds for basic and clinical growth research.

Publications: *Fourth Friday* (monthly newsletter); Growth Series (brochures).

Hypoglycemia Support Foundation, Inc.
3822 NW 122nd Terrace
Sunrise, FL 33323
(954) 742-3098
Roberta Ruggiero, President
http://www.hypoglycemia.org

Purpose: Seeks to inform, support, and encourage people with hypoglycemia about diet and hypoglycemia.

Publications: *The Hypoglycemia Support Foundation Newsletter* (quarterly); *The Dos & Don'ts of Low Blood Sugar* (book).

Indian Health Service (IHS)
IHS Headquarters West
Central Diabetes Program
5300 Homestead Road NE
Albuquerque, NM 87110
(505) 837-4182
http://www.tucson.ihs.gov

An agency of the Public Health Service, Department of Health and Human Services, IHS supports 17 model Diabetes Health Care Programs serving Native Americans and Alaskans. These programs develop and evaluate effective and culturally accepted prevention and treatment methods for diabetes and its complications. Diabetes control officers in each IHS region provide surveillance, training, and other services to promote the use of techniques recommended by the program.

Publications: The model programs and the IHS produce culturally relevant publications for native populations, including nutrition guides, complication-specific educational materials, and guides for professionals. Publications are available only to persons working with Native American or Alaskan populations.

International Diabetes Center (IDC)
5000 West 39th Street
Minneapolis, MN 55416
(612) 927-3393
http://www.hsmnet.com/hsm/mhms/idc.htm

A division of the Park Nicollet Medical Foundation, IDC offers education classes for people with diabetes and training programs for health professionals. The programs for health professionals focus on team management of diabetes. IDC also provides inpatient and outpatient treatment services in adult and pediatric clinics, supports clinical research to assess new diabetes care systems and approaches, conducts psychosocial research, and supports a network of IDC satellite centers that offer specialized programs in diabetes. The IDC has been designated as a World Health Organization Collaborating Center for Diabetes Education and Training.

Publications: The organization publishes *Living Well With Diabetes*, a quarterly magazine for people with diabetes. Other publications include management and nutrition guides for patients, low-literacy patient education booklets, guides for health professionals, audiovisuals, and general publications related to chronic health problems and nutrition. For publications/mail order pharmacy services:

Chronimed
P.O. Box 47945
Minneapolis, MN 55447-9727
(800) 876-6540
or (800) 477-6388 (In MN)
(612) 546-1146

International Diabetes Federation (IDF)
40 Rue Washington
1050 Brussels, Belgium
322/647-4414

IDF collaborates with more than 100 member associations in over 80 countries, the World Health Organization, and other affiliated organizations and individuals to ensure that people with diabetes receive quality treatment and education services.

Publications: IDF publishes a newsletter, a journal entitled *IDF Bulletin*, the *Directory 1991: A Guide to the Activities of Member Diabetes Associations*, as well as other publications.

International Diabetic Athletes Association (IDAA)
1647 West Bethany Home Road #B
Phoenix, AZ 85015
(602) 433-2113 or 1-800-898-IDAA (800-898-4322)
(602) 433-9331 Fax
e-mail: idaa@getnet.com
http://www.getnet.com/~idaa

IDAA is a nonprofit, membership organization for persons with diabetes who participate in fitness activities at all levels. The organization sponsors workshops, conferences, and other events. It offers educational programs for active individuals with diabetes, their families, and friends. IDAA also offers educational programs to diabetes educators, coaches, school nurses, recreation workers, and other professionals who interact with people with diabetes in a recreational setting. The organization's board of directors includes well-known athletes with diabetes, physicians, and other health professionals who are experts in diabetes and sports.

Publications: IDAA publishes the quarterly newsletter, *The Challenge*, which includes helpful articles about managing diabetes during athletic activities and stories about people with diabetes who participate in sports events.

Iron Overload Diseases Association, Inc.
433 Westwind Drive
N. Palm Beach, FL 33408-5123
(561) 840-8512
Roberta Crawford, President
http://www.emi.net/~iron_iod

Purpose: Serves and counsels hemochromatosis patients and families and offers doctor referral, as well as patient advocacy with insurance, Medicare, blood banks, and the FDA; encourages research and public information; emphasizes early diagnosis and encourages research.

Publications: *Ironic Blood: Information on Iron Overload* (bimonthly newsletter); *Overload: An Ironic Disease* (booklet); Iron Overload Alert (information brochure).

Joslin Diabetes Center

One Joslin Place
Boston, MA 02215
(617) 732-2400
http://www.joslin.harvard.edu

The Joslin Diabetes Center offers inpatient and outpatient treatment, education, and other support services to adults and children with diabetes; provides professional medical education; sponsors camps for children with diabetes; and supports research to improve treatment and find a cure for diabetes and its complications. The center is affiliated with Harvard Medical School and a number of hospitals in the Boston area and operates affiliated clinics in several states. The Joslin Diabetes Center is one of six Diabetes Endocrinology Research Centers supported by the National Institute of Diabetes and Digestive and Kidney Diseases.

Publications: Joslin produces a variety of educational materials for patients and professionals, including manuals, nutrition guides, materials for children with diabetes, and films. *The Joslin Magazine* is issued quarterly to members of the Joslin Society.

Juvenile Diabetes Foundation (JDF) International

120 Wall Street
New York, NY 10005-4001
(212) 785-9500
(800) JDF-CURE
(212) 785-9595 Fax
http://www.jdfcure.com

JDF is a private, nonprofit, voluntary organization with chapters throughout the world. JDF raises funds to support research on the cause, cure, treatment, and prevention of diabetes and its complications. The organization awards research grants for laboratory and clinical investigations and sponsors a variety of career development and research training programs for new and established investigators. JDF also sponsors international workshops and conferences for biomedical researchers. Individual chapters offer support groups and other activities for families.

Publications: JDF publishes the quarterly journal *Countdown* and a series of patient education brochures about insulin-dependent and noninsulin-dependent diabetes.

March of Dimes
1275 Mamaroneck Avenue
White Plains, NY 10605
(914) 428-7100
Jennifer Howe, Ph.D., President
http://modimes.org

Purpose: Promotes education and research on genetic and environmental causes of birth defects.

Publications: Information pamphlets.

Metabolic Information Network
P.O. Box 670847
Dallas, TX 75367-0847
(214) 696-2188
1-800-945-2188
Susan G. Mize, Project Director

Purpose: Provides a system for sharing reported data on inborn errors of metabolism that may be useful to professionals caring for patients, to research investigators, and to patients seeking access to treatment.

Disorders: The 10 groups of disorders in MIN's working database of inborn errors of metabolism are: biotin defects, galactosemias, glycogen storage diseases, hereditary tyrosine disorders, homocystinurias, hyperphenyla-laninemias, maple syrup urine diseases, mucopolysaccharidoses, organic acidurias, and urea cycle disorders.

National Adrenal Diseases Foundation
505 Northern Boulevard, Suite 200
Great Neck, NY 11021
(516) 487-4992
Joyce Mullen, Executive Director
http://medhlp.netusa.net/www/nadf.htm#Nadfpubs

Purpose: Provides a national self-help network for educational and emotional support for patients and their families.

Publications: *NADF Newsletter* (periodic); educational materials.

National Brain Tumor Foundation
785 Market Street, Suite 1600
San Francisco, CA 94103
Toll-Free: (800) 934-CURE
Fax: (415) 284-0208
http://www.braintumor.org

Patient Services: Research to save lives; a national network of support services to help patients and families combat brain tumors; hope for adults and children.

National Center for the Study of Wilson's Disease
432 West 58th Street
Suite 614
New York, NY 10091
(212) 523-8717
I. Herbert Scheinberg, M.D., President

Purpose: Encourages and supports research concerning hereditary diseases of copper metabolism (Wilson's disease and Menkes' disease). Seeks to increase doctors' awareness of these diseases; and sponsors a diagnostic and treatment center for Wilson's disease.

Disorder: Wilson's disease is a genetic disorder in which excessive amounts of copper collect in the liver, brain, and kidneys. Menkes' disease is the reverse of Wilson's disease and is characterized by a defect in intestinal absorption of copper that leads to copper deficiency.

Publications: Information brochures.

National Diabetes Information Clearinghouse (NDIC)
One Information Way
Bethesda, MD 20892-3560
http://www.aerie.com/nihdb/dmtest.html

NDIC is a service of the National Institute of Diabetes and Digestive and Kidney Diseases, which is the government's lead agency for diabetes research. The clearinghouse functions as an information, educational, and referral resource for health professionals, people with diabetes, and the general public.

Publications: NDIC offers a variety of publications for use by the general public, people with diabetes, and health professionals. Publications include guides for patients and professionals, bibliographies, reports, and fact sheets. The clearinghouse also publishes the newsletter *Diabetes Dateline* and maintains the diabetes subfile of the Combined Health Information Database, available through BRS Online.

National Eye Institute (NEI)
National Eye Health Education Program
Box 20/20
Bethesda, MD 20892
(800) 869-2020 or (301) 496-5248
http://www.nei.nih.gov

NEI, one of the National Institutes of Health, supports basic and clinical research to develop effective treatments for diabetic eye disease. The institute's National Eye Health Education Program promotes public and professional awareness of the importance of early diagnosis and treatment of diabetic eye disease.

Publications: NEI produces patient and professional education materials related to diabetic eye disease and its treatment, including literature for patients, guides for health professionals, and education kits for community health workers and for pharmacists.

National Graves' Disease Foundation
2 Tsitsi Court
Brevard, NC 28712
(704) 877-5251
Nancy Patterson, Ph.D., Executive Director
http://www.ngdf.org

Purpose: Provides medical information, referral, and resource information to patients; aids in the development of support groups; provides professional education through lectures and forums; and sponsors, develops, participates in, and supports research on Graves' disease.

Publications: Newsletter (quarterly); information brochures.

The National Institute of Diabetes and Digestive and Kidney Diseases
National Institutes of Health
9000 Rockville Pike, Building 31, Room 9A04
Bethesda, MD 20892
(301) 496-3583
http://www.niddk.nih.gov

The National Institute of Diabetes and Digestive and Kidney Diseases (NIDDK) conducts and supports research on many of the most serious diseases affecting the public health. NIDDK conducts a broad range of basic research studies that rely on the principles and tools of genetics, chemistry, biochemistry, chemical physics, pharmacology, pathology, physiology, and molecular biology. NIDDK conducts clinical research on diabetes, other metabolic diseases such as cystic fibrosis, endocrine disorders, digestive diseases, nutrition, kidney diseases, and blood disorders.

The NIDDK's three extramural research divisions—the Division of Diabetes, Endocrinology, and Metabolic Diseases; the Division of Digestive Diseases and Nutrition; and the Division of Kidney, Urologic, and Hematologic Diseases—support basic and clinical research and research training through investigator-initiated grants, program project and center grants, and career development and research training awards.

National MPS Society, Inc.
17 Kraemer Street
Hicksville, NY 11801
(516) 931-6338
Marie Capobianco, President
http://members.aol.com/mpssociety.index.html

Purpose: Acts as a support group for families of children with MPS (mucopolysaccharidoses) and ML (mucolipidoses); increases professional and public awareness; facilitates diagnosis and treatment through referrals to doctors and hospitals; and raises funds to further research on MPS and ML.

Disorders: MPS and ML are rare hereditary disorders caused by the body's inability to produce certain enzymes, resulting in an abnormal deposit of complex sugars in tissues and cells. This causes progressive damage that can range in severity from bone and joint involvement to massive complications in all organ systems.

Publications: *Courage* (quarterly newsletter); information booklets.

National Organization for Rare Disorders
P.O. Box 8923
New Fairfield, CT 06812-8923
(203) 746-6518
Abbey S. Meyers, Executive Director
http://199.249.196.59/nord

Purpose: Acts as a clearinghouse for information about orphan diseases and as a network for families with similar disorders; encourages and promotes increased scientific research on the cause, control and ultimate cure of rare disorders, including inherited metabolic diseases; accumulates and disseminates information about orphan drugs and devices; and educates the general public and medical profession about the existence, diagnosis, and treatment of rare disorders.

Publications: *Orphan Disease Update* (quarterly newsletter).

National Osteoporosis Foundation
1150 17th Street NW
Suite 500
Washington, DC 20036
(202) 223-2226
Sandra C. Raymond, Executive Director
http://www.nof.org

Purpose: Increases public awareness and knowledge about osteoporosis; provides information to patients and their families; educates physicians and allied health professionals; and supports basic biomedical, epidemiological, clinical, behavioral, and social research and research training.

Publications: *Osteoporosis Report* (quarterly newsletter); *Osteoporosis: A Woman's Guide*, and *Boning Up on Osteoporosis: A Guide to Prevention and Treatment*; information brochures and other educational materials.

Organic Acidemia Association, Inc.
2287 Cypress Avenue
San Pablo, CA 94806
(510) 724-0297
Carol Barton, President
http://just4u.com/oaa

Purpose: Fosters communication among parents and professionals; acts as a support group. Members include dietitians, researchers, and geneticists; clinics; parents and relatives of children with organic acidemia disorders.

Disorder: Organic acidemia is the collective name for a class of genetic metabolic disorders that lead to enzyme deficiencies and require protein-restricted diets. Organic acidemia disorders include: propionic acidemia, arginino succinic aciduria, isovaleric acidemia, and methylmalonic aciduria.

Publications: *Organic Acidemia Association Newsletter* (quarterly).

The Oxalosis and Hyperoxaluria Foundation
P.O. Box 1632
Kent, WA 98035
(508) 461-0614
Ann Dayton, Director

Purpose: Informs patients, their families, physicians, and medical professionals about hyperoxaluria and related conditions, oxalosis and calcium oxalate kidney stones. Provides support network to patients and supports and encourages research efforts to find the cure for hyperoxaluria.

Disorder: Primary hyperoxaluria is an inherited disorder characterized by a missing enzyme from the liver that causes calcium oxalate crystals to form, which leads to kidney failure.

Publications: *In Touch* (quarterly newsletter); *Understanding Oxalosis and Hyperoxaluria* and information on low oxalate diet.

The Paget Foundation for Paget's Disease of Bone and Related Disorders
200 Varick Street
Suite 1004
New York, NY 10014-4810
(212) 229-1582
1-800-23-PAGET
Charlene Waldman, Executive Director

Purpose: Serves patients with Paget's disease of bone, primary hyperparathyroidism, and other related disorders; and assists the medical community that treats these patients.

Publications: Newsletter (quarterly); Primary Hyperparathyroidism (patient education brochure).

Pennsylvania Diabetes Academy
777 East Park Drive
Box 8820
Harrisburg, PA 17105-8820
(717) 558-7750, ext 271
(800) 228-7823 (AA Medical Society)

The academy is a nonprofit organization affiliated with the Pennsylvania Medical Society. It operates as a cooperative venture with the state's Department of Health and the Pennsylvania Diabetes Task Force offering education, training, and consultation services to health care professionals in the state of Pennsylvania.

Publications: Materials available from the academy include a newsletter, self-study modules for physicians, and low-literacy teaching aids for diabetes educators.

The Pituitary Foundation
17/18 The Courtyard, Woodlands
Almondsbury, Bristol
BS12 4NQ, UK
Phone: 44 (454) 616046
Fax: 44 (454) 616071

Publication: *Treating Acromegaly*

41

Pituitary Tumor Network Association

16350 Ventura Boulevard, Suite 231
Encino, CA 91436
(805) 499-9973
1-800-642-9211
Robert Knutzen, Chairman, CEO
http://pituitary.com

Purpose: Promotes early diagnosis; encourages research and pursues the cure of diseases caused by pituitary tumors; serves patients with diseases caused by pituitary tumors; and provides a telephone network of people with pituitary tumors in all age groups.

Publications: *Network* (quarterly newsletter); information pamphlets. *The Pituitary Patient Resource Guide*; for pituitary patients, their families, physicians and all health care providers.

Patient Contacts

West
Sheree Jones-Pistol
Encino-Tarzana Medical Center
Tarzana, California
Phone: (818) 708-5598
Fax: (818) 708-5443

James & Connie Greenwald
El Cajon, California
Phone: (619) 588-0969

Jane Horner
San Jose, California
Phone: (408) 288-9565

Midwest
Melissa Napier, P.A.
Grand Blanc, Michigan
Phone & Fax: (810) 694-0262

Kathryn Pearson
4930 S.66th St.
Lincoln, Nebraska
Phone: (402) 489-3510

East
Lisa Kaufman
New York, New York
Phone: (212) 865-5319

The Thyroid Foundation of America, Inc.
Room 350, Ruth Sleeper Hall
40 Parkman Street
Boston, MA 02114-2698
(617) 726-8500
1-800-832-8321
Ilia Stacy, Executive Director
http://clark.net/pub/tfa

Purpose: Provides public education programs, patient informa-tion, and support. Refers patients to qualified endocrinologists. Please send a business sized self-addressed stamped envelope.

Publications: *The Bridge* (quarterly newsletter); information bro-chures.

Thyroid Society for Education and Research
7515 South Main Street
Suite 545
Houston, TX 77030
(713) 799-9909
1-800-THYROID
Kathy Kobos, Executive Director

Purpose: Pursues the prevention, treatment, and cure of thyroid disease. Participates in and raises funds for patient and community education programs, professional education, and scientific research.

Publications: Patient education brochures.

Turner's Syndrome Society of the United States
15500 Wayzata Boulevard
#768-214
Wayzata, MN 55391
Phone: (612) 475-9944
Fax: (612) 475-9949
http://turner-syndrome-us.org

United Leukodystrophy Foundation
2304 Highland Drive
Sycamore, IL 60178
(815) 895-3211
Paula Braazeal, President
http://www.ulf.org

Purpose: Acts as a support group for parents and families of patients with various forms of inherited leukodystrophy.

Disorder: The leukodystrophies are a group of genetically determined neurologic disorders in which progressive degeneration occurs, primarily affecting white matter. The leukodystrophies include: Krabbe's leukodystrophy (globoid cell leukodystrophy or GLD), metachromatic leukodystrophy (MLD), adrenoleukodystrophy, Pelizaeus-Merzbacher disease, spongy degeneration of the brain, and Alexander's disease.

United Way
http://www.unitedway.org

There is no national hotline number. Please check your local telephone directory for the nearest chapter.

Wilson's Disease Association
4 Navaho Drive
Brookfield, CT 06804
800-399-0266
H. Ascher Sellner, President
http://www.medhelp.org/wda/wil.htm

Purpose: Promotes and sponsors research concerning the cause, treatment, and cure of Wilson's and Menkes' diseases; stresses the importance of public awareness, early diagnosis, and treatment; provides financial aid and moral support to needy individuals and organizations sharing the association's goals; collects and disseminates information to members and the public concerning developments, current research, and legislation; and acts as a clearinghouse.

Publications: The Wilson's Disease Association publishes brochures on Wilson's disease. Serial publication: *Wilson's Disease Association Newsletter*, quarterly—tips for patients and reports about current research and legislation.

Part Two

Pancreatic and Diabetic Disorders

Chapter 5

The Pancreas

The pancreas is an elongated organ that generally measures six inches in length and lies sideways slightly below the stomach. As an exocrine organ, the pancreas produces enzymes that influence digestion. Our present concern with the pancreas, however, is with a tiny fraction of the organ that is composed of a cluster of hormone-producing cells referred to as the islets of Langerhans.

The hormone-producing cells of the pancreas are named for Paul Langerhans. It was Langerhans who in the late 1860s first described the existence of cells within the pancreas that were not connected to ducts. Later scientists discovered that these scattered cells actually operated as an endocrine gland. Estimates of the number of Langerhans' islets occupying a normal pancreas vary, but some go as high as 1 million. You can imagine how small they must be if all together they make up less than 2% of the entire pancreas.

Scientists have identified three types of cells within each of these minuscule islets. They are known as alpha, beta, and delta cells. Delta cells secrete somatostatin, but no one is quite sure what its purpose is. For now, it is enough to realize it exists. The beta cells, which comprise approximately 80% of the islets, manufacture and secrete insulin. This hormone helps remove glucose from the blood by binding to receptor cells and increasing its target tissue's ability to take up and use glucose. Glucagon, the hormone produced by the alpha cells, works in direct opposition to insulin—it increases blood sugar. Unlike many other hormones, neither insulin nor glucagon is controlled by the pituitary gland. Both alpha and beta cells receive signals directly from the circulating blood and the nervous system. With a balance of insulin and glucagon secretions, the body is able to constantly adjust its level of circulating glucose.

Breaking Down and Building Up

Meeting the daily needs of every organ in the body requires an enormous amount of energy. Even when a person is sleeping or sitting perfectly still, billions of cells continue to function, and they all have to be fed. To add to the complexity, different organs have different requirements. The brain demands a constant diet of pure glucose and is the largest consumer of glucose in the entire body. Whether you are puzzling through a homework assignment in advanced trigonometry or playing with your cat, your brain's appetite stays at nearly the exact same level. If supplies of blood sugar fall too low, the brain will stop functioning at full capacity almost immediately. In comparison, muscles like a mixture of glucose, fat, and protein. The heart thrives on mostly fat, some glucose, and just a dash of protein.

Much of the body's blood sugar is derived from carbohydrates. After a meal, glucose levels in the blood rise. This triggers the release of insulin from the pancreas. The insulin circulates through the body and attaches itself to receptors on the appropriate cells. Muscle cells are particularly well supplied with insulin receptors. Once the insulin is in place, it allows glucose to enter the cell, where it is used as energy. When levels of insulin are high, glucose that is not metabolized or used right away is turned into glycogen and stored in the liver. Some is also converted into fat and stored in the adipose, or "fatty," tissues. These fat cells are known as triglycerides. Excess carbohydrate molecules are used in this conversion. Adipose tissue insulates the body from cold and heat and serves as a convenient reserve bank for energy. Thus, insulin lowers blood sugar levels both by getting glucose into the cells that need it and by converting it into products for storage.

Glucagon, the hormone produced by the alpha cells, has the reverse function. It increases the amount of glucose in circulation. When sugar levels fall too low, alpha cells are stimulated. Glucagon production rises, and glycogen stored in the liver is converted back into glucose. The liver releases the glucose into the blood, and blood sugar increases. Amino acids can also be converted into glucose if necessary. Glucagon can affect its secretion, as well as that of adrenaline and cortisol from the adrenal gland and growth hormone from the pituitary.

Diabetes

When insulin supplies are deficient, or when the body is unable to use supplies of insulin, blood sugar levels rise to dangerous levels. This condition is known as hyperglycemia, and recognition of its symptoms led to identification and, eventually, to treatment of the disease called diabetes mellitus.

This disease has been known for several thousand years, and the original meaning of its name accurately describes its most prevalent, observable symptoms. The ancient Greeks referred to it as diabetes, meaning "siphon," and in the late 17th century the Latin word mellitus, meaning "honey-sweet," was added. The siphoning, or excretion, of vast quantities of urine containing extremely high concentrations of sugar is an early sign of diabetes mellitus.

Excessive amounts of sugar in the blood reduce the kidneys' ability to absorb water. This results in polyuria, a drastic increase in urination. In turn, this creates polydipsia, a desperate thirst. At the same time, although the sugar level is high, it is not reaching the cells that need it. The body is starving for energy, and polyphagia, or excessive eating, is common. Unable to use glucose—its main source of energy—the body will begin using stores of protein as an alternative fuel. This causes protein deficiencies. As a result, healing and infection fighting become more difficult.

When there is a lack of insulin, or if insulin is not able to perform, the liver begins to break down reserve stores of fat. This causes weight loss and also releases an acidic product called ketones. Ketones give the breath a peculiar odor that can be mistaken for alcohol. In some unfortunate cases, diabetics have gone into a coma and died because bystanders assumed they were drunk rather than in need of immediate medical attention. Most doctors encourage their diabetic patients to wear medical alert bracelets. These have saved hundreds of thousands of lives. In the United States alone there are currently over 4 million diabetics; over 100,000 new cases of diabetes mellitus are diagnosed each year. And the number is rising. Diabetes is the third leading cause of death in the United States, behind only heart disease and cancer. Having diabetes doubles the chance of having a fatal heart attack or stroke. It causes at least 20% of all kidney failures, and it is the leading cause of blindness in adults.

Unfortunately, there is no cure for diabetes. There are, however, many excellent treatments currently available that allow most diabetic patients to lead a fairly normal life. In many cases, effective therapy depends directly on the patients' ability to take an active interest in monitoring and treating themselves.

Early detection of diabetes is now often possible. A laboratory test called a glucose tolerance test (GTT) is used to identify the prediabetic, and recent advances in at-home blood tests now offer easy, accurate, and safe testing of glucose levels. Susceptibility to diabetes mellitus increases in adults over the age of 45, and after the age of 30 it is more commonly found in women than in men. Obese people are more likely to get diabetes than are people of normal weight. Diabetes also tends to be genetically transmitted, so those whose families have a history of diabetes should be exceptionally aware that its early diagnosis can mean the difference between life and death.

Chapter 6

Pancreatitis

Your pancreas is a large gland behind your stomach and close to your duodenum. The pancreas secretes powerful digestive enzymes that enter the small intestine through a duct. These enzymes help you digest fats, proteins, and carbohydrates. The pancreas also releases the hormones insulin and glucagon into the bloodstream. These hormones play an important part in metabolizing sugar.

Pancreatitis is a rare disease in which the pancreas becomes inflamed. Damage to the gland occurs when digestive enzymes are activated and begin attacking the pancreas. In severe cases, there may be bleeding into the gland, serious tissue damage, infection, and cysts. Enzymes and toxins may enter the bloodstream and seriously injure organs, such as the heart, lungs, and kidney.

There are two forms of pancreatitis. The acute form occurs suddenly and may be a severe, life-threatening illness with many complications. Usually, the patient recovers completely. If injury to the pancreas continues, such as when a patient persists in drinking alcohol, a chronic form of the disease may develop, bringing severe pain and reduced functioning of the pancreas that affects digestion and causes weight loss.

What Is Acute Pancreatitis?

An estimated 50,000 to 80,000 cases of acute pancreatitis occur in the United States each year. This disease occurs when the pancreas

National Institute of Diabetes and Digestive and Kidney Diseases, National Institutes of Health. NIH Pub. No. 95-1596, July 1992.

51

suddenly becomes inflamed and then gets better. Some patients have more than one attack but recover fully after each one. Most cases of acute pancreatitis are caused either by alcohol abuse or by gallstones. Other causes may be use of prescribed drugs, trauma or surgery to the abdomen, or abnormalities of the pancreas or intestine. In rare cases, the disease may result from infections, such as mumps. In about 15 percent of cases, the cause is unknown.

What Are the Symptoms of Acute Pancreatitis?

Acute pancreatitis usually begins with pain in the upper abdomen, that may last for a few days. The pain is often severe. It may be constant pain, just in the abdomen, or it may reach to the back and other areas. The pain may be sudden and intense, or it may begin as a mild pain that is aggravated by eating and slowly grows worse. The abdomen may be swollen and very tender. Other symptoms may include nausea, vomiting, fever, and an increased pulse rate. The person often feels and looks very sick.

About 20 percent of cases are severe. The patient may become dehydrated and have low blood pressure. Sometimes the patient's heart, lungs, or kidneys fail. In the most severe cases, bleeding can occur in the pancreas, leading to shock and sometimes death.

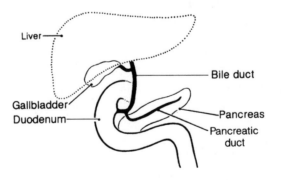

Figure 6.1. The pancreas and nearby organs.

How Is Acute Pancreatitis Diagnosed?

During acute attacks, high levels of amylase (a digestive enzyme formed in the pancreas) are found in the blood. Changes may also occur in blood levels of calcium, magnesium, sodium, potassium, and bicarbonate. Patients may have high amounts of sugar and lipids (fats) in their blood too. These changes help the doctor diagnose pancreatitis. After the pancreas recovers, blood levels of these substances usually return to normal.

What Is the Treatment for Acute Pancreatitis?

The treatment a patient receives depends on how bad the attack is. Unless complications occur, acute pancreatitis usually gets better on its own, so treatment is supportive in most cases. Usually the patient goes into the hospital. The doctor prescribes fluids by vein to restore blood volume. The kidneys and lungs may be treated to prevent failure of those organs. Other problems, such as cysts in the pancreas, may need treatment too.

Sometimes a patient cannot control vomiting and needs to have a tube through the nose to the stomach to remove fluid and air. In mild cases, the patient may not have food for 3 or 4 days but is given fluids and pain relievers by vein. An acute attack usually lasts only a few days, unless the ducts are blocked by gallstones. In severe cases, the patient may be fed through the veins for 3 to 6 weeks while the pancreas slowly heals.

Antibiotics may be given if signs of infection arise. Surgery may be needed if complications such as infection, cysts, or bleeding occur. Attacks caused by gallstones may require removal of the gallbladder or surgery of the bile duct.

Surgery is sometimes needed for the doctor to be able to exclude other abdominal problems that can simulate pancreatitis or to treat acute pancreatitis. When there is severe injury with death of tissue, an operation may be done to remove the dead tissue.

After all signs of acute pancreatitis are gone, the doctor will determine the cause and try to prevent future attacks. In some patients the cause of the attack is clear, but in others further tests need to be done.

What If the Patient Has Gallstones?

Ultrasound is used to detect gallstones and sometimes can provide the doctor with an idea of how severe the pancreatitis is. When gallstones are found, surgery is usually needed to remove them. When they are removed depends on how severe the pancreatitis is. If it is mild, the gallstones often can be removed within a week or so. In more severe cases, the patient may wait a month or more, until he improves, before the stones are removed. The CAT (computer axial tomography) scan may also be used to find out what is happening in and around the pancreas and how severe the problem is. This is important information that the doctor needs to determine when to remove the gallstones.

After the gallstones are removed and inflammation subsides, the pancreas usually returns to normal. Before patients leave the hospital, they are advised not to drink alcohol and not to eat large meals.

What Is Chronic Pancreatitis?

Chronic pancreatitis usually follows many years of alcohol abuse. It may develop after only one acute attack, especially if there is damage to the ducts of the pancreas. In the early stages, the doctor cannot always tell whether the patient has acute or chronic disease. The symptoms may be the same. Damage to the pancreas from drinking alcohol may cause no symptoms for many years, and then the patient suddenly has an attack of pancreatitis. In more than 90 percent of adult patients, chronic pancreatitis appears to be caused by alcoholism. This is more common in men than women and often develops between 30 and 40 years of age. In other cases, pancreatitis may be inherited. Scientists do not know why the inherited form occurs. Patients with chronic pancreatitis tend to have three kinds of problems: pain, malabsorption of food leading to weight loss, or diabetes.

Some patients do not have any pain but most do. Pain may be constant in the back and abdomen, and for some patients, the pain attacks are disabling. In some cases, the abdominal pain goes away as the condition advances. Doctors think this happens because pancreatic enzymes are no longer being made by the pancreas.

Patients with this disease often lose weight, even when their appetite and eating habits are normal. This occurs because the body does not secrete enough pancreatic enzymes to break down food, so nutrients are not absorbed normally. Poor digestion leads to loss of fat, protein, and sugar into the stool. Diabetes may also develop at this stage if the insulin-producing cells of the pancreas (islet cells) have been damaged.

How Is Chronic Pancreatitis Diagnosed?

Diagnosis may be difficult but is aided by a number of new techniques. Pancreatic function tests help the physician decide if the pancreas still can make enough digestive enzymes. The doctor can see abnormalities in the pancreas using several techniques (ultrasonic imaging, endoscopic retrograde cholangiopancreatography (ERCP), and the CAT scan). In more advanced stages of the disease, when diabetes and malabsorption (a problem due to lack of enzymes) occur, the doctor can use a number of blood, urine, and stool tests to help in the diagnosis of chronic pancreatitis and to monitor the progression of the disorder.

How Is Chronic Pancreatitis Treated?

The doctor treats chronic pancreatitis by relieving pain and managing the nutritional and metabolic problems. The patient can reduce the amount of fat and protein lost in stools by cutting back on dietary fat and taking pills containing pancreatic enzymes. This will result in better nutrition and weight gain. Sometimes insulin or other drugs must be given to control the patient's blood sugar.

In some cases, surgery is needed to relieve pain by draining an enlarged pancreatic duct. Sometimes, part or most of the pancreas is removed in an attempt to relieve chronic pain.

Patients must stop drinking, adhere to their prescribed diets, and take the proper medications in order to have fewer and milder attacks.

Additional Reading

Banks PA, Frey CF, Greenberger NJ. The spectrum of chronic pancreatitis. *Patient Care,* 1989; 23(9): 163-96. This review article for physicians is written in technical language. Available in medical libraries.

Facts and Fallacies About Digestive Diseases. 1991. This fact sheet discusses commonly held beliefs about digestive diseases, including pancreatitis and gallbladder disease. Available from the National Digestive Diseases Information Clearinghouse, Box NDDIC, 2 Information Way, Bethesda, MD 20892-3570. (301) 654-3810.

Clayman CB, ed. *The American Medical Association Encyclopedia of Medicine.* New York: Random House. 1989. Authoritative reference guide for patients with sections on irritable bowel syndrome and other disorders of the digestive system. Widely available in libraries and bookstores.

Frey CF, et al. Progress in acute pancreatitis. *Patient Care,* 1989; 23(5): 38-53. This review article for physicians is written in technical language. Available in medical libraries.

National Digestive Diseases Information Clearinghouse
2 Information Way
Bethesda, MD 20892-3570
(301) 654-3810

The National Digestive Diseases Information Clearinghouse (NDDIC) is a service of the National Institute of Diabetes and Digestive and Kidney Diseases, part of the National Institutes of Health, under the U.S. Public Health Service. The clearinghouse, authorized by Congress in 1980, provides information about digestive diseases and health to people with digestive diseases and their families, health care professionals, and the public. The NDDIC answers inquiries; develops, reviews, and distributes publications; and works closely with professional and patient organizations and government agencies to coordinate resources about digestive diseases.

Publications produced by the clearinghouse are reviewed carefully for scientific accuracy, content, and readability. Materials produced by other sources are also reviewed for scientific accuracy and are used, along with clearinghouse publications, to answer requests.

Chapter 7

Pancreatic Cancer

What Is Cancer of the Pancreas?

Cancer of the pancreas is a disease in which cancer (malignant) cells are found in the tissues of the pancreas. The pancreas is about 6 inches long and is shaped something like a thin pear, wider at one end and narrowing at the other. The pancreas lies behind the stomach, inside a loop formed by part of the small intestine. The broader right end of the pancreas is called the head, the middle section is called the body, and the narrow left end is the tail.

The pancreas has two basic jobs in your body. It produces juices that help you break down (digest) your food, and hormones (such as insulin) that regulate how your body stores and uses food. The area of the pancreas that produces digestive juices is called the exocrine pancreas. About 95% of pancreatic cancers begin in the exocrine pancreas. The hormone-producing area of the pancreas is called the endocrine pancreas. Only about 5% of pancreatic cancers start here. This text has information on cancer of the exocrine pancreas. For more information on cancer of the endocrine pancreas (also called islet cell cancer) see the PDQ Patient Information Statement on Islet Cell Carcinoma [in the next chapter].

How Pancreatic Cancer Is Diagnosed

Cancer of the pancreas is hard to find (diagnose) because the organ is hidden behind other organs. Organs around the pancreas in-

National Cancer Institute (NCI) Document #208/00046, CancerNet (cancernet. nci.nih.gov) last modified September 1997.

clude the stomach, small intestine, bile ducts (tubes through which bile, a digestive juice made by the liver, flows from the liver to the small intestine), gallbladder (the small sac below the liver that stores bile), the liver, and the spleen (the organ that stores red blood cells and filters blood to remove excess blood cells). The signs of pancreatic cancer are like many other illnesses, and there may be no signs in the first stages. You should see your doctor if you have any of the following: nausea, loss of appetite, weight loss without trying to lose weight, pain in the upper or middle of your abdomen, or yellowing of your skin (jaundice).

If you have symptoms, your doctor will examine you and order tests to see if you have cancer and what your treatment should be. You may have an ultrasound, a test that uses sound waves to find tumors. A CT scan, a special type of x-ray that uses a computer to make a picture of the inside of your abdomen, may also be done. Another special scan called magnetic resonance imaging (MRI), which uses magnetic waves to make a picture of the inside of your abdomen, maybe done as well.

A test called an ERCP (endoscopic retrograde cholangiopancreatography) may also be done. During this test, a flexible tube is put down the throat, through the stomach, and into the small intestine. Your doctor can see through the tube and inject dye into the drainage tube (duct) of the pancreas so that the area can be seen more clearly on an x-ray. During ERCP, your doctor may also put a fine needle into the pancreas to take out some cells. This is called a biopsy. The cells can then be looked at under a microscope to see if they contain cancer.

PTC (percutaneous transhepatic cholangiography) is another test that can help find cancer of the pancreas. During this test, a thin needle is put into the liver through your right side. Dye is injected into the bile ducts in the liver so that blockages can be seen on x-rays.

In some cases, a needle can be inserted into the pancreas during an x-ray or ultrasound so that cells can be taken out to see if they contain cancer. You may need surgery to see if you have cancer of the pancreas. If this is the case, your doctor will cut into the abdomen and look at the pancreas and the tissues around it for cancer. If you have cancer and it looks like it has not spread to other tissues, your doctor may remove the cancer or relieve blockages caused by the tumor.

Stages of Cancer of the Pancreas

Once cancer of the pancreas is found, more tests will be done to find out if the cancer has spread from the pancreas to the tissues around it or to other parts of the body. This is called staging. The following stages are used for cancer of the pancreas:

Stage I. Cancer is found only in the pancreas itself, or has started to spread just to the tissues next to the pancreas, such as the small intestine, the stomach, or the bile duct.

Stage II. Cancer has spread to nearby organs such as the stomach, spleen, or colon, but has not entered the lymph nodes. (Lymph nodes are small, bean-shaped structures that are found throughout the body; they produce and store infection-fighting cells).

Stage III. Cancer has spread to lymph nodes near the pancreas. The cancer may or may not have spread to nearby organs.

Stage IV. Cancer has spread to places far away from the pancreas, such as the liver or lungs.

Recurrent. Recurrent disease means that the cancer has come back (recurred) after it has been treated. It may come back in the pancreas or in another part of the body.

How Cancer of the Pancreas Is Treated

There are treatments for all patients with cancer of the pancreas. Three kinds of treatment are used: surgery (taking out the cancer or relieving symptoms caused by the cancer), radiation therapy (using high-dose x-rays or other high-energy rays to kill cancer cells), chemotherapy (using drugs to kill cancer cells).

The use of biological therapy (using the body's immune system to fight cancer)is being tested for pancreatic cancer.

Surgery

Surgery may be used to take out the tumor. Your doctor may take out the cancer using one of the following operations:

- A *Whipple procedure* removes the head of the pancreas, part of the small intestine, and some of the tissues around it. Enough of the pancreas is left to continue making digestive juices and insulin.

- *Total pancreatectomy* takes out the whole pancreas, part of the small intestine, part of the stomach, the bile duct, the gallbladder, spleen, and most of the lymph nodes in the area.

- *Distal pancreatectomy* takes out the body and tail of the pancreas.

If your cancer has spread and it cannot be removed, your doctor may do surgery to relieve symptoms. If the cancer is blocking the small intestine and bile builds up in the gallbladder, your doctor may do surgery to go around (bypass) all or part of the small intestine. During this operation, your doctor will cut the gallbladder or bile duct and sew it to the small intestine. This is called biliary bypass. Surgery or x-ray procedures may also be done to put in a tube (catheter) to drain bile that has built up in the area. During these procedures, your doctor may make the catheter drain through a tube to the outside of the body or the catheter may go around the blocked area and drain the bile to the small intestine. In addition, if the cancer is blocking the flow of food from the stomach, the stomach may be sewn directly to the small intestine so you can continue to eat normally.

Radiation Therapy

Radiation therapy uses high-energy x-rays to kill cancer cells and shrink tumors. Radiation may come from a machine outside the body (external radiation therapy) or from putting materials that produce radiation (radioisotopes) through thin plastic tubes in the area where the cancer cells are found (internal radiation therapy).

Chemotherapy

Chemotherapy uses drugs to kill cancer cells. Chemotherapy may be taken by pill, or it may be put into the body by a needle in the vein or muscle. Chemotherapy is called a systemic treatment because the drug enters the bloodstream, travels through the body, and can kill cancer cells outside the pancreas.

Biological Therapy

Biological therapy tries to get your own body to fight cancer. It uses materials made by your own body or made in a laboratory to boost, direct, or restore your body's natural defenses against disease. Biological therapy is sometimes called biological response modifier (BRM) therapy or immunotherapy. Biological therapy is being tested in clinical trials.

Treatment by Stage

Treatment for cancer of the pancreas depends on the stage of your disease, your age, and your overall condition.

You may receive treatment that is considered standard based on its effectiveness in a number of patients in past studies, or you may choose to go into a clinical trial. Most patients with cancer of the pancreas are not cured with standard therapy and some standard treatments may have more side effects than are desired. For these reasons, clinical trials are designed to find better ways to treat cancer patients and are based on the most up-to-date information. Clinical trials are going on in most parts of the country for all stages of cancer of the pancreas. If you wish to know more about clinical trials, call the Cancer Information Service at 1-800-4-CANCER (1-800-422-6237); TTY at 1-800-332-8615.

Stage I Pancreatic Cancer

Your treatment may be one of the following:

1. Surgery to remove the head of the pancreas, part of the small intestine, and some of the surrounding tissues (Whipple procedure).

2. Surgery to remove the entire pancreas and the organs around it (total pancreatectomy).

3. Surgery to remove the body and tail of the pancreas (distal pancreatectomy).

4. Surgery followed by chemotherapy and radiation therapy.

5. Clinical trials of radiation therapy with or without chemotherapy given before, during, or after surgery.

Stage II Pancreatic Cancer

Your treatment may be one of the following:

1. Surgery or other treatments to reduce symptoms.

2. External radiation therapy with or without chemotherapy.

3. Surgery to remove all or part of the pancreas with or without chemotherapy and radiation therapy.

4. Clinical trials of radiation therapy and chemotherapy given before surgery.

5. Clinical trials of radiation therapy plus drugs to make cancer cells more sensitive to radiation (radiosensitizers).

6. Clinical trials of chemotherapy.

7. Clinical trials of radiation therapy given during surgery with or without internal radiation therapy.

Stage III Pancreatic Cancer

Your treatment may be one of the following:

1. Surgery or other treatments to reduce symptoms.

2. External radiation therapy with or without chemotherapy.

3. Surgery to remove all or part of the pancreas with or without chemotherapy and radiation therapy.

4. Clinical trials of radiation therapy given before surgery.

5. Clinical trials of surgery plus radiation therapy plus drugs to make cancer cells more sensitive to radiation (radiosensitizers).

6. Clinical trials of chemotherapy.

7. Clinical trials of radiation therapy given during surgery, with or without internal radiation therapy.

Stage IV Pancreatic Cancer

Your treatment may be one of the following:

1. Surgery or other treatments to reduce symptoms.

2. Treatments for pain.

3. Chemotherapy.

4. Clinical trials of chemotherapy or biological therapy.

Recurrent Pancreatic Cancer

Your treatment may be one of the following:

1. Chemotherapy.

2. Surgery or other treatments to reduce symptoms.

3. External radiation therapy to reduce symptoms.

4. Treatments for pain.

5. Other medical care to reduce symptoms.

6. Clinical trials of chemotherapy or biological therapy.

To Learn More

To learn more about cancer of the pancreas, call the National Cancer Institute's Cancer Information Service at 1-800-4-CANCER (1-800-422-6237); TTY at 1-800-332-8615. By dialing this toll-free number, you can speak with someone who can answer your questions.

The Cancer Information Service can also send you booklets. The following booklets about cancer of the pancreas may be helpful to you:

- What You Need To Know About Cancer of the Pancreas
- Research Report: Cancer of the Pancreas

The following general booklets on questions related to cancer may also be helpful:

- What You Need To Know About Cancer
- Taking Time: Support for People with Cancer and the People Who Care About Them
- What Are Clinical Trials All About?
- Chemotherapy and You: A Guide to Self-Help During Treatment
- Radiation Therapy and You: A Guide to Self-Help During Treatment
- Eating Hints for Cancer Patients
- Advanced Cancer: Living Each Day
- When Cancer Recurs: Meeting the Challenge Again

There are many other places you can get material about cancer treatment and services to help you. You can check the social service office at your hospital for local and national agencies that help with your finances, getting to and from treatment, care at home, and dealing with your problems.

You can also write to the National Cancer Institute at this address:

National Cancer Institute
Office of Cancer Communications
31 Center Drive, MSC 2580
Bethesda, MD 20892-2580

What Is PDQ?

PDQ is a computer system that gives up-to-date information on cancer and its prevention, detection, treatment, and supportive care. It is a service of the National Cancer Institute (NCI) for people with cancer and their families and for doctors, nurses, and other health care professionals.

To ensure that it remains current, the information in PDQ is reviewed and updated each month by experts in the fields of cancer treatment, prevention, screening, and supportive care. PDQ also provides information about research on new treatments (clinical trials), doctors who treat cancer, and hospitals with cancer programs. The treatment information in this summary is based on information in the PDQ summary for health professionals on this cancer.

How to use PDQ

PDQ can be used to learn more about current treatment of different kinds of cancer. You may find it helpful to discuss this information with your doctor, who knows you and has the facts about your disease. PDQ can also provide the names of additional health care professionals who specialize in treating patients with cancer.

Before you start treatment, you also may want to think about taking part in a clinical trial. PDQ can be used to learn more about these trials. A clinical trial is a research study that attempts to improve current treatments or finds information on new treatments for patients with cancer. Clinical trials are based on past studies and information discovered in the laboratory. Each trial answers certain scientific questions in order to find new and better ways to help patients with cancer. Information is collected about new treatments, their risks, and how well they do or do not work. When clinical trials show that a new treatment is better than the treatment currently used as "standard" treatment, the new treatment may become the standard treatment. Listings of current clinical trials are available on PDQ. Many cancer doctors who take part in clinical trials are listed in PDQ.

To learn more about cancer and how it is treated, or to learn more about clinical trials for your kind of cancer, call the National Cancer Institute's Cancer Information Service. The number is 1-800-4-CANCER (1-800-422-6237); TTY at 1-800-332-8615. The call is free and a trained information specialist will be available to answer cancer-related questions.

PDQ is updated whenever there is new information. Check with the Cancer Information Service to be sure that you have the most up-to-date information.

Chapter 8

Islet Cell Carcinoma

What Is Islet Cell Cancer?

Islet cell cancer, a rare cancer, is a disease in which cancer (malignant) cells are found in certain tissues of the pancreas. The pancreas is about 6 inches long and is shaped like a thin pear, wider at one end and narrower at the other. The pancreas lies behind the stomach, inside a loop formed by part of the small intestine. The broader right end of the pancreas is called the head, the middle section is called the body, and the narrow left end is the tail.

The pancreas has two basic jobs in your body. It produces juices that help you break down (digest) your food, and hormones (such as insulin) that regulate how your body stores and uses food. The area of the pancreas that produces digestive juices is called the exocrine pancreas. About 95% of pancreatic cancers begin in the exocrine pancreas. The hormone-producing area of the pancreas has special cells called islet cells and is called the endocrine pancreas. Only about 5% of pancreatic cancers start here. This text has information on cancer of the endocrine pancreas (islet cell cancer). For more information on cancer of the exocrine pancreas, see the PDQ patient information statement on cancer of the pancreas. [Included in the previous chapter.]

The islet cells in the pancreas make many hormones, including insulin, which help your body store and use sugars. When islet cells

National Cancer Institute (NCI) #208/00790, June 1996; NCI's CancerNet is available at cancernet.nci.nih.gov in the pancreas become cancerous, they may make too many hormones. Islet cell cancers that make too many hormones are called functioning tumors. Other islet cell cancers may not make extra hormones and are called non-functioning tumors. Tumors that do not spread to other parts of the body can also be found in the islet cells. These are called benign tumors and are not cancer. Your doctor will need to determine whether your tumor is cancer or a benign tumor.

Like most cancer, islet cell cancer is best treated when it is found (diagnosed) early. You should see your doctor if you have pain in your abdomen, diarrhea, stomach pain, a tired feeling all the time, fainting, or weight gain without eating too much.

If you have symptoms, your doctor will order blood and urine tests to see whether the amounts of hormones in your body are normal. Other tests, including x-rays and special scans, may also be done.

Your chance of recovery (prognosis) depends on the type of islet cell cancer you have, how far the cancer has spread, and your overall health.

Stages of Islet Cell Cancer

Once islet cell cancer is found, more tests will be done to find out if cancer cells have spread to other parts of the body. This is called staging. The staging system for islet cell cancer is still being developed. These tumors are most often divided into one of three groups:

- islet cell cancers occurring in one site within the pancreas
- islet cell cancers occurring in several sites within the pancreas
- islet cell cancers that have spread to lymph nodes near the pancreas or to distant sites

Your doctor also needs to know the type of islet cell tumor you have to plan treatment. The following types of islet cell tumors are found.

Gastrinoma. The tumor makes large amounts of a hormone called gastrin, which causes too much acid to be made in the stomach. There may be ulcers in the stomach because of the increased acid.

Insulinoma. Thee tumor makes too much of the hormone insulin and causes the body to store sugar instead of burning the sugar as energy. This causes too little sugar in the blood, a condition called hypoglycemia.

Miscellaneous. Other types of islet cell cancer can affect the pancreas and/or small intestine. Each type of tumor may affect different hormones in the body and cause different symptoms.

Recurrent. Recurrent disease means that the cancer has come back (recurred) after it has been treated. It may come back in the pancreas or in another part of the body.

How Islet Cell Cancer Is Treated

There are treatments for all patients with islet cell cancer. Three types of treatment are used:

- surgery (taking out the cancer)

- chemotherapy (using drugs to kill cancer cells)

- hormone therapy (using hormones to stop cancer cells from growing).

Surgery is the most common treatment for islet cell cancer. Your doctor may take out the cancer and most or part of the pancreas. Sometimes the stomach is taken out (gastrectomy) because of ulcers. Lymph nodes in the area may also be removed and looked at under a microscope to see if they contain cancer.

Chemotherapy uses drugs to kill cancer cells. Chemotherapy may be taken by pill, or it may be put into the body by a needle in the vein or muscle. Chemotherapy is called a systemic treatment because the drug enters the bloodstream, travels through the body, and can kill cancer cells throughout the body.

Hormone therapy uses hormones to stop the cancer cells from growing or to relieve symptoms caused by the tumor.

Hepatic arterial occlusion or embolization uses drugs or other agents to reduce or block the flow of blood to the liver in order to kill cancer cells growing in the liver.

Treatment by Type

Treatment for islet cell cancer depends on the type of tumor, the stage, and your overall health.

You may receive treatment that is considered standard based on its effectiveness in a number of patients in past studies, or you may choose to go into a clinical trial. Not all patients are cured with standard therapy and some standard treatments may have more side effects than are desired. For these reasons, clinical trials are designed to find better ways to treat cancer patients and are based on the most up-to-date information. Clinical trials are going on in many parts of the country for patients with islet cell cancer. If you want more information, call the Cancer Information Service at 1-800-4-CANCER (1-800-422-6237); TTY at 1-800-332-8615.

Gastrinoma

Your treatment may be one of the following:

1. Surgery to remove the cancer.
2. Surgery to remove the stomach (gastrectomy).
3. Surgery to cut the nerve that stimulates the pancreas.
4. Chemotherapy.
5. Hormone therapy.
6. Hepatic arterial occlusion or embolization to kill cancer cells growing in the liver.

Insulinoma

Your treatment may be one of the following:

1. Surgery to remove the cancer.
2. Chemotherapy.
3. Hormone therapy.
4. Drugs to relieve symptoms.
5. Hepatic arterial occlusion or embolization to kill cancer cells growing in the liver.

Miscellaneous Islet Cell Cancer

Your treatment may be one of the following:

1. Surgery to remove the cancer.
2. Chemotherapy.
3. Hormone therapy.
4. Hepatic arterial occlusion or embolization to kill cancer cells growing in the liver.

Recurrent Islet Cell Carcinoma

Your treatment depends on many factors, including what treatment you had before and where the cancer has come back. Your treatment may be chemotherapy, or you may want to consider taking part in a clinical trial.

To Learn More

To learn more about islet cell cancer, call the National Cancer Institute's Cancer Information Service at 1-800-4-CANCER (1-800-422-6237); TTY at 1-800-332-8615. By dialing this toll-free number, you can speak with someone who can answer your questions.

The Cancer Information Service can also send you booklets. The following booklets about pancreatic cancer may be helpful to you:

- What You Need To Know About Cancer of the Pancreas
- Research Report: Cancer of the Pancreas

The following general booklets on questions related to cancer may also be helpful:

- What You Need To Know About Cancer
- Taking Time: Support for People with Cancer and the People Who Care About Them
- What Are Clinical Trials All About?
- Chemotherapy and You: A Guide to Self-Help During Treatment
- Radiation Therapy and You: A Guide to Self-Help During Treatment
- Eating Hints for Cancer Patients
- Advanced Cancer: Living Each Day
- When Cancer Recurs: Meeting the Challenge Again

There are other places where you can get material about cancer treatment and information about services to help you. You can check the social service office at your hospital for local and national agencies that help with your finances, getting to and from treatment, receiving care at home, and dealing with your problems. The American Cancer Society, for example, has many free services. Their local offices are listed in the white pages of the telephone book.

You can also write to the National Cancer Institute at this address:

National Cancer Institute
Office of Cancer Communications
31 Center Drive, MSC 2580
Bethesda, MD 20892

If you want to know more about cancer and how it is treated, or if you wish to know about clinical trials for your type of cancer, you can call the NCI's Cancer Information Service at 1-800-422-6237, toll free. A trained information specialist can talk with you and answer your questions.

Overview of PDQ

PDQ is a computer system that gives up-to-date information on cancer treatment. It is a service of the National Cancer Institute (NCI) for people with cancer and their families, and for doctors, nurses, and other health care professionals.

PDQ tells about the current treatments for most cancers. The information in PDQ is reviewed each month by cancer experts. It is updated when there is new information. The patient information in PDQ also tells about warning signs and how the cancer is found. PDQ also lists information about research on new treatments (clinical trials), doctors who treat cancer, and hospitals with cancer programs. The treatment information in this summary is based on information in the PDQ treatment summary for health professionals on this cancer.

How to Use PDQ

You can use PDQ to learn more about current treatment for your kind of cancer. Bring this material from PDQ with you when you see your doctor. You can talk with your doctor, who knows you and has the facts about your disease, about which treatment would be best for you. Before you start your treatment, you might also want to seek a second opinion from a doctor who treats cancer.

Before you start treatment, you also may want to think about taking part in a clinical trial. A clinical trial is a study that uses new treatments to care for patients. Each study is based on past studies and what has been learned in the laboratory. Each trial answers certain scientific questions in order to find new and better ways to help cancer patients. During clinical trials, more and more information is collected about new treatments, their risks, and how well they do or do not work. If clinical trials show that the new treatment is better than the treatment currently being used, the new treatment may become the "standard" treatment. Listings of clinical trials are a part of PDQ. Many cancer doctors who take part in clinical trials are listed in PDQ.

If you want to know more about cancer and how it is treated, or if you wish to learn about clinical trials for your kind of cancer, you can call the National Cancer Institute's Cancer Information Service. The number is 1-800-4-CANCER (1-800-422-6237); TTY at 1-800-332-8615. The call is free and a trained information specialist will talk with you and answer your questions.

PDQ may change when there is new information. Check with the Cancer Information Service to be sure that you have the most up-to-date information.

Chapter 9

Insulin-Dependent Diabetes

What Is Diabetes?

Diabetes is a group of conditions in which glucose (sugar) levels are abnormally high. Diabetes occurs when the pancreas stops making enough insulin, which is necessary for the proper metabolism of digested foods.

About 14 million people in the United States have some form of diabetes, although only half are diagnosed. The three main types of diabetes are insulin-dependent, also known as Type I diabetes; noninsulin-dependent, also called Type II diabetes; and gestational diabetes, which occurs during pregnancy.

Insulin-dependent diabetes mellitus (IDDM) most often develops in children and young adults. Sometimes people over age 40 get IDDM, but it usually begins at younger ages. For this reason, IDDM used to be known as "juvenile" diabetes. IDDM is one of the most common chronic disorders in U.S. children. Each year, from 11,000 to 12,000 children are diagnosed with IDDM. Among the more than 7 million people in the United States who are being treated for diabetes, about 5 to 10 percent have IDDM.

Noninsulin-dependent diabetes mellitus (NIDDM) is the most common type of diabetes. It accounts for 90 to 95 percent of diagnosed diabetes and almost all of undiagnosed diabetes. NIDDM usually develops

U.S. Department of Health and Human Services, National Institute of Diabetes and Digestive and Kidney Diseases, NIH Pub. No. 95-2098, September 1994.

73

in adults over age 40 and is most common in those who are overweight. People with NIDDM usually produce some insulin, but the body cells cannot use it efficiently because the cells are resistant to the insulin. By losing weight, exercising, or taking oral medications, most people with NIDDM can overcome this resistance to insulin. However, some people with NIDDM require daily insulin injections.

Gestational diabetes occurs in some women during pregnancy. It usually ends after the baby is born, but women with gestational diabetes may develop NIDDM when they get older. Gestational diabetes results from the body's resistance to the action of insulin. This resistance is caused by hormones the placenta produces during pregnancy. The condition develops about midway through the pregnancy. Gestational diabetes is usually treated with diet. Some women may need insulin. Gestational diabetes cannot be treated with pills that lower blood glucose as these medicines can cause harm to the baby.

Note about Terminology in This Chapter

This chapter is about insulin-dependent diabetes, or IDDM for short. The word "diabetes" in the text refers to insulin-dependent diabetes unless otherwise noted. This chapter does not replace the advice of a doctor. However, it can help you learn about diabetes and suggest questions to ask a doctor. Local diabetes organizations and clinics that sponsor meetings and educational programs about diabetes can also be helpful. Groups that have information about diabetes programs are listed at the end of this chapter.

What Causes Diabetes?

When we eat, foods containing proteins, fats, and carbohydrates are broken down into simpler, easily absorbed chemicals. One of these is a form of simple sugar called glucose. Glucose circulates in the blood stream where it is available for body cells to use. The body relies on glucose as a source of fuel for important organs such as the brain.

The pancreas, a large gland located behind the stomach, produces the hormone insulin. In people without diabetes, the pancreas makes the correct amount of insulin needed to allow glucose to enter body cells. In people with diabetes, however, not enough insulin is produced. As a result, glucose builds up in blood, overflows into the urine, and passes out of the body unused. Thus, the body loses an important source of fuel—even though the blood contains large amounts of glucose.

Insulin also allows the body to store excess glucose as fat, proteins as muscle protein, and important enzymes that control metabolism. A severe deficiency of insulin causes excess breakdown of stored fats and proteins.

What Are the Causes and Symptoms of IDDM?

Causes of IDDM

In people with insulin-dependent diabetes (IDDM), the pancreas produces too little or no insulin at all. The pancreas is not able to produce insulin because the body's immune system has destroyed the insulin-producing cells.

Scientists do not know why the body's immune system, which allows it to fight disease and other "foreign" substances that may invade the body, attacks and destroys insulin-producing cells. A combination of factors may be involved, including exposure to common viruses or other substances early in life, as well as an inherited risk for IDDM.

Researchers can now test family members of people with IDDM to identify those at increased risk for diabetes. Scientists hope to find a way to prevent the disease through a study called the Diabetes Prevention Trial-Type 1. This study is described in the research section of this chapter.

Early Symptoms of IDDM

The early symptoms of IDDM can be gradual or sudden. They include frequent urination (particularly at night), increased thirst, unexplained weight loss (in spite of increased appetite), and extreme tiredness. These symptoms are caused by the build-up of sugar in the blood and its loss in the urine.

To eliminate sugar in the urine, the kidney "borrows" water from the body. The loss of this extra sugar and water in the urine results in dehydration, which causes increased thirst.

In addition to causing high blood glucose, the lack of insulin causes the body to break down stored fats and proteins. As fats are broken down, the body can convert these fats into waste products called ketones. If ketone production is excessive, abnormal amounts of ketones in the blood can spill into the urine. If blood ketone levels rise too high, a life-threatening condition called ketoacidosis can develop, which requires immediate medical attention. Symptoms of ketoacidosis include

75

abdominal pain, vomiting, rapid breathing, extreme tiredness, and drowsiness.

Points to Remember

The symptoms of IDDM include:

- Frequent urination
- Increased thirst
- Increased hunger
- Unexplained weight loss
- Extreme tiredness

How Does a Person Live with Diabetes?

Diabetes requires constant attention and daily care to keep blood sugar levels in balance. Injecting insulin, following a diet, exercising, and testing blood sugar are some of the day-to-day requirements. To feel good and stay healthy, a person with IDDM must follow a daily management routine. For this reason, diabetes is often referred to as a "24-hour" disease. This section provides general guidelines for diabetes management and explains the roles of various health care professionals who can help you manage your diabetes. The treatment recommendations are based on a 10-year study recently completed by the Federal Government called the Diabetes Control and Complications Trial (DCCT).

The Diabetes Control and Complications Trial

Diabetes can affect many parts of the body. Over time, it can damage a person's kidneys, eyes, nerves, and heart. These long-term complications can result in kidney disease, vision loss, nerve damage, heart attack, and other problems. The DCCT proved that lowering blood sugar levels delayed or prevented diabetes complications by 50 to 80 percent.

The DCCT compared two approaches to managing IDDM: intensive and standard treatment. People in the intensive treatment group learned how to adjust their insulin according to food intake and exercise. They injected insulin three to four times a day or used an insulin pump and tested their blood sugar at least four times a day and once a week at 3 a.m. They also followed a diet and exercise plan and met once a month with a health care team composed of a physician, nurse educator, dietitian, and mental health professional.

People in the standard treatment group followed a plan that was not as strict. They took one or two insulin injections a day, tested sugar levels once or twice a day, and met with the doctor or nurse every 3 months.

At the end of the DCCT, volunteers on intensive treatment had lower rates of kidney, eye, and nerve damage than volunteers in the standard treatment group. The study showed that efforts to improve control of blood sugar made a major difference. In fact, the study found that any long-term lowering of blood sugar levels will reduce the risk of complications, even in people with poor control of their diabetes and early complications of diabetes. For this reason, people with IDDM are encouraged to do the best they can to keep their blood sugar levels as close to the normal range as possible.

However, intensive treatment does increase the risk of low blood sugar episodes, or hypoglycemia, and is not recommended for everyone, particularly older adults, children under age 13, people with heart problems or advanced complications, and people with a history of frequent severe hypoglycemia. Your doctor should help you decide if intensive control is right for you.

Points to Remember

The DCCT showed that intensive control of blood sugar levels can help reduce the risk of complications associated with diabetes. The study showed that any sustained lowering of blood sugar levels is helpful.

Health Care Providers

Diabetes requires daily attention, and you need to learn how to care for your diabetes. A number of people can help you:

A doctor experienced in treating diabetes. These doctors are called endocrinologists or diabetologists. They will work with you to develop an individualized management routine and help you determine your ideal blood sugar range and ways to stay within that range.

"People with IDDM should be under the care of, or have regular contact with, a diabetes specialist who is up to date on diabetes and its management," advises Dr. Julio Santiago, an endocrinologist with the DCCT Center at Washington University in St Louis. "During the last 10 years, diabetes care has greatly improved and become more complex. Services offered by diabetes specialists help people

77

with IDDM learn the nuts and bolts of modern care and its benefits," he says.

A diabetes educator. Diabetes educators specialize in teaching people how to manage their diabetes. Most are registered nurses, pharmacists, dietitians, or physician assistants with advanced training and experience. They help you and your physician develop a management plan based on your age, school or work schedule, daily activities, and eating habits. They can teach you the importance of good nutrition, exercising regularly, and testing your blood sugar. These professionals can also help you adjust to having diabetes. Diabetes educators who use the initials C.D.E. (Certified Diabetes Educator) after their names have passed an examination qualifying them to provide health education to people with diabetes.

A nutritionist or dietitian. Nutritionists or dietitians trained in diabetes care provide diet guidelines and meal planning advice. They can teach you how to balance food intake and insulin requirements and how to handle special situations such as low blood sugar (hypoglycemia) and sick days. Some dietitians are also C.D.E.s.

A mental health professional. A person with diabetes can never take a vacation from daily management chores. For this and other reasons, diabetes can affect the way a person feels. If you need advice on managing diabetes during stressful or difficult times, or if having diabetes makes you feel sad or depressed, talking to a social worker, psychologist, or psychiatrist may be helpful.

"These professionals are trained to help people cope with chronic conditions that require constant care," says Dr. Alan Jacobson, a psychiatrist at the Joslin Diabetes Center in Boston. Dr. Jacobson, who counseled volunteers at the DCCT center at Joslin, says "Discussing their problems and anxieties with a professional helped DCCT volunteers feel emotionally and physically in control."

If a mental health professional is not available to you, Dr. Jacobson suggests joining a local diabetes support group. "Talking with someone else who has IDDM may help," he advises. Information about support groups is available from your physician or C.D.E. and local offices of the American Diabetes Association (ADA) and Juvenile Diabetes Foundation (JDF) International. These organizations also can provide suggestions on how to form a support group if one does not exist in your community. The addresses of these organizations are located at the end of this chapter.

Daily Insulin

People with IDDM must give themselves insulin every day. Insulin cannot be taken in pill form. It can be injected, which involves use of a needle and syringe, or it can be given by an insulin pump. Insulin pumps are worn outside the body on a belt or in a pocket. They deliver a steady supply of insulin through a tube that connects to a needle placed under the skin. Extra amounts of insulin are taken before meals, depending on the blood glucose level and food to be eaten.

Another injection aid is an insulin pen. This device contains a replaceable insulin cartridge and a sterile, disposable needle. Insulin pens are handy because they eliminate the need for carrying extra syringes and insulin bottles. Jet injectors can also be used to give insulin, but these devices are expensive. A jet injector uses high pressure rather than a needle to propel insulin through the skin and into the tissue. Researchers are exploring the use of implantable pumps and other devices for giving insulin. Talk to your doctor about the insulin delivery system that is best for you.

The amount of insulin you need depends on your height, weight, age, food intake, and activity level. Insulin doses must be balanced with meal times and activities, and dosage levels can be affected by illness, stress, or unexpected events. Your doctor or diabetes educator will calculate how much insulin you should take each day to keep your blood sugar levels from rising too high or falling too low. They also will advise you about handling special situations. Most people with newly diagnosed IDDM can begin to inject their own insulin and estimate their insulin dosage needs within the first few days after instruction by a diabetes educator.

Points to Remember

All people with IDDM need insulin. Ways to give insulin include:

- A needle and syringe
- An insulin pump
- An insulin pen
- A jet injector

Blood Glucose Monitoring

Since the early 1980's, self-monitoring of blood glucose (SMBG) has been shown to be the best way to determine if the blood sugar levels of a person with IDDM are too high or too low. The measurement helps you monitor your diabetes control to determine if adjustments in diet, insulin, or exercise are needed. Although SMBG may at first seem difficult and adds to the expense of treatment, diabetes management has improved greatly since this testing method became widely available.

SMBG involves taking a drop of blood, usually from the tip of a finger, and placing it on a specially coated strip. Strips are "read" either visually or by a meter. Visually read strips change color according to the amount of sugar in the blood. The color is then compared to a color chart provided with the strips. To use a glucose meter, you insert the strip into the meter and it gives a digital reading of your blood sugar level, usually within a minute.

Using a blood glucose meter is a more accurate way to test blood sugar. SMBG meters available since the early 1990s offer many features. Some are small and lightweight, and some can store blood sugar readings for a few days or weeks. Meters are sold in drug stores or in diabetes supply stores. You should consult your diabetes educator about which meter would be most appropriate for your lifestyle. Before using a meter, you should receive instructions from a health care professional on how to operate and maintain the device. Correct use of the meter is necessary to obtain accurate readings.

It is important to follow the manufacturer's recommendations for testing the accuracy of your meter (called calibrating the meter). Failure to do so could cause inaccurate test readings, leading to errors in management.

Results of blood sugar measurements should be recorded in a diabetes diary available through pharmacies and doctors' offices. The books have space for recording events such as extra activities or sickness that may affect blood sugar levels. This information will help you and your doctor adjust insulin doses or make other changes in care, if necessary. Sometimes the diary may show patterns in blood sugar levels that indicate a need to contact a health professional between office visits.

Frequent SMBG was an important tool in the DCCT. "For volunteers in the intensive management group, blood glucose testing results served as a guidepost to making decisions about food intake and insulin doses in order to achieve better control," says Ms. Patricia Callahan, a DCCT diabetes nurse educator at the International Diabetes Center in Minneapolis. "Blood glucose testing should be done at least four times a day or as often as necessary to achieve optimal control," she advises. "The idea is to use your SMBG to make adjustments in your food, exercise, and insulin so that your blood sugar stays in a range that is best for you."

Another blood test, the hemoglobin A1c test, shows the average level of blood sugar for the past 2 to 3 months. Your blood sample is sent to a laboratory for analysis. You should have a hemoglobin A1c test at least every 3 months. Based on the results, you and your physician will know how well you have been doing in controlling your diabetes over the last few months.

Points to Remember

Blood glucose testing is very important for monitoring daily care.

- SMBG shows current blood sugar levels.
- Hemoglobin A1c tests average blood sugar levels over the past 2 to 3 months.

Meal Plans

Like everyone else, people with IDDM should follow a healthy eating plan. Your meal plan should be low in fat and cholesterol because these foods have been linked to heart disease, a common problem in people with diabetes. Children and pregnant women with diabetes may have additional nutritional needs. Guidelines for nutrition are available from your dietitian, diabetes educator, or the ADA. Organizations that can help you find resources for nutritional guidance are listed at the end of this chapter.

Different foods have different effects on blood sugar. Therefore, you should try to be as consistent as possible in your food choices and eating times. Some foods raise blood sugar quickly; others have a more gradual effect. By testing your blood sugar after eating, you can learn how particular foods affect your blood sugar levels.

Timing of meals and coordinating them according to your insulin injections is important. Regular insulin, for example, has its peak glucose-lowering effect approximately 2 hours after injection and acts for 4 to 6 hours. It is usually given before meals. Other insulin preparations are absorbed more slowly and have a longer duration of action.

Insulin regimens should be designed to fit a person's eating habits and lifestyle and should be as consistent as possible on a day-to-day basis. A dietitian can personalize a meal plan to include foods you like. Your physician and diabetes educator can also help.

The DCCT volunteers on intensive treatment learned about the relationship between food choices and blood sugar levels. "Each individual's insulin needs were adjusted to fit his or her lifestyle and diet, rather than trying to match the diet to fit the insulin," says Ms. Linda Delahanty, a dietitian with the DCCT Center at Massachusetts General Hospital in Boston. By understanding the relationship between food choices and blood sugar levels, she notes, volunteers in the intensive therapy group had more flexibility in their daily lives and could adjust their insulin doses to changes in their food intake and activity levels.

Points to Remember

- Consult with a dietician to develop a meal plan for you.
- Learn how different foods affect your blood sugar levels.
- Try to keep insulin injections, meals, and activities as consistent as possible on a day-to-day basis.

Exercise

People with IDDM are encouraged to exercise for the same reasons as people without diabetes. Exercise keeps the body in tone and is good for the heart and lungs. Before exercising you should check your blood sugar levels because exercise tends to lower blood sugar. If your blood sugar is too low or if some time has passed since you ate, you should eat a snack before exercising. Sometimes exercise can cause very high blood sugar to rise even higher. If your blood sugar is over 300 mg/dl (before eating), you should give yourself insulin or wait until your blood sugar level falls before beginning to exercise.

"Exercise is an important part of the patient's management plan. Participation in sports and regular exercise helps to improve overall physical fitness," says Dr. Santiago. An exercise program should be planned with the help of a doctor or an experienced physical therapist or trainer.

Points to Remember

Exercise can lower blood sugar levels quickly. Before beginning exercise:

- Check your blood sugar levels.
- If your blood sugar is on the low side, eat a snack.
- If your blood sugar is very high, you should bring it under control before beginning to exercise.
- It may also be necessary to lower your insulin dose before planned exercise.

How Should Diabetic Emergencies Be Handled?

People with diabetes must always balance food, exercise, and insulin to control blood sugar levels. When this balance is disrupted, certain emergency conditions, including low blood sugar (hypoglycemia) or high blood sugar (hyperglycemia) may result. People with IDDM should always wear a medical identification bracelet, necklace, or watch band. These tags state that the wearer has IDDM and list a telephone number to call for help.

Hypoglycemia

Very low blood sugar, called hypoglycemia, is sometimes referred to as an "insulin reaction." This condition can be caused by too much insulin, too little or delayed food, exercise, alcohol, or any combination of these factors. When hypoglycemia occurs, a person can become cranky, tired, sweaty, hungry, confused, and shaky. If blood sugar levels drop too low, a person can lose consciousness or experience a seizure.

Hypoglycemia can usually be treated quickly by eating or drinking something with sugar in it, such as a sweetened drink or orange juice. You should always carry a high-sugar snack that can be used to treat an insulin reaction. Special products to treat insulin reactions, including glucose tablets and gels, are available in drugstores.

If a person loses consciousness or cannot swallow because of hypoglycemia, medical help is necessary. Dial 911 or take the person to a hospital emergency room. An injectable medication called glucagon, available by prescription in drugstores, raises blood sugar quickly. A family member or friend should learn when and how to inject glucagon in an emergency. Your doctor, diabetes educator, or dietitian can give advice about treating hypoglycemia.

In the DCCT, volunteers on intensive treatment had three times as many episodes of hypoglycemia severe enough to require help from another person as the volunteers on standard therapy. Because of this potential danger, intensive management is not recommended for everyone, particularly older adults, children under age 13, or people with heart problems or advanced complications. People who do not experience the usual symptoms of low blood sugar, a condition known as hypoglycemia unawareness, need to take extra care to avoid hypoglycemia. They should measure their blood glucose more often, particularly before driving or operating dangerous machinery.

Points to Remember

- Hypoglycemia is low blood sugar.
- Hypoglycemia can develop quickly, especially with exercise.
- Always carry a high-sugar snack to treat low blood sugar.
- Hypogycemia, if not treated in time, can lead to unconsciousness.
- Test blood sugar levels to avoid hypoglycemia, particularly before driving or exercising.

Hyperglycemia

Hyperglycemia is the opposite of hypoglycemia. Hyperglycemia occurs when the body has too much sugar in the blood. This condition may be caused by insufficient insulin, overeating, inactivity, illness, stress, or a combination of these factors. The symptoms of hyperglycemia include extreme thirst, frequent urination, fatigue, blurred vision, vomiting, and weight loss.

If your blood sugar levels are above 250 mg/dl before meals, you should test your urine for ketones. Ketones are chemicals that the body makes when insulin levels are very low and excessive amounts of fat are being burned. Ketone buildup over several hours can lead to serious illness and coma, a condition called ketoacidosis. Ketone testing kits are available in drugstores or at doctors' offices. They should be available for you to use at home when you are ill or when your blood sugar is very high. Signs of ketoacidosis include vomiting, weakness, rapid breathing, and a sweet breath odor.

Points to Remember

- Hyperglycemia is high blood sugar.
- Hyperglycemia develops more slowly than hypoglycemia.
- Hyperglycemia can indicate that ketoacidosis may be present.
- If blood sugar is high, test urine for ketones.

How Does Diabetes Affect Your Body?

Diabetes can cause damage to both large and small blood vessels, resulting in complications affecting the kidneys, eyes, nerves, heart, and gums. The DCCT showed that maintaining blood sugar levels as close to normal as possible prevents or slows the development of many of these complications.

Kidney Disease

Diabetic kidney disease, called diabetic nephropathy, can be a life-threatening complication of IDDM in about 40 percent of people who have had diabetes for 20 or more years. The kidneys are vital to good health because they serve as a filtering system to clean waste products from the blood. Diabetic nephropathy develops when the small blood vessels that filter these wastes are damaged. Sometimes this damage causes the kidneys to stop working. This condition is called kidney failure or end-stage renal disease. People with kidney failure must either have their blood cleaned by a dialysis machine or have a kidney transplant.

High blood pressure (hypertension) also increases a person's chance of developing kidney disease. People with diabetes are more likely to develop high blood pressure than people without diabetes. Therefore, keeping blood pressure under control is especially important for someone with IDDM. Your doctor should check your blood pressure at every visit.

Blood pressure tests measure how hard your heart is working to pump blood to the organs and vessels in your body. If blood pressure is too high, it can be treated with a doctor's help. Left untreated, bladder and kidney infections can also harm the kidneys. Consult your doctor if symptoms such as painful urination occur.

An early sign of kidney disease is albumin or protein in the urine. A doctor should test your urine for protein or albumin once a year. The doctor should also do an annual blood test to evaluate kidney function. More frequent tests may be necessary if findings are not normal.

The DCCT proved that intensive therapy can prevent the development and slow the progression of early diabetic kidney disease. Another recent study has shown that a type of medication called an ACE inhibitor can help protect the kidneys from damage.

Eye Disease

Diabetes can affect the small blood vessels in the back of the eye, a condition called diabetic retinopathy. Retinopathy means disease of the retina, the tissue at the back of the eye that is sensitive to light. Diabetes eventually causes changes in the tiny vessels that supply the retina with blood. These small changes are called background retinopathy. Most people who have had diabetes for a number of years have background retinopathy, which usually does not affect sight.

85

Over time, the blood vessels may rupture or leak fluid. In a minority of patients, most often those with higher blood sugar, retinopathy becomes more severe and new blood vessels may grow on the retina. These vessels may bleed into the clear gel, or vitreous, that fills the eye or detach the retina from its normal position because of bleeding or scar formation.

Laser treatment can help restore vision impaired by diabetic retinopathy. If you have had IDDM for 5 years or more, you should see an eye doctor at least once a year for an examination through dilated pupils. An annual exam is the best way to detect and treat eye damage before the condition becomes severe. Laser treatment, as well as surgical procedures performed by eye doctors who specialize in diabetic problems, can often help preserve useful vision even in cases of advanced retinopathy.

In the DCCT, intensive management reduced the risk of diabetic eye disease by 76 percent in participants with no eye damage at the beginning of the study. In those with early retinopathy, intensive therapy slowed the progression of eye damage by 50 percent.

Nerve Disease

Nerve disease caused by diabetes is called diabetic neuropathy. There are three types of nerve disease: peripheral, autonomic, and mononeuropathy. Peripheral neuropathy affects the hands, feet, legs, toes, or fingers. A person's feet, legs, and fingertips may lose feeling, burn, or become painful. To relieve the pain, doctors prescribe pain-killing drugs and sometimes antidepressant drugs. Scientists are studying other substances to help relieve pain associated with diabetic peripheral neuropathy.

Because of the loss of feeling associated with peripheral neuropathy, feet are especially vulnerable. You should check your feet carefully each day for cuts, bruises, and sores. If you notice anything unusual, see a doctor as soon as possible because foot infections and open sores can be difficult to treat in people with diabetes. Your doctor should check your feet at every visit. At least once a year, the doctor should check your neurological function by testing how well you sense temperature, pinprick, and vibration in your feet and changes of position in your toes. Your doctor may recommend that you see a foot care specialist, called a podiatrist.

Another type of nerve disease that may occur after several years of diabetes is called autonomic neuropathy. Autonomic neuropathy affects the internal organs such as the heart, stomach, sexual organs, and urinary tract. It can cause digestive problems and lead to incontinence (a loss of ability to control urine or bowel movements), and sexual impotence. A doctor can help diagnose problems associated with internal organs and may prescribe medication to help relieve pain and other problems associated with autonomic neuropathy.

Mononeuropathy is a form of nerve disease that affects specific nerves, most often in the torso, leg, or head. Mononeuropathy may cause pain in the lower back, chest, abdomen, or in the front of one thigh. Sometimes, this nerve disease can cause aching in the eye, an inability to focus the eye, or double vision. Mononeuropathy may also cause facial paralysis, a condition called Bell's palsy, or problems with hearing. Mononeuropathies occur most often in older people and can be quite painful. Usually the symptoms improve in weeks or months without causing long-term damage.

Lowering blood sugar levels may help prevent or reduce early neuropathy. DCCT study results showed the risk of significant nerve damage was reduced by 60 percent in persons on intensive treatment.

Cardiovascular Disease

As with high blood pressure, heart disease is more common in people with diabetes than in people without diabetes. People with diabetes tend to have more fat and cholesterol in their arteries. The arteries are the large blood vessels that keep the heart beating and the blood flowing. When too much fat and cholesterol build up in the arteries, the arteries and heart must work harder. Over time, this extra work can lead to a heart attack. To help avoid heart problems, you should have your blood cholesterol and triglyceride levels checked once a year. Other risk factors that may cause the heart to become overworked include high blood pressure, smoking, age, extra weight, and lack of exercise.

People with diabetes are also at greater risk for stroke and other forms of large blood vessel disease. A stroke is the result of damage to the blood vessels that circulate blood in the brain. Blockage of major blood vessels in the feet, legs, or arms is called peripheral vascular disease. Peripheral vascular disease causes poor circulation and can contribute to foot and leg ulcers.

DCCT participants were checked regularly for heart disease and related problems, although they were not expected to have many heart-related problems because of their young age. Volunteers in the intensive treatment group had fewer heart attacks and significantly lower risks of developing high blood cholesterol, which causes heart disease. The risk was 35 percent lower in these volunteers, suggesting that intensive treatment can help prevent heart disease. The DCCT volunteers on intensive therapy are being followed closely for the next 10 years to see if their risk of heart disease is reduced.

Points to Remember

To reduce the risk of heart disease:

- Do not smoke.
- Eat a diet low in fat and high in fruits and vegetables.
- Have your blood pressure checked regularly.
- Have your cholesterol checked regularly.

Periodontal (Gum) Disease

People with diabetes, especially those with poor control of their blood sugar, are at risk for developing infections of the gum and bone that hold the teeth in place. Like all infections, gum infections can cause blood sugar to rise and make diabetes harder to control.

Periodontal disease starts as gingivitis, which causes sore, bleeding gums. If not stopped, gingivitis can lead to serious periodontal disease that can damage the bone that holds the tooth in its socket. Without treatment, teeth may loosen and fall out.

Good blood sugar control lowers the risk of gum disease. People with good control have no more gum disease than people without diabetes. Good blood sugar control, daily brushing and flossing, and regular dental checkups are the best defense against gum problems.

Points to Remember

Take special care of your teeth and gums.

- Visit your dentist every 6 months.
- Brush and floss teeth at least twice daily.
- Practice other dental care guidelines recommended by the dentist or dental hygienist.

How Should Special Situations Be Handled?

Illness, Stress, and Surgery

Illness and stress can affect blood sugar levels in people with diabetes. Therefore, during times of illness and stress, you need to be extra careful about keeping blood sugar levels in control. If you develop an illness such as the flu or strep throat, keep in touch with your doctor, test your blood sugar levels often, and check your urine for ketones. Even if you are feeling too sick to eat or have trouble keeping food down, you should continue giving yourself some insulin. In such situations, your doctor will tell you how much insulin to take as well as liquid diets to follow.

A doctor or diabetes nurse educator can also provide guidelines on how to handle stress. If you need hospitalization for an illness or require surgery, doctors and hospital personnel should know that you have diabetes. Your diabetes doctor should also be informed about the hospitalization and should be part of the team that monitors your care. Your doctor will give you advice regarding who to call in case of illness, vomiting, or very high blood sugar levels. In many cases, an early telephone call can prevent lengthy hospitalization.

Pregnancy

Before the 1950s, most pregnant women with diabetes had little chance of having a normal baby. Since the 1960s major advances in diabetes treatment have taken place in Europe and North America. Today, with careful planning, most women with diabetes can become pregnant and deliver a healthy baby with the help of their doctors. Women with diabetes need to discuss their plans with their physicians before they become pregnant. Several studies show that excellent blood glucose control is important at the time a women becomes pregnant. Careful control during the first 2 months of pregnancy can reduce the risk of major birth defects. Later, during the third to ninth months of pregnancy, excellent blood glucose control is essential to protect the health of the baby and reduce complications related to premature delivery.

If you are a pregnant woman with IDDM, you should be treated by a team of doctors or at a center that specializes in the treatment of diabetic pregnancies. The center can provide guidelines for handling such pregnancy-related problems as morning sickness as well as closely monitor your baby before, during, and after delivery.

Because pregnancy sometimes can affect the eyes, kidneys, and blood pressure, your doctors will need to check your eyes, kidneys, and blood pressure before and throughout the pregnancy.

Points to Remember

- Most women with IDDM can have successful pregnancies.

89

- Blood sugar levels should be in good control before a woman becomes pregnant.
- Women with IDDM must be under the close care of specialists experienced in diabetic pregnancies.

School Activities

Children with IDDM can attend school, do homework, play with friends, and participate in clubs or sports. However, special attention should be paid to diabetes care while the child is in school and involved in daily activities. If old enough, children may keep a blood glucose meter at school or with the school nurse. To safeguard against hypoglycemia, the child can carry extra snacks, or snacks can be given to the teacher for use in case the child's blood sugar level drops. Teachers, friends, club leaders, school nurses, or coaches should be aware that a child has diabetes and should know the signs of low blood sugar and how to treat it in case of emergency.

Points to Remember

- Inform teachers and school staff that your child has diabetes and how to treat hypoglycemia.
- Always bring extra snacks in case hypoglycemia occurs with exercise.

Social Activities

Just like people without diabetes, people with diabetes can go to parties and participate in social activities. Some helpful tips are:

- Call ahead to see what foods the host or hostess will serve and at approximately what time. This will help you keep track of how much food you should eat or how much insulin you will need.

- If there does not seem to be food you should eat, offer to bring a snack that everyone, including you, can enjoy.

- Make sure you bring your blood glucose meter to the party to check blood sugar levels before participating in any physical activities, such as strenuous dancing.

Adults with diabetes, even those with IDDM, can drink alcohol safely in moderation. Moderation usually means one or two occasional drinks taken with food. Drinking on an empty stomach and at bedtime can cause blood sugar levels to drop quickly, causing hypoglycemia, with symptoms of shakiness, dizziness, and confusion. People who do not know that someone has diabetes may mistake these symptoms for drunkenness. A dietitian can give guidelines about using alcohol and how to include it in a meal plan. People with nerve damage due to diabetes should avoid frequent alcohol use.

Points to Remember

- Alcohol can lower blood glucose.
- Always eat when drinking alcohol.
- Drink in moderation.
- If you have nerve damage due to diabetes, avoid regular alcohol use.

What Is Happening in Diabetes Research?

The DCCT was one of many recent research programs supported by the Federal Government and by nongovernment organizations to improve the health and well-being of people with diabetes and to find ways to prevent and cure the disorder. A 10-year follow-up to the DCCT, the Epidemiology of Diabetes Intervention and Complications Study, is focusing on the development of macrovascular and renal complications in DCCT volunteers.

The National Institute of Diabetes and Digestive and Kidney Diseases (NIDDK) conducts basic and clinical research in its own laboratories and supports research at centers and hospitals throughout the United States. Other institutes of the National Institutes of Health support studies on diabetic eye, heart, vascular, and nerve disease; pregnancy and diabetes; dental complications; and the immunological aspects of diabetes. This research has led to improved treatments for the complications of diabetes and ways to prevent complications from occurring.

Preventing Diabetes

Researchers are searching diligently for the causes of all forms of diabetes and ways to delay or prevent the disorder. Much progress has been made. Scientists have identified antibodies in the blood that make a person susceptible to IDDM, making it possible to screen relatives of people with diabetes and determine their risk for developing the disease.

A new NIDDK clinical trial, the Diabetes Prevention Trial-Type 1 (DPT-1), began in 1994. It is identifying relatives at risk for developing IDDM and treating them with low doses of insulin or with oral

91

insulin-like agents in the hope of preventing IDDM. Similar research is being conducted at other medical centers throughout the world. These studies are based on encouraging results in laboratory animals with IDDM and on pilot studies in relatives of people with IDDM.

Advances in Managing Diabetes

In the past 15 years, many advances have improved treatment for people with diabetes:

- **Genetically engineered insulin.** Because it is identical to in-sulin produced by the human body, genetically engineered insu-lin is less apt to cause skin and other allergic reactions. Supplies of genetically engineered insulin are readily available.

- **Self-monitoring of blood glucose.** By testing your own blood sugar, you enable your doctor to offer you much better treatment than was available before 1980 when testing urine for glucose was the only way of estimating diabetes control.

- **Hemoglobin A1c testing.** Using one blood test, doctors can now monitor your average blood sugar control over a period of 2 to 3 months. This test tells you how well you are doing and whether any changes are needed in your management routine.

- **Insulin pumps, insulin pens, and other aids for adminis-tering insulin.** Insulin pumps, including implantable pumps now under development, can supply insulin in a more natural pattern, similar to the way the pancreas in a person without diabetes makes insulin. Other injection aids make giving insu-lin easier and more convenient than in the past, even in young children and people who are visually impaired.

Other improvements in diabetes management being developed include insulin in the form of nasal sprays, patches, or pills and devices to test blood sugar levels without having to prick a finger to get a blood sample. Perhaps one of the most important advances has been the development of an entirely new approach to diabetes management in which IDDM patients take responsibility for much of their own care.

Curing Diabetes

Transplantation of the pancreas or of the insulin-producing islets of the pancreas offer a hope for a cure for IDDM. Many people with

IDDM have had successful pancreas transplants, and a few have had islet transplants. Unfortunately, pancreas and islet transplants cannot be offered to everyone with diabetes as yet. The body's immune system rejects "foreign" or transplanted tissue, and people who have transplants must take powerful drugs to prevent rejection. These drugs are costly and may cause serious health problems. Therefore, pancreas or islet transplants are usually given only to people who have had or require a kidney transplant because of advanced complications and are already taking drugs to prevent rejection.

Researchers are working to develop less harmful drugs and better methods of transplanting pancreatic tissue to prevent rejection by the body, such as encapsulating the islet cells in a semi-permeable membrane that offers protection from immune attack, implanting the cells in the thymus gland to induce tolerance by the immune system, and using bioengineering techniques to create artificial islet cells that secrete insulin in response to increased sugar levels in the blood.

Clinical Trials

Clinical trials are one way to test new treatments that emerge from basic research. NIDDK plans and supports clinical trials related to diabetes, such as the DCCT and DPT-Type 1. For information about NIDDK-supported clinical trials, contact the National Diabetes Information Clearinghouse (NDIC), at the address and telephone number on given in the Resources section below.

Other medical centers also conduct clinical studies. The best way to find out about studies in progress is to contact a nearby university-affiliated hospital or large medical center. Additional information can also be obtained from a local chapter of the American Diabetes Association or Juvenile Diabetes Foundation.

Other Resources

The following organizations offer educational materials about diabetes and can help you find support groups and education programs in your community, including family activities and camp programs for children. Local affiliates and chapters of these organizations often can identify health professionals such as diabetologists, certified diabetes educators, and dietitians in the community. To locate affiliates and chapters of these organizations, consult your local telephone directory, or contact the following national offices:

American Association of Diabetes Educators
444 N. Michigan Avenue, Suite 1240
Chicago, IL 60611
(800) 832-6874

American Diabetes Association
ADA National Service Center
1660 Duke Street
Alexandria, VA 22314
(800) 232-3472

Juvenile Diabetes Foundation International
432 Park Avenue South
New York, NY 10016-8013
(800) 223-1138

American Dietetic Association
216 W. Jackson Blvd.
Chicago, IL 60606-6995
(800) 366-1655

Additional publications about diabetes are available from the National Diabetes Information Clearinghouse. The clearinghouse can also provide information about research and clinical trials supported by the National Institutes of Health. The address and telephone number are:

National Diabetes Information Clearinghouse
1. Information Way
Bethesda, MD 20892-3560
(301) 654-3327

For more information about improving blood sugar control, write:

National Diabetes Outreach Program
1 Diabetes Way
Bethesda, MD 20892-3600

Acknowledgments

Our thanks to: Julio Santiago, M.D., of Washington University for his careful review of this text.

We also wish to acknowledge the contributions of: Patricia Callahan, R.N., B.S., C.D.E., Linda Delahanty, M.S., R.D., and Alan Jacobson, M.D.

Chapter 10

Noninsulin-Dependent Diabetes

Introduction

This chapter is about **noninsulin-dependent diabetes**. The word "diabetes" in the text of this chapter refers to noninsulin-dependent diabetes unless otherwise specified.

Of the estimated 13 to 14 million people in the United States with diabetes, between 90 and 95 percent have **noninsulin-dependent or type II diabetes.** Formerly called adult-onset, this form of diabetes usually begins in adults over age 40, and is most common after age 55. Nearly half of people with diabetes don't know it because the symptoms often develop gradually and are hard to identify at first. The person may feel tired or ill without knowing why. Diabetes can cause problems that damage the heart, blood vessels, eyes, kidneys, and nerves.

Although there is no cure for diabetes yet, daily treatment helps control blood sugar, and may reduce the risk of complications. Under a doctor's supervision, treatment usually involves a combination of weight loss, exercise and medication.

This chapter isn't a guide to treatment and it doesn't replace the advice of a doctor. It's one of many sources of extra information about diabetes. Local diabetes groups and clinics sponsor meetings and educational programs about diabetes that also can be helpful. At the end of this chapter is a list of groups that have information on diabetes programs.

U.S. Department of Health and Human Services, National Institute of Diabetes and Digestive and Kidney Diseases. NIH Pub. No. 95-241. September 1992.

Points to Remember

- Only a doctor can treat diabetes.
- Treatment usually involves weight loss, exercise and medication.
- Daily treatment helps control diabetes and may reduce the risk of complications.

What Is Diabetes?

The two types of diabetes, insulin-dependent and noninsulin-dependent, are different disorders. While the causes, short-term effects, and treatments for the two types differ, both can cause the same long-term health problems. Both types also affect the body's ability to use digested food for energy. Diabetes doesn't interfere with digestion, but it does prevent the body from using an important product of digestion, glucose (commonly known as sugar), for energy.

After a meal the digestive system breaks some food down into glucose. The blood carries the glucose or sugar throughout the body, causing blood glucose levels to rise. In response to this rise the hormone insulin is released into the bloodstream to signal the body tissues to metabolize or burn the glucose for fuel, causing blood glucose levels to return to normal. A gland called the pancreas, found just behind the stomach, makes insulin. Glucose the body doesn't use right away goes to the liver, muscle or fat for storage.

In someone with diabetes, this process doesn't work correctly. In people with insulin-dependent diabetes, the pancreas doesn't produce insulin. This condition usually begins in childhood and is also known as type I (formerly called juvenile-onset) diabetes. People with this kind of diabetes must have daily insulin injections to survive.

In people with noninsulin-dependent diabetes the pancreas usually produces some insulin, but the body's tissue don't respond very well to the insulin signal and therefore, don't metabolize the glucose properly, a condition called insulin resistance. Insulin resistance is an important factor in noninsulin-dependent diabetes.

Points to Remember

- Diabetes interferes with the body's use of food for energy.
- While noninsulin-dependent diabetes and insulin-dependent diabetes are different disorders, they can cause the same complications.

Symptoms

The symptoms of diabetes may begin gradually and can be hard to identify at first. They may include fatigue, a sick feeling, frequent urination, especially at night, and excessive thirst. When there is extra glucose in blood, one way the body gets rid of it is through frequent urination. This loss of fluids causes extreme thirst. Other symptoms may include sudden weight loss, blurred vision, and slow healing of skin, gum and urinary tract infections. Women may notice genital itching.

A doctor also may suspect a patient has diabetes if the person has health problems related to diabetes. For instance, heart disease, changes in vision, numbness in the feet and legs or sores that are slow to heal, may prompt a doctor to check for diabetes. These symptoms do not mean a person has diabetes, but anyone who has these problems should see a doctor.

Points to Remember

- The symptoms of diabetes can develop gradually and may be hard to identify at first.
- Symptoms may include feeling tired or ill, excessive thirst, frequent urination, sudden weight loss, blurred vision, slow healing of infections, and genital itching.

What Causes Noninsulin-Dependent Diabetes?

There is no simple answer to what causes noninsulin-dependent diabetes. While eating sugar, for example, doesn't cause diabetes, eating large amounts of sugar and other rich, fatty foods, can cause weight gain. Most people who develop diabetes are overweight. Scientists do not fully understand why obesity increases someone's chances of developing diabetes, but they believe obesity is a major factor leading to noninsulin-dependent diabetes. Current research should help explain why the disorder occurs and why obesity is such an important risk factor.

A major cause of diabetes is insulin resistance. Scientists are still searching for the causes of insulin resistance, but they have identified two possibilities. The first could be a defect in insulin receptors on cells. Like an appliance that needs to be plugged into an electrical outlet, insulin has to bind to a receptor to function. Several things can go wrong with receptors. There may not be enough receptors for insulin to bind to, or a defect in the receptors may prevent insulin from binding.

A second possible cause involves the process that occurs after insulin plugs into the receptor. Insulin may bind to the receptor, but the cells don't read the signal to metabolize the glucose. Scientists are studying cells to see why this might happen.

Points to Remember

- In people with noninsulin-dependent diabetes, insulin doesn't lower blood sugar, a condition called insulin resistance.
- Obesity is a risk factor for diabetes.

Who Develops Noninsulin-Dependent Diabetes?

Age, sex, weight, physical activity, diet, lifestyle, and family health history all affect someone's chances of developing diabetes. The chances that someone will develop diabetes increase if the person's parents or siblings have the disease. Experts now know that diabetes is more common in African Americans, Hispanics, Native Americans and Native Hawaiians than whites. They believe this is the result of both heredity and environmental factors, such as diet and lifestyle. The highest rate of diabetes in the world is in an Arizona community of American Indians called the Pimas. While the chances of developing diabetes increase with age, gender isn't a risk factor, although African American women are more likely to develop diabetes than African American men.

While people can't change family history, age, or race, it is possible to control weight and physical fitness. A doctor can decide if someone is at risk for developing diabetes and offer advice on reducing that risk.

Points to Remember

- The following factors increase someone s chances of developing diabetes: obesity, family history of diabetes, and advancing age.

Diagnosing Diabetes

A doctor can diagnose diabetes by checking for symptoms such as excessive thirst and frequent urination and by testing for glucose in blood or urine. When blood glucose rises above a certain point, the kidneys pass the extra glucose in the urine. However, a urine test alone is not sufficient to diagnose diabetes.

A second method for testing glucose is a blood test usually done in the morning before breakfast (fasting glucose test) or after a meal (postprandial glucose test).

The oral glucose tolerance test is a second type of blood test used to check for diabetes. Sometimes it can detect diabetes when a simple blood test does not. In this test, blood glucose is measured before and after a person has consumed a thick, sweet drink of glucose and other sugars. Normally, the glucose in a person's blood rises quickly after the drink and then falls gradually again as insulin signals the body to metabolize the glucose. In someone with diabetes, blood glucose rises and remains high after consumption of the liquid.

A doctor can decide, based on these tests and a physical exam, whether someone has diabetes. If a blood test is borderline abnormal, the doctor may want to monitor the person's blood glucose regularly. If a person is overweight, he or she probably will be advised to lose weight. The doctor also may monitor the patient's heart, since diabetes increases the risk of heart disease.

Points to Remember

A doctor will diagnose diabetes by looking for four kinds of evidence:

- risk factors like excess weight and a family history of diabetes
- symptoms such as thirst and frequent urination
- complications like heart trouble
- signs of excess glucose or sugar in blood and urine tests.

Treating Diabetes

The goals of diabetes treatment are to keep blood glucose within normal range and to prevent long-term complications. Why control blood glucose? In the first place, diabetes can cause short-term effects: some are unpleasant and some are dangerous. These include thirst, frequent urination, weakness, lack of ability to concentrate, loss of coordination, and blurred vision. Loss of consciousness is possible with very high or low blood sugar levels, but is more of a danger in insulin-dependent than in noninsulin-dependent diabetes.

In the second place, the long-term complications of diabetes may result from many years of high blood glucose. Research is under way to find out if this is true and to learn if careful control can help prevent complications. Meanwhile, most doctors feel that if people with diabetes keep their blood glucose levels under control, they will reduce the risk of complications.

In 1986, a National Institutes of Health panel of experts recommended that the best treatment for noninsulin-dependent diabetes is a diet that helps the person maintain normal weight. In people who are overweight, losing weight is the one treatment that is clearly effective in controlling diabetes.

In some people, exercise can help keep weight and diabetes under control. However, when diet and exercise alone can't control diabetes, two other kinds of treatment are available: oral diabetes medications and insulin. The treatment a doctor suggests depends on the person's age, lifestyle, and the severity of the diabetes.

Points to Remember

- Diabetes treatment can reduce symptoms, like thirst and weakness, and the chances of long-term problems, like heart and eye disease.

- If treatment with diet and exercise isn't effective, a doctor may prescribe oral medications or insulin.

- There is no known cure for diabetes, daily treatment must continue throughout a person's lifetime.

Diabetes Diet

The proper diet is critical to diabetes treatment. It can help someone with diabetes:

- Achieve and maintain desirable weight. Many people with diabetes can control their blood glucose by losing weight and keeping it off.

- Maintain normal blood glucose levels.

- Prevent heart and blood vessel diseases, conditions that tend to occur in people with diabetes.

A doctor will usually prescribe diet as part of diabetes treatment. A dietitian or nutritionist can recommend a diet that is healthy, but also interesting and easy to follow. No one has to be limited to a pre-printed, standard diet. Someone with diabetes can get assistance in the following ways:

- A doctor can recommend a local nutritionist or dietitian.

- The local American Diabetes Association, American Heart Association, and American Dietetic Association can provide names of qualified dietitians or nutritionists and information about diet planning.

- Local diabetes centers at large medical clinics, hospitals, or medical universities usually have dietitians and nutritionists on staff.

The guidelines for diabetes diet planning include the following:

- Many experts, including the American Diabetes Association, recommend that 50 to 60 percent of daily calories come from carbohydrates, 12 to 20 percent from protein, and no more than 30 percent from fat.

- Spacing meals throughout the day, instead of eating heavy meals once or twice a day, can help a person avoid extremely high or low blood glucose levels.

- With few exceptions, the best way to lose weight is gradually: one or two pounds a week. Strict diets **must never** be undertaken without the supervision of a doctor.

- People with diabetes have twice the risk of developing heart disease as those without diabetes, and high blood cholesterol levels raise the risk of heart disease. Losing weight and reducing intake of saturated fats and cholesterol, in favor of unsaturated and monounsaturated fats, can help lower blood cholesterol.

  For example, meats and dairy products are major sources of saturated fats, which should be avoided; most vegetable oils are high in unsaturated fats, which are fine in limited amounts; and olive oil is a good source of monounsaturated fat, the healthiest type of fat. Liver and other organ meats and egg yolks are particularly high in cholesterol. A doctor or nutritionist can advise someone on this aspect of diet.

- Studies show that foods with fiber, such as fruits, vegetables, peas, beans, and whole-grain breads and cereals may help lower blood glucose. However, it seems that a person must eat much more fiber than the average American now consumes to get this benefit. A doctor or nutritionist can advise someone about adding fiber to a diet.

- Exchange lists are useful in planning a diabetes diet. They place foods with similar nutrients and calories into groups. With the help of a nutritionist, the person plans the number of servings from each exchange list that he or she should eat throughout the day. Diets that use exchange lists offer more choices than preprinted diets. More information on exchange lists is available from nutritionists and from the American Diabetes Association.

Continuing research may lead to new approaches to diabetes diets. Because one goal of a diabetes diet is to maintain normal blood glucose levels, it would be helpful to have reliable information on the effects of foods on blood glucose. For example, foods that are rich in carbohydrates, like breads, cereals, fruits, and vegetables break down into glucose during digestion, causing blood glucose to rise. However, scientists don't know how each of these carbohydrates affect blood glucose levels. Research is also under way to learn whether foods with sugar raise blood glucose higher than foods with starch. Experts do know that cooked foods raise blood glucose higher than raw, unpeeled foods. A person with diabetes can ask a doctor or nutritionist about using this kind of information in diet planning.

Alcoholic Beverages

Most people with diabetes can drink alcohol safely if they drink in moderation (one or two drinks occasionally), because in higher quantities alcohol can cause health problems:

- Alcohol has calories without the vitamins, minerals, and other nutrients that are essential for maintaining good health. A doctor can discuss whether it's safe for an individual with diabetes to drink. People who are trying to lose weight need to account for the calories in alcohol in diet planning. A dietitian also can provide information about the sugar and alcohol content of various alcoholic drinks.

- Alcohol on an empty stomach can cause low blood glucose or hypoglycemia. Hypoglycemia is a particular risk in people who use oral medications or insulin for diabetes. It can cause shaking, dizziness, and collapse. People who don't know someone has diabetes may mistake these symptoms for drunkenness and neglect to seek medical help.

- Oral diabetes medications—tolbutamide and chlorpropamide—can cause dizziness, flushing, and nausea when combined with alcohol. A doctor can advise patients on the safety of drinking when taking these and other diabetes medications.

- Frequent, heavy drinking can cause liver damage over time. Because the liver stores and releases glucose, blood glucose levels may be more difficult to control in a person with liver damage from alcohol.

- Frequent heavy drinking also can raise the levels of fats in blood, increasing the risk of heart disease.

Points to Remember

- A diabetes diet should do three things: achieve ideal weight, maintain normal blood glucose levels, and limit foods that contribute to heart disease.

- A nutritionist or dietitian can help plan a diabetes diet.

Exercise

Exercise has many benefits, and for someone with diabetes regular exercise combined with a good diet can help control diabetes. Exercise not only burns calories, which can help with weight reduction, but it also can improve the body's response to the hormone insulin. As a result, following a regular exercise program can make oral diabetes medications and insulin more effective and can help control blood glucose levels.

Exercise also reduces some risk factors for heart disease. For example, exercise can lower fat and cholesterol levels in blood which increase heart disease risk. It also can lower blood pressure and increase production of a cholesterol, called HDL, that protects against heart disease.

However, infrequent, strenuous exercise can strain muscles and the circulatory system and can increase the risk of a heart attack during exercise. A doctor can decide how much exercise is safe for an individual. The doctor will consider how well controlled a person's diabetes is, the condition of the heart and circulatory system, and whether complications require that the person avoid certain types of activity.

Walking is great exercise, especially for an inactive person, and it's easy to do. A person can start off walking for 15 or 20 minutes, three or four times a week, and gradually increase the speed or distance of the walks. The purpose of a good exercise program is to find an enjoyable activity and do it regularly. Doing strenuous exercise for six months and then stopping isn't as effective. People taking oral drugs or insulin need to remember that strenuous exercise can cause dangerously low blood glucose and they should carry a food or drink high in sugar for medical emergencies. Signs of hypoglycemia include hunger, nervousness, shakiness, weakness, sweating, headache, and blurred vision. As a precaution, a person with diabetes should wear an identification bracelet or necklace to alert a stranger that the wearer has diabetes and may need special medical help in an emergency.

A doctor may advise someone with high blood pressure or other complications to avoid exercises that raise blood pressure. For example, lifting heavy objects and exercises that strain the upper body raise blood pressure.

People with diabetes who have lost sensitivity in their feet also can enjoy exercise. They should choose shoes carefully and check their feet regularly for breaks in skin that could lead to infection. Swimming or bicycling can be easier on the feet than running.

Points to Remember

- Exercise has three major benefits: it burns calories, improves the body's response to insulin, and reduces risk factors for heart disease.

- An exercise program should be started slowly and with the advice of a doctor.

Oral Medications

Oral diabetes medicines, or oral hypoglycemics, can lower blood glucose in people who have diabetes, but are able to make some insulin. They are an option if diet and exercise don't work. Oral diabetes medications are not insulin and are not a substitute for diet and exercise. Although experts don't understand exactly how each oral medicine works, they know that they increase insulin production and affect how insulin lowers blood glucose. These medications are most effective in people who developed diabetes after age 40, have had diabetes less than 5 years, are normal weight, and have never received insulin or have taken only 40 units or less of insulin a day. Pregnant and nursing women shouldn't take oral medications because their effect on the fetus and newborn is unknown, and because insulin provides better control of diabetes during pregnancy.

There is also some question about whether oral diabetes medications increase the risk of a heart attack. Experts disagree on this point and many people with noninsulin-dependent diabetes use oral medicines safely and effectively. The Food and Drug Administration (FDA), the agency of the Federal Government that approves medications for use in this country, requires that oral diabetes medicines carry a warning concerning the increased risk of heart attack. Whether someone uses a medication depends on its benefits and risks, something a doctor can help the patient decide.

Six FDA-approved oral diabetes medications are now on the market. Their generic names are tolbutamide, chlorpropamide, tolazamide, acetohexamide, glyburide, and glipizide. The generic name refers to the chemical that gives each medicine its particular effect. Some of these medications are made by more than one pharmaceutical company and have more than one brand name. All six are different types of one class of medication, called sulfonylureas, but each affects metabolism differently. A doctor will choose a patient's medication based on the person's general health, the amount his or her blood glucose needs to be lowered, the person's eating habits, and the medicine's side effects.

The purpose of oral medications is to lower blood glucose. Therefore, the person taking them must eat regular meals and engage in only light to moderate exercise, to prevent blood glucose from dipping too low. Medications taken for other health problems, including illness, also can lower blood sugar and may react with the diabetes medicine. Therefore, a doctor needs to know all the medications a person is taking to prevent a harmful interaction. Lowering blood sugar too much can cause hypoglycemia with symptoms such as headache, weakness, shakiness, and if the condition is severe enough, collapse.

Oral diabetes medications usually don't cause side effects. However, a few people do experience nausea, skin rashes, headache, either water retention or diuresis (increased urination), and sensitivity to direct sunlight. These effects should gradually subside, but a person should see a doctor if they persist. For reasons that aren't always clear, sometimes oral diabetes medications don't help the person for whom they're prescribed. Investigations are under way to learn why this happens.

Points to Remember

- Oral diabetes medications may be used when diet and exercise alone don't control diabetes.

- Oral diabetes medicines aren't a substitute for diet and exercise.

Insulin

Like oral diabetes medications, insulin is an alternative for some people with noninsulin-dependent diabetes who can't control their blood glucose levels with diet and exercise. In special situations, such as surgery and pregnancy, insulin is a temporary but important means of controlling blood glucose. A section of this chapter called "special situations" discusses insulin use during pregnancy and surgery.

Sometimes it's unclear whether insulin or oral medications are more effective in controlling blood-glucose; therefore, a doctor will consider a person's weight, age, and the severity of the diabetes before prescribing a medicine. Experts do know that weight control is essential for insulin to be effective. A doctor is likely to prescribe insulin if diet, exercise, or oral medications don't work, or if someone has a bad reaction to oral medicines. A person also may have to take insulin if his or her blood glucose fluctuates a great deal and is difficult to control. A doctor will instruct a person with diabetes on how to purchase, mix, and inject insulin. Various types of insulin are available that differ in purity, concentration, and how quickly they work. They also are made differently. In the past, all commercially available insulin came from the pancreas glands of cows and pigs. Today, human insulin is available in two forms: one uses genetic engineering and the other involves chemically changing pork insulin into human insulin. The best sources of information on insulin are the company that makes it and a doctor.

Points to Remember

- Insulin may be used when diet, exercise, or oral medications don't control diabetes.

- Weight control is important when taking insulin.

- Insulin is taken in special situations such as surgery and pregnancy.

Checking Blood Glucose Levels

When a person's body is operating normally, it automatically checks the level of glucose in blood. If the level is too high or too low, the body will adjust the sugar level to return it to normal. This system operates in much the same way that cruise control adjusts the speed of a car. With diabetes, the body doesn't do the job of controlling blood glucose automatically. To make up for this, someone with diabetes has to check blood sugar regularly and adjust treatment accordingly.

A doctor can measure blood glucose during an office visit. However, levels change from hour to hour and someone who visits the doctor only every few weeks won't know what his or her blood glucose is daily. Do-it-yourself tests enable people with diabetes to check their blood sugar daily.

The easiest test someone can do at home is a urine test. When the level of glucose in blood rises above normal, the kidneys eliminate the excess glucose in urine. Glucose in urine, therefore, reflects an excess of glucose in blood.

Urine testing is easy. Tablets or paper strips are dipped in urine. The color change that occurs indicates whether blood glucose is too high. However, urine testing is not completely accurate because the reading reflects the level of blood glucose a few hours earlier. In addition, not everyone's kidneys are the same. Even when the amount of glucose in two people's urine is the same, their sugar levels may be different. Certain drugs and vitamin C also can affect the accuracy of urine tests.

It's more accurate to measure blood glucose directly. Kits are available that allow people with diabetes to test their blood glucose at home. The test involves pricking a finger to draw a drop of blood. A spring-operated "lancet" does this automatically. The drop of blood is placed on a strip of specially coated plastic or into a small machine that "reads" how much glucose is in the blood. A doctor may suggest that someone test his or her blood glucose several times a day. Self blood glucose monitoring can show how the body responds to meals, exercise, stress, and diabetes treatment.

Another test that measures the effectiveness of treatment is a "glycosylated hemoglobin" test. It measures the glucose that has become attached to hemoglobin, the molecule in red blood cells that gives blood its red color. Over time, hemoglobin absorbs glucose, according to its concentration in blood. Once glucose is absorbed by hemoglobin it remains there until the blood cells die and new ones replace them. With the "glycosylated hemoglobin" test, a doctor can tell whether blood glucose has been very high over the last few months.

Points to Remember

- Testing blood glucose levels regularly can show whether treatment is working.

Diabetes Complications

A key goal of diabetes treatment is to prevent complications because, over time, diabetes can damage the heart, blood vessels, eyes, kidneys, and nerves, although the person may not know damage is taking place. It's important to diagnose and treat diabetes early, because it can cause damage even before it makes someone feel ill.

How diabetes causes long-term problems is unclear. However, changes in the small blood vessels and nerves are common. These changes may be the first step toward many problems that diabetes causes. Scientists can't predict who among people with diabetes will develop complications, but complications are most likely to occur in someone who has had diabetes for many years. However, because a person can have diabetes without knowing it, a complication may be the first sign.

Heart Disease

Heart disease is the most common life-threatening disease linked to diabetes, and experts say diabetes doubles a person's risk of developing heart disease. In heart disease, deposits of fat and cholesterol build-up in the arteries that supply the heart with blood. If this buildup blocks blood from getting to the heart, a potentially fatal heart attack can occur.

Other risk factors include hypertension or high blood pressure, obesity, high amounts of fats and cholesterol in blood, and cigarette smoking. Eliminating these risk factors, along with treating diabetes, can reduce the risk of heart disease. The American Heart Association has literature that explains what heart disease is and how to prevent it. The association's address is in the resources section of this chapter.

Kidney Disease

People with diabetes are also more likely to develop kidney disease than other people. The kidneys filter waste products from the blood and excrete them in the form of urine, maintaining proper fluid balance in the body. While people can live without one kidney, those without both must have special treatment, called dialysis. Most people with diabetes will never develop kidney disease, but proper diabetes treatment can further reduce the risk. High blood pressure also can add to the risk of kidney disease. Therefore, regular blood pressure checks and early treatment of the disorder can help prevent kidney disease.

Urinary tract infections are also a cause of kidney problems. Diabetes can affect the nerves that control the bladder, making it difficult for a person to empty his or her bladder completely. Bacteria can form in the unemptied bladder and the tubes leading from it, eventually causing infection. The symptoms of a urinary tract infection include frequent, painful urination, blood in the urine, and pain in the lower abdomen and back. Without prompt examination and treatment by a doctor, the infection can reach the kidneys, causing pain, fever, and possibly kidney damage. A doctor may prescribe antibiotics to treat the infection and may suggest that the person drink large amounts of water.

Kidney problems are one cause of water retention, or edema, a condition in which fluid collects in the body, causing swelling, often in the legs and hands. A doctor can decide if swelling or water retention relates to kidney function.

A nephrologist, a doctor specially trained to diagnose and treat kidney problems, can identify the cause of problems and recommend ways to reduce the risk of kidney disease.

Eye Problems

Diabetes can affect the eyes in several ways. Frequently, the effects are temporary and can be corrected with better diabetes control. However, long-term diabetes can cause changes in the eyes that threaten vision. Stable blood glucose levels and yearly eye examinations can help reduce the risk of serious eye damage.

Blurred vision is one effect diabetes can have on the eyes. The reason may be that changing levels of glucose in blood also can affect the balance of fluid in the lens of the eye, which works like a flexible camera lens to focus images. If the lens absorbs more water than normal and swells, its focusing power changes. Diabetes also may affect the function of nerves that control eyesight, causing blurred vision.

Cataract and glaucoma are eye diseases that occur more frequently in people with diabetes. Cataract is a clouding of the normally clear lens of the eye. Glaucoma is a condition in which pressure within the eye can damage the optic nerve that transmits visual images to the brain. Early diagnosis and treatment of cataract and glaucoma can reduce the severity of these disorders.

Diabetic Retinopathy

Retinopathy, a disease of the retina, the light sensing tissue at the back of the eye, is a common concern among people with diabetes.

Diabetic retinopathy damages the tiny vessels that supply the retina with blood. The blood vessels may swell and leak fluid. When retinopathy is more severe, new blood vessels may grow from the back of the eye and bleed into the clear gel that fills the eye, the vitreous.

While most people with diabetes may never develop serious eye problems, people who have had diabetes for 25 years are more likely to develop retinopathy. Experts think high blood pressure may contribute to diabetic retinopathy, and that smoking can cause the condition to worsen. If someone experiences blurred vision that lasts longer than a day or so, sudden loss of vision in either eye, or black spots, lines, or flashing lights in the field of vision, a doctor should be alerted right away.

Treatment for diabetic retinopathy can help prevent loss of vision and can sometimes restore vision lost because of the disease. A yearly eye examination with dilated pupils makes it possible for an ophthalmologist, an eye doctor, to notice changes before the illness becomes harder to treat. Scientists are testing new means of treating diabetic retinopathy. For more information on eye complications of diabetes and the treatment of these conditions, see the resource list at the end of this chapter.

Legs and Feet

Leg and foot problems can arise in people with diabetes due to changes in blood vessels and nerves in these areas. Peripheral vascular disease is a condition in which blood vessels become narrowed by fatty deposits, reducing blood supply to the legs and feet. Diabetes also can dull the sensitivity of nerves. Someone with this condition, called peripheral neuropathy, might not notice a sore spot caused by tight shoes or pressure from walking. If ignored, the sore can become infected, and because blood circulation is poor, the area may take longer to heal.

Proper foot care and regular visits to a doctor can prevent foot and leg sores and ensure that any that do appear don't become infected and painful. Helpful measures include inspecting the feet daily for cuts or sore spots. Blisters and sore spots are not as likely when shoes fit well and socks or stockings aren't tight. A doctor also may suggest washing feet daily, with warm, not hot water; filing thick calluses; and using lotions that keep the feet from getting too dry. Shoe inserts or special shoes can be used to prevent pressure on the foot.

Diabetic neuropathy, or nerve disease, dulls the nerves and can be extremely painful. A person with neuropathy also may be depressed. Scientists aren't sure whether the depression is an effect of neuropathy, or if it's simply a response to pain. Treatment, aimed at relieving pain and depression, may include aspirin and other pain-killing drugs.

Any sore on the foot or leg, whether or not it's painful, requires a doctor's immediate attention. Treatment can help sores heal and prevent new ones from developing. Problems with the feet and legs can cause life-threatening problems that require amputation—surgical removal of limbs—if not treated early.

Other Effects of Diabetic Neuropathy

Nerves provide muscle tone and feeling and help control functions like digestion and blood pressure. Diabetes can cause changes in these nerves and the functions they control. These changes are most frequent in people who have had other complications of diabetes, like problems with their feet. Someone who has had diabetes for some years and has other complications, may find that spells of indigestion or diarrhea are common. A doctor may prescribe drugs to relieve these symptoms. Diabetes also can affect the nerves that control penile erection in men, which can cause impotence that shows up gradually, without any loss of desire for sex. A doctor can find out whether impotence is the result of physical changes, such as diabetes, or emotional changes, and suggest treatment or counseling.

Skin and Oral Infections

People with diabetes are more likely to develop infections, like boils and ulcers, than the average person. Women with diabetes may develop vaginal infections more often than other women. Checking for infections, treating them early, and following a doctor's advice can help ensure that infections are mild and infrequent.

Infections also can affect the teeth and gums, making people with diabetes more susceptible to periodontal disease, an inflammation of tissue surrounding and supporting the teeth. An important cause of periodontal disease is bacterial growth on the teeth and gums. Treating diabetes and following a dentist's advice on dental care can help prevent periodontal disease.

Emergencies

Very high blood glucose levels cause symptoms that are hard to ignore: frequent urination and excessive thirst. However, in someone who is elderly or in poor health these symptoms may go unnoticed.

Without treatment, a person with high blood glucose or hyperglycemia can lose fluids, become weak, confused, and even unconscious. Breathing will be shallow and the pulse rapid. The person's lips and tongue will be dry, and his or her hands and feet will be cool. A doctor should be called immediately.

The opposite of high blood glucose, very low blood glucose or hypoglycemia, is also dangerous. Hypoglycemia can occur when someone hasn't eaten enough to balance the effects of insulin or oral medicine. Prolonged, strenuous exercise in someone taking oral diabetes drugs or insulin also can cause hypoglycemia, as can alcohol.

Someone whose blood glucose has become too low may feel nervous, shaky, and weak. The person may sweat, feel hungry, and have a headache. Severe hypoglycemia can cause loss of consciousness. A person with hypoglycemia who begins to feel weak and shaky should eat or drink something with sugar in it immediately, like orange juice. If the person is unconscious, he or she should be taken to a hospital emergency room right away. An identification bracelet or necklace that states that the wearer has diabetes will let friends know that these symptoms are a warning of illness that requires urgent medical help.

Points to Remember

- Diabetes can cause long-term complications such as heart, kidney, eye, and nerve disease.

- Careful treatment of diabetes and checking for signs of complications can lower the chances that someone will be troubled by these conditions.

- An identification bracelet or necklace stating that the wearer has diabetes can help ensure that friends or strangers won't ignore symptoms that signal a medical emergency.

Special Situations

Surgery

Surgery is stressful, both physically and mentally. It can raise blood glucose levels even in someone who is careful about control. To make sure that surgery and recovery are successful for someone with diabetes, a doctor will test blood glucose and keep it under careful control, usually with insulin. Careful control makes it possible for someone with diabetes to have surgery with little or no more risk than someone without diabetes.

To plan a safe and successful surgery, the surgeon and attending physicians must know that the person they're treating has diabetes. While tests done before surgery can detect diabetes, the patient should inform the doctor of his or her condition. A surgical team also will evaluate the possible effect of complications of diabetes, such as heart or kidney problems.

Pregnancy

Bearing a child places extra demands on a woman's body. Diabetes makes it more difficult for her body to adjust to these demands and it can cause problems for both mother and baby. Some women may develop a form of diabetes during pregnancy called gestational diabetes. Gestational diabetes develops most frequently in the middle and later months of pregnancy, after the time of greatest risk for birth defects. Although this kind of diabetes often disappears after the baby's birth, treatment is necessary during pregnancy to make sure the diabetes doesn't harm the mother or fetus.

A woman who knows she has diabetes should keep her condition under control before she becomes pregnant, so that her diabetes won't increase the risk of birth defects. A woman whose diabetes isn't well-controlled may have an unusually large baby. Diabetes also increases the risk of premature birth and problems in the baby, such as breathing difficulties, low blood sugar and occasionally, death.

Blood glucose monitoring and treatment with insulin can ensure that a baby born to a mother with diabetes will be healthy. Oral diabetes drugs aren't given during pregnancy because the effects of these drugs on the unborn baby aren't known. By following the advice of a doctor trained to treat gestational diabetes, the mother can make sure her blood glucose is normal and her baby is well nourished.

Approximately half of women with gestational diabetes will no longer have abnormal blood glucose tests shortly after giving birth. However, many women with gestational diabetes will develop noninsulin-dependent diabetes later in their lives. Regular check-ups can ensure that if a woman does develop diabetes later, it will be diagnosed and treated early.

Is Diabetes Hereditary?

Scientists estimate that the child of a parent with noninsulin-dependent diabetes has approximately a 10 to 15 percent chance of developing noninsulin-dependent diabetes. If both parents have diabetes, the child's risk of having the disease increases. The child's health habits throughout his or her life will affect the risk of developing diabetes. Obesity, for example, may increase the risk of diabetes or cause it to occur earlier in life.

Noninsulin-dependent diabetes in a parent has no effect on the chances that his or her child will have insulin-dependent diabetes, the more severe form of diabetes.

Stress and Illness

One way the body responds to stress is to increase the level of blood glucose. In a person with diabetes, stress may increase the need for treatment to lower blood glucose levels. Illnesses such as colds and flu are forms of physical stress that a doctor can treat. The doctor will advise the person to drink plenty of fluids. When blood glucose is high, the body gets rid of glucose through urine, and this fluid needs to be replaced.

If nausea makes eating or taking oral diabetes drugs a problem, a doctor should be consulted. Not eating can increase the risk of low blood glucose, while stopping oral medications or insulin during illness can lead to very high blood glucose. A doctor may prescribe insulin temporarily for someone with diabetes who can't take medicine by mouth.

Great thirst, rapid weight loss, high fever, or very high urine or blood glucose are signs that blood sugar is out of control. If a person has these symptoms, a doctor should be called immediately.

Like illness, stress that results from losses or conflicts at home or on the job can affect diabetes control. Urine and blood glucose checks can be clues to the effects of stress. If someone finds that stress is making diabetes control difficult, a doctor can advise treatment and suggest sources of help.

Points to Remember

- Special situations such as pregnancy, surgery, and illness call for extra careful diabetes control.

- Special control may require the use of insulin, even in people who don't normally use insulin.

Dealing with Diabetes

Good diabetes care requires a daily effort to follow a diet, stay active, and take medicine when necessary. Talking to people who have diabetes or who treat diabetes may be helpful for someone who needs emotional support. The list of organizations at the end of this chapter can help patients find discussion groups or counselors familiar with diabetes. It's very important for people with diabetes to understand how to stay healthy, follow a proper diet, exercise, and be aware of changes in their bodies. People with diabetes can live long, healthy lives if they take care of themselves.

Points to Remember

- Good diabetes care is a daily responsibility.

- Local diabetes organizations offer programs so people with diabetes can share experiences and support.

- The good health care urged for people with diabetes is beneficial to anyone who wishes to stay healthy.

Finding Help

A person with diabetes is responsible for his or her daily care and a doctor is the best source of information on that care. A doctor in family practice or internal medicine can diagnose and treat diabetes, and may refer the patient to a doctor who specializes in treating diabetes. "Endocrinologists" and "diabetologists" are doctors with advanced training and experience in diabetes treatment. The local chapters of the American Diabetes Association or the Juvenile Diabetes Foundation have lists of doctors who specialize in diabetes. Another alternative is to contact a university-based medical center. These centers may have special diabetes clinics or may be able to suggest diabetes doctors who practice in the community.

Points to Remember

- Medical guidance is available from a variety of sources such as diabetes groups, local medical societies and hospitals, and diabetes clinics.

Printed Information

While information in books and magazines can't replace a doctor's personal advice, it can provide a clear explanation of diabetes and describe advancements in diabetes treatment. The American Diabetes Association and Juvenile Diabetes Foundation have brochures about diabetes and diabetes treatment. These publications are for people without a medical background. The addresses of these organizations are in the resources section at the back of this chapter.

Brochures and books about diabetes also are available from public libraries and bookstores. Local chapters of the American Diabetes Association, hospitals, and medical centers frequently sponsor educational programs on diabetes and diabetes treatment. Information about diabetes programs is also available from a doctor's office, a local hospital or health department, or a local diabetes organization.

Points to Remember

- Information on diabetes is available from local bookstores, libraries, and local diabetes programs and groups.

Resources on Diabetes

Agency for Health Care Policy and Research (AHCPR)
Medical Treatment Effectiveness Program
2101 East Jefferson Avenue
Rockville, MD 20852
(301) 227-8364—Division of Information and Publications

The Agency supports grant and contract research on the relationship between the use of medical services and procedures and patient outcomes.

American Association of Diabetes Educators (AADE)
444 N. Michigan Avenue
Suite 1240
Chicago, IL 60611
(312) 644-2233 or (800) 338-3633

The AADE is a multidisciplinary organization, with state and regional chapters, for health professionals involved in diabetes education. It sponsors continuing education programs on both beginning and advanced levels and a certification program for diabetes educators, and provides grants, scholarships, and awards for educational research and teaching activities. The AADE publishes a monthly journal, curriculum guides, consensus statements, self-study programs, and other resources for diabetes educators.

American Diabetes Association National Service Center
1660 Duke Street
P.O. Box 25757
Alexandria, VA 22313
(703) 549-1500 or (800) 232-3472

A private, voluntary organization that fosters public awareness of diabetes and supports and promotes diabetes research. It publishes information on many aspects of diabetes, and local affiliates sponsor community programs. Local affiliates can be found in the telephone directory or through the national office.

American Dietetic Association
430 North Michigan Avenue
Chicago, IL 60611
(312) 822-0330

A professional organization that can help someone find a nutritionist in the community.

American Heart Association
7320 Greenville Avenue
Dallas, TX 75231
(800) 242-1793

A private, voluntary organization that has literature on heart disease and how to prevent it. Contact the local affiliate of the American Heart Association listed in telephone directories.

Centers for Disease Control (CDC)
National Center for Chronic Disease Prevention
and Health Promotion
1600 Clifton Road
The Rodes Building
MS K-13
Atlanta, GA 30333
Technical Information Services Branch
(404) 488-5080

The CDC is an agency of the Federal Government that has information on the surveillance and prevention of diabetes for health care professionals and people with diabetes.

117

Juvenile Diabetes Foundation International
432 Park Avenue, South
New York, NY 10016
(212) 889-7575 or (800) 223-1138

A private, voluntary organization with an interest in type I or insulin-dependent diabetes. Local affiliates are found across the country. It also has information on noninsulin-dependent diabetes.

National Diabetes Information Clearinghouse
Box NDIC
Bethesda, MD 20892
(301) 468-2162

The National Diabetes Information Clearinghouse has a variety of publications for distribution to the public and to health professionals. The clearinghouse is a program of the National Institute of Diabetes and Digestive and Kidney Diseases, a component of the National Institutes of Health, leading the Federal Government's research on diabetes.

National Eye Health Education Program
National Eye Institute
National Institutes of Health
Box 20/20
Bethesda, MD 20892
(301) 496-5248

Information about how diabetes affects the eyes is available from the National Eye Institute, a component of the Federal Government's National Institutes of Health.

National Heart, Lung, and Blood Institute
Building 31, Room 4A21
National Institutes of Health
Bethesda, MD 20892
(301) 496-4236

Information on heart disease is available from this component of the Federal Government's National Institutes of Health.

Chapter 11

Insulin Resistance

A Multifaceted Syndrome Responsible for NIDDM, Obesity, Hypertension, Dyslipidemia, and Atherosclerotic Cardiovascular Disease

Diabetes mellitus is commonly associated with systolic/diastolic hypertension [high blood pressure] and a wealth of epidemiological data suggest that this association is independent of age and obesity. Much evidence indicates that the link between diabetes and essential hypertension is hyperinsulinemia [elevated levels of insulin in the blood]. Thus when hypertensive patients, whether obese or of normal body weight, are compared with age- and weight-matched normotensive [normal blood pressure] control subjects a heightened plasma insulin response to a glucose challenge is consistently found. A state of cellular resistance to insulin action subtends [underlies] the observed hyperinsulinism. With the insulin/glucose clamp technique in combination with tracer glucose infusion and indirect calorimetry [a technique for measuring calories/heat used], it has been demonstrated that the insulin resistance of essential hypertension is located in peripheral tissues (muscle), is limited to nonoxidative pathways of glucose

DeFronzo, Ralph A. and Eleuterio Ferrannini. "Insulin Resistance: A Multifaceted Syndrome Responsible for NIDDM, Obesity, Hypertension, Dyslipidemia, and Atherosclerotic Cardiovascular Disease," *Diabetes Care*, Vo. 14. No. 3, March 1991; reprinted with permission. Bracketed comments have been added to assist the layreader.

disposal (glycogen synthesis), and correlates directly with the severity of hypertension. The reasons for the association of insulin resistance and essential hypertension can be sought in at least four general types of mechanisms: Na [sodium] retention, sympathetic nervous system overactivity, disturbed membrane ion transport, and proliferation of vascular smooth muscle cells. Physiological maneuvers, such as calorie restriction (in the overweight patient) and regular physical exercise, can improve tissue sensitivity to insulin; evidence indicates that these maneuvers can also lower blood pressure in both normotensive and hypertensive individuals. Insulin resistance and hyperinsulinemia are also associated with an atherogenic [causing hardening of the arteries] plasma lipid profile. Elevated plasma insulin concentrations enhance very-low-density lipoprotein (VLDL) synthesis, leading to hypertriglyceridemia [high levels of fatty acids in the blood]. Progressive elimination of lipid [fats in the blood] and apolipoproteins [part of the lipid-protein combinations in the blood] from the VLDL particle leads to an increased formation of intermediate-density and low-density lipoproteins both of which are atherogenic. Last, insulin, independent of its effects on blood pressure and plasma lipids, is known to be atherogenic. The hormone enhances cholesterol transport into arteriolar smooth muscle cells and increases endogenous lipid synthesis by these cells. Insulin also stimulates the proliferation of arteriolar smooth muscle cells, augments collagen synthesis in the vascular wall, increases the formation of and decreases the regression of lipid plaques and stimulates the production of various growth factors. In summary, insulin resistance appears to be a syndrome that is associated with a clustering of metabolic disorders, including non-insulin-dependent diabetes mellitus, obesity, hypertension, lipid abnormalities, and atherosclerotic cardiovascular disease. *Diabetes Care* 14:173-94, 1991.

Background

Obesity, non-insulin-dependent diabetes mellitus (NIDDM), hypertension, and atherosclerotic cardiovascular disease (ASCVD) are common metabolic disorders that affect the majority of individuals who live in westernized societies. Moreover, all of these common medical disorders occur with increasing incidence as the population ages. In young individuals, obesity, NIDDM, hypertension, and ASCVD are uncommon. However, by 70 years of age, the incidence of these metabolic disorders reaches epidemic proportions (Table 11.1). Over half of such elderly individuals have evidence of ASCVD, and 45-50% are

Table 11.1. Age-related prevalence of non-insulin-dependent diabetes mellitus, obesity, essential hypertension, and atherosclerotic cardiovascular disease in the general population

	Overall Prevalence (%)	Age-related prevalence (%)	
		20 yr	70 yr
NIDDM	~7	< 1	~10
Obesity	~30	~5	~50
Essential hypertension	~20	~5	~50
ASCVD	~25	<1	~50

NIDDM: Non-insulin-dependent diabetes mellitus
~ about
< less than
ASCVD: Atherosclerotic cardiovascular disease

Table 11.2. Syndrome of insulin resistance

Obesity
Non-insulin-dependent diabetes mellitus
Hypertension
Atherosclerotic cardiovascular disease
Dyslipidemia
Hyperinsulinemia

obese and hypertensive. The incidence of NIDDM is somewhat lower (about 10 to 12%), although in some populations it is much higher. Because obesity, NIDDM, hypertension, and ASCVD occur frequently in the population at large, it is not surprising that any given individual, especially if he or she is more than 60-70 years of age, might manifest two or more of these common medical problems. In the subsequent discussion, we provide evidence that the common occurrence of the pentad [five elements]—obesity, NIDDM, hypertension, ASCVD, and dyslipidemia—in the same individual is more than a chance occurrence and is related in part to a gene or set of genes for insulin resistance (Table 11.2). Moreover, it is now recognized that this pentad is commonly associated with hyperinsulinemia and a specific abnormal lipid profile, i.e., elevated plasma triglycerides, low high-density lipoprotein cholesterol (HDL-chol), and increased low-density lipoprotein cholesterol (LDL-chol), all of which can predispose to the development of atherosclerosis (Table 11.2). In the following sections, we review a considerable amount of published data that suggest that insulin resistance, with its compensatory hyperinsulinemia and associated lipid abnormalities, is etiologically related to the high prevalence of NIDDM, obesity, hypertension, and ASCVD in the general population.

Obesity and NIDDM: What Do They Share in Common?

When a nondiabetic person consumes excessive calories and gains weight, the body becomes markedly resistant to the action of insulin. With the euglycemic insulin-clamp technique, many investigators have shown that tissue sensitivity to insulin declines by about 30-40% when an individual becomes more than 35-40% over ideal body weight. The insulin resistance primarily affects muscle and involves both the oxidative and nonoxidative pathways of glucose disposal. Despite the severe impairment in insulin action, however, glucose tolerance remains normal because the pancreatic ß-cells are able to augment their insulin secretory capacity to offset the insulin resistance. The net result is a well-compensated metabolic state in which the insulin resistance is closely counterbalanced by an increase in insulin secretion such that glucose tolerance remains normal or only slightly impaired. The trade-off is hyperinsulinemia. With advancing duration of obesity or with further weight gain, the excessive rates of insulin secretion cannot be maintained. Because of the presence of severe insulin resistance, even the slightest decline in insulin secretion will lead to the development of frank diabetes mellitus. Nonetheless, both the fasting and meal-stimulated plasma insulin levels remain 1.5- to 2-fold elevated compared with age-matched and weight-matched control subjects. Only much later in the natural history of obesity and diabetes do we see a significant decline in insulin secretion. At this stage, plasma insulin levels return to or below normal, and severe glucose intolerance ensues. The sequence of events for obese diabetic individuals has been confirmed by a prospective follow-up of the same subjects who were subsequently restudied 10 years later. Similar results have been published by Saad et al. in a prospective study carried out in Pima Indians. It is important to underscore, however, that, during most of his/her lifetime, the obese person—whether he/she maintains normal glucose tolerance, becomes glucose intolerant, or develops frank diabetes—will be exposed to a persistent state of hyperinsulinemia.

Normal-weight NIDDM individuals are also characterized by insulin-resistance. However, as opposed to obesity, where the defect in insulin action is acquired, the insulin resistance is genetically transmitted in NIDDM. In identical twins and in the offspring of two diabetic parents, the incidence of diabetes ranges from 70 to 90%, whereas in first-degree relatives, the incidence of diabetes is 30-40%.

The severity of the insulin resistance in NIDDM is of similar magnitude to that observed in nondiabetic obese subjects and involves both the oxidative and nonoxidative (glycogen synthesis) pathways of glucose disposal. Thus, from the standpoint of insulin action, it is difficult to distinguish between the nondiabetic obese individual and the normal-weight NIDDM person. What distinguishes the two groups is the plasma insulin concentration. In normal-weigh NIDDM patients, the plasma insulin response, although elevated compared with the normal-weight control subjects, is significantly decreased compared with the nondiabetic obese subjects despite a similar degree of insulin resistance. Early in the evolution of NIDDM all subjects are hyperinsulinemic both in the fasting state and in response to insulin. In a group of 77 normal-weight NIDDM patients both the fasting and glucose-stimulated plasma insulin concentrations rose progressively as fasting plasma glucose increased from 4.4 to 6.6 mM. Thereafter the augmented rate of insulin secretion could not be maintained and there was a progressive decline in both the fasting and glucose-stimulated plasma insulin concentrations. Nonetheless up to fasting glucose levels of 8.8-10 mM (i.e., moderately severe diabetes) diabetic patients remained hyperinsulinemic compared with normal-weight control subjects even though they were less hyperinsulinemic than nondiabetic obese subjects.

From the above discussion the following scenario can be constructed—Syndrome of insulin resistance: An excessive caloric intake leads to obesity which leads to insulin resistance, or an inherited genetic defect leads to NIDDM which leads to insulin resistance. Insulin resistance leads to hyperinsulinemia which can lead to hypertension, hypertriglyceridemia, hypercholesterolemia, decreased HDL-chol, and/or atherosclerosis. The metabolic cascade leads from acquired (obesity) or inherited (non-insulin-dependent diabetes mellitus) insulin resistance to hyperinsulinemia and eventually to hypertension, abnormal plasma lipid profile, and atherosclerosis.

Insulin resistance is a characteristic feature of both obesity and NIDDM. In the former it is acquired due to excessive calorie intake whereas in the later the diabetic patient inherits a gene or set of genes that confer insulin resistance. The normal ß-cell is able to recognize the presence of insulin resistance and to augment its secretion of insulin. In the obese nondiabetic person, the compensatory response is nearly perfect and no alteration in glucose tolerance ensues. In the diabetic individual the ß-cell response is less than perfect and glucose intolerance ensues. In both groups however day-long hyperinsulinemia is present. Only in the severely diabetic patient (fasting plasma glucose concentration greater than 10-11 mM) does insulinopenia develop. There is now mounting evidence that persistently elevated plasma insulin levels can contribute to the development of hypertension plasma lipid abnormalities and atherosclerosis. These associations will be discussed at length subsequently.

In summary, the results reviewed in this section clearly demonstrate that insulin resistance is a characteristic feature of both obesity and NIDDM involves the pathways of glucose oxidation and nonoxidative glucose disposal and is compensated for at least in part by augmented insulin secretion by the pancreas.

Hypertension, Obesity, and Diabetes: Common Metabolic Defect?

For many years it has been recognized that hypertension is very common in obese and diabetic individuals. It is also known that weight loss and physical training, interventions that improve the body's sensitivity to insulin, are effective in lowering the blood pressure in obese and diabetic patients. Moreover the improvement in insulin sensitivity and resultant lowering of the elevated plasma insulin concentration are closely related to the decline in systolic/diastolic blood pressure in nondiabetic obese subjects. Similar observations have been made by Krotkiewski et al., who demonstrated that after a chronic physical training program both systolic and diastolic blood pressure fell even though body weight remained unchanged. Significant decreases in blood pressure were observed only in obese subjects with elevated fasting plasma insulin concentrations and correlated closely with the decline in fasting plasma insulin levels. Several prospective epidemiological studies have also shown that the fasting plasma insulin concentration is closely related to the elevation in blood pressure in obese and diabetic subjects.

Based on the above observations Manicardi et al. examined the relationship between blood pressure and oral glucose tolerance in age-matched obese hypertensive (174/104 mmHg) and obese normotensive (124/80 mmHg) individuals. Compared with the normotensive group, the obese hypertensive subjects were glucose intolerant despite a plasma insulin response that was approximately threefold greater. These results strongly suggest the presence of insulin resistance in the obese hypertensive group. Most important, the plasma insulin response during the oral glucose tolerance test was strongly correlated ($r = 0.75$, $P < 0.001$) to the elevated systolic/diastolic blood pressure in the obese hypertensive group; no correlation between blood pressure and insulin was observed in the normotensive group. As discussed earlier the plasma insulin response provides an indirect measure of the severity of insulin resistance. Thus the results of Manicardi et al. suggest that insulin resistance per se or acting through hyperinsulinemia is linked to the increase in systolic/diastolic blood pressure.

Because obesity can lead to insulin resistance, Ferrannini et al. studied a group of normal-weight young essential hypertensive individuals with the quantitatively more precise euglycemic insulin-clamp technique. Insulin-mediated total-body glucose uptake was reduced by about 30-40% in the essential hypertensive group and the severity of insulin resistance was closely related ($r = 0.76$, $P < 0.001$) to the increase in blood pressure. The impairment in insulin-mediated glucose disposal was entirely accounted for by a defect in nonoxidative glucose uptake (i.e., glycogen synthesis); stimulation of glucose oxidation by insulin was not diminished. With the forearm-catheterization technique, Ferrannini has documented that muscle is the primary site of the insulin resistance in patients with essential hypertension (unpublished observations).

In summary, essential hypertension, like obesity and NIDDM, is an insulin-resistant state. Note however that not all essential hypertensive subjects are insulin resistant and it would be unreasonable to think that insulin resistance and/or its compensatory hyperinsulinemia can explain the development of essential hypertension in all individuals. Nonetheless, in most subjects with essential hypertension, insulin resistance and hyperinsulinemia are present and in this group it is plausible to suggest that these metabolic abnormalities may contribute in a causal fashion to the pathogenesis of hypertension.

Insulin and Hypertension

From the preceding discussion, it is obvious that hypertension obesity and NIDDM are insulin-resistant states, and their frequent occurrence in the same individual is probably more than a chance association. It is reasonable to ask what then is the link between insulin resistance and hypertension? One potential explanation is that cellular insulin resistance per se is responsible for the development of hypertension by some unidentified mechanism. For instance, it is possible that insulin resistance alters the substrate supply or energy needs of the cell, and the resultant changes in substrate/energy requirements sensitize, either directly or by altering ion fluxes into the cell, the vascular smooth muscle response to pressor amines [organic compounds containing nitrogen that tend to increase blood pressure] such as norepinephrine [a hormone] and angiotensin II [a blood component that stimulates muscle contractions in arteries and capillaries]. Unfortunately, little is known about such interactions, and they are deserving of further investigation.

An alternative explanation for the link between hypertension and insulin resistance is the development of hyperinsulinemia. The normal ß-cell response to insulin resistance is to augment its secretion of insulin, and individuals with essential hypertension, obesity, and NIDDM clearly have been shown to be hyperinsulinemic. There are several potential mechanisms by which elevated plasma insulin levels can lead to hypertension:

Kidney sodium handling. It long has been recognized that total-body sodium content is increased in obese and NIDDM subjects with hypertension. Moreover, weight loss is associated with natriuresis [abnormal amounts of sodium in the urine], reduction in blood pressure, and decline in fasting/meal-stimulated plasma insulin levels. Conversely, acute carbohydrate ingestion is associated with hyperinsulinemia and sodium retention. Similarly, refeeding edema [excessive fluid in the tissues] with its associated antinatriuresis has been shown to be related to hyperinsulinemia. All of these observations point to an important role for insulin in kidney salt and water reabsorption.

To examine the relationship between insulin and kidney sodium excretion in more detail, euglycemic insulin-clamp studies have been performed in healthy young subjects. Within 30-60 minutes after a physiological increment in the plasma insulin concentration, urinary sodium excretion declined, eventually reaching a nadir that was about 50% lower than the basal rate. Using micropuncture and micro-perfusion techniques, the antinatriuretic [reducing the excretion of sodium in the urine] effect of insulin has been shown to be exerted on both the proximal and distal parts of the nephron [kidney]. It is important to emphasize that an increment in the plasma insulin concentration of as little as 30-40 μU/ml is capable of eliciting this antinatriuretic effect. Such insulin concentrations are within the range of fasting insulin concentrations observed in the obese individuals and are considerably less than meal-stimulated insulin levels. For the compensatory hyperinsulinemia to induce kidney sodium retention, expansion of the extracellular fluid volume, and ultimately hypertension, it is necessary that the kidneys of obese, diabetic, and hypertensive subjects maintain normal sensitivity to the antinatriuretic effect of insulin, even though severe resistance exists regarding carbohydrate metabolism. One study has shown this to be true in obese insulin-resistant subjects. The effect of insulin on kidney sodium excretion in patients with NIDDM and essential hypertension has yet to be studied.

Sypathetic nervous system (SNS). A second mechanism by which insulin can cause hypertension involves stimulation of the sympathetic nervous system [the part of the nervous system that regulates cardiovascular functions]. Various studies in humans and animals have demonstrated that changes in dietary intake have a profound influence on SNS activity. Thus, fasting decreases whereas feeding activates the SNS. In these studies, the change in SNS activity was closely correlated with the change in plasma insulin concentration. With the insulin/glucose-clamp technique, Rowe et al. demonstrated that insulin caused a dose-related increase in the plasma norepinephrine level, whereas hyperglycemia was without effect. The increase in plasma norepinephrine concentration was closely related to an increase in pulse and blood pressure. Note that an active-transport system in the neural synapse [the place where an impulse is transferred from one neuron to an adjacent neuron] recaptures the major fraction of norepinephrine released from nerve terminals. Thus, the increase in plasma norepinephrine observed by Rowe et al. grossly under estimates the magnitude of SNS activation by insulin. Studies in dogs, humans, and rats have provided additional evidence for the role of insulin in stimulation of the SNS.

The SNS can influence the blood pressure by augmenting the cardiac output (increased cardiac contractibility and heart rate), by increasing cardiopulmonary blood volume (constriction of the great veins), by directly vasoconstricting resistant vessels, and by enhancing kidney sodium reabsorption (direct stimulation of renal tubular sodium reabsorption, renal vasoconstriction, and stimulation of renin secretion) with expansion of the extracellular fluid volume. In addition to the effects of catecholamines [a group of compounds, including epinephrine and norepinephrine, that mimic the impulses of the sympathetic nervous system] on the cardiovascular system, it is well recognized that epinephrine is a powerful insulin antagonist. It inhibits insulin-mediated glucose uptake by muscle and blocks the suppressive action of insulin on hepatic glucose production. Both of these defects are characteristic of obesity and NIDDM.

The relationship between insulin resistance, plasma insulin concentration, SNS activity, and hypertension is summarized as follows:

Primary insulin resistance leads to
>   hyperinsulinemia which can lead to adrenergic overactivity or
>>   sodium retention which leads to
>>>   hypertension

Adrenergic overactivity leads to secondary insulin resistance, hypertension, or
>   sodium retention which leads to
>>   hypertension

Primary CNS overdrive leads to
>   adrenergic overactivity which can lead to secondary insulin resistance, hypertension, or
>>   sodium retention which leads to
>>>   hypertension

If insulin resistance represents the primary metabolic defect that is inherited (NIDDM, essential hypertension) or acquired (obesity, aging), the ß-cell will respond to this by augmenting its secretion of insulin. The resultant hyperinsulinemia has two important effects: first, insulin directly enhances kidney sodium reabsorption, leading to extracellular volume expansion and hypertension; second, insulin activates the SNS, and this in turn causes hypertension through various mechanisms (enhanced kidney sodium reabsorption and volume expansion, peripheral vasoconstriction, increased cardiac output). Of particular importance, SNS activation can induce or worsen preexisting insulin resistance, closing a feedback loop, which ensures the perpetuation of both the insulin resistance and hypertension. It should be emphasized that we need not assume that the primary metabolic abnormality that initiates the sequence of events outlined above is insulin resistance. It is possible that the basic disturbance is primary central nervous system overdrive, leading to excessive SNS activity. This in turn can lead to hypertension and, secondarily, to insulin resistance.

Altered cellular electrolyte transport and composition. For insulin to act, it first must bind to specific receptors present on the cell surface of all insulin target tissues. Once insulin has bound to its receptor, the second messenger for insulin action is activated. There is considerable controversy concerning the precise identification of the second messenger for insulin's many varied effects. However, many authorities believe that tyrosine kinase, which is an integral part of the ß-subunit of the insulin receptor, is a prime candidate for insulin's second messenger. Once the second messenger has been generated, it stimulates glucose transport via a complex mechanism that involves the translocation of glucose-transport units from within the cell and their insertion into the cell membrane. Once inserted into the cell membrane, the glucose-transport units are activated by insulin, and glucose fluxes into the cell. However, free glucose does not accumulate intracellularly because it is rapidly oxidized or converted to glycogen. The basic cellular metabolic defects responsible for the insulin resistance of NIDDM, obesity, aging, and hypertension remain unknown. However, considerable evidence suggests that a defect in glucose transport per se or in coupling of the insulin receptor with the glucose-transport system is responsible for the impairment in insulin action, although several publications implicate a primary abnormality in glycogen synthesis in NIDDM. Whatever genetic defect represents the inherited metabolic disturbance responsible for the insulin resistance in these common disorders (diabetes, obesity, hypertension, normal aging), the pancreatic ß-cell responds by augmenting its secretion of insulin. The resultant hyperinsulinemia can in turn alter the activity of several sodium pumps, which are present in all cell membranes, including the arteriolar smooth muscle cells. This will lead to the intracellular accumulation of sodium, which in turn sensitizes the arteriolar smooth muscle cells to the pressor effects of norepinephrine and angiotensin II. Such a sequence of events could explain the frequent association between hyperinsulinemia and hypertension.

Na^+-K^+-ATPase represents a key insulin-regulated enzyme, which plays a critical role in maintaining the normal intracellular electrolyte milieu. This pump extrudes Na^+ in exchange for K^+ in a ratio of 3:2 and is thus electrogenic. Obesity, diabetes, and hypertension all represent insulin-resistant states with respect to glucose metabolism. If this insulin resistance were to extend to the enzyme Na^+-K^+-ATPase, Na^+ would be expected to accumulate within the cell. In patients with essential hypertension, there is evidence that both the intracellular Na^+ content and transmembrane Na^+ transport rate are diminished in leukocytes [white blood cells]; similar but less consistent results have been reported in erythrocytes [red blood cells]. An excellent review of this subject has been published by Hilton [Hilton PJ: Cellular sodium transport in essential hypertension. *New England Journal of Medicine* 314:229, 1986]. The activity of the Na^+-K^+-ATPase also has been reported to be reduced in various cell systems in both human essential hypertension and experimental animal models of hypertension. Reduced activity of the Na^+ pump also has been reported in other insulin-resistant states, including obesity, human insulin-dependent-diabetes mellitus, and experimental models of diabetes. Consistent with this, the ability of insulin to enhance K^+ uptake in human obesity has been shown to be reduced. We are unaware of studies that have examined Na^+-K^+-ATPase activity in NIDDM in humans. The studies reviewed above are consistent with the hypothesis that in certain insulin-resistant states (i. e., obesity and some types of diabetes) in humans and animals, the Na^+-K^+ pump may not be normally responsive to insulin.

Several recent observations, however, suggest that an abnormality in the Na^+-K^+-ATPase pump is unlikely to explain the elevation in blood pressure in patients with essential hypertension. First, with the euglycemic insulin-clamp technique, it has been shown that the ability of a physiological increment in the plasma insulin concentration to promote K^+ uptake is normal in essential hypertensive subjects. Second, it is well established that insulin-stimulated K^+ uptake *in vivo* and *in vitro* is unrelated to its stimulatory effect on glucose metabolism in muscle and other insulin-dependent tissues. This latter issue has been evaluated more directly with the forearm-catheterization technique combined with intra-arterial insulin infusion to quantitate glucose and K^+ uptake by muscle. In healthy subjects, physiological hyperinsulinemia markedly enhanced both glucose and K^+ uptake by muscle. When oubain, a potent inhibitor of the Na^+-K^+-ATPase pump, was infused with insulin, forearm muscle K^+ uptake was completely abolished, whereas glucose uptake remained unaffected. These results demonstrate that, *in vivo* in humans, the effects of insulin on K^+ and glucose uptake by muscle, the primary tissue responsible for glucose and K^+ disposal, are readily dissociable. There is therefore no a priori reason to expect that the insulin resistance documented with respect to glucose metabolism should extend to K^+. Third, forearm K^+ and glucose uptake have been directly quantitated in patients with essential hypertension over a wide range of plasma insulin concentrations. Although insulin-mediated glucose uptake by forearm muscle was reduced by 30-40% at all insulin doses spanning the physiological and pharmacological range, K^+ uptake was normal (E.F., unpublished observations). Fourth, it is uncertain whether changes in leukocyte/erythrocyte (as opposed to muscle) Na^+ and K^+ content can be causally related to the development of hypertension. On the contrary, most authorities believe that such changes are genetic, rather than pathogenetic [causing disease] markers.

Another cell membrane pump that has received considerable attention in the pathogenesis of essential hypertension is the Na^+-H^+ exchanger, which is considered to be equivalent to the Na^+-Li^+-cotransport system. This transport system is found in various cell types, has a 1:1 stoichiometry for $Na^+ H^+$ (i.e., it is electrically neutral), and is specifically inhibited by amiloride. Significantly, insulin has been shown to stimulate the activity of the Na^+-proton exchanger in skeletal muscle and adipocytes [fat cells]. This Na^+-H^+ pump has also been shown to be linked to Ca^{2+} exchange and to play a critical role in the maintenance of intracellular pH.

The physiological functions of the Na^+-proton exchanger make it an attractive candidate to explain the elevation in blood pressure observed in insulin-resistant states such as essential hypertension, diabetes mellitus and obesity. As discussed previously, a primary defect in insulin action will be counterbalanced by enhanced secretion of insulin. The resultant hyperinsulinemia will augment Na^+-H^+ exchange, assuming that this pump retains normal sensitivity to insulin. The intracellular accumulation of Na^+ and Ca^{2+} would be expected to enhance the sensitivity of the vascular smooth musculature to the pressor [blood-pressure raising] effects of norepinephrine, angiotensin, and NaCl loading. Enhanced Na^+-H^+ exchange also will lead to an increase in cell pH. Intracellular alkalosis [the accumulation of a base or the loss of acid] is a known stimulator of protein synthesis and cell proliferation and eventually could lead to the characteristic hypertrophy [enlargement] of resistance vessel walls that is observed in established hypertension. Intracellular alkalinization [creating reactions with fatty acids] also is known to directly increase smooth muscle contractility. Consistent with this, Ng et al. have demonstrated increased leukocyte intracellular pH and Na^+-Ha^{+-}-antiport activity in patients with essential hypertension. In addition, Na^+-H^+ exchange has been implicated as a transmembrane signal for various growth factors known to be stimulated by insulin.

Several clinical observations are consistent with the above hypothesis. First, the Na^+-H^+ exchanger is the only known genetic marker for essential hypertension. Second, many investigators have demonstrated increased erythrocyte Na^+-H^+ countertransport in hypertensive versus nonhypertensive individuals. Third, increased Na^+-H^+ activity has also been demonstrated in platelets and leukocytes of patients with essential hypertension. Fourth, intracellular free Ca^{2+} has been shown to be increased in erythrocytes of patients with essential hypertension. Fifth, increased Na^+-Li^+ countertransport activity has been reported in erythrocytes of hypertensive versus normotensive insulin-dependent diabetic subjects and in normotensive children of hypertensive diabetic parents. Similar studies have yet to be carried out in NIDDM subjects.

Note that the sequence of events discussed above was initiated with a single primary cellular defect: insulin resistance. In this scheme, the Na^+-H^+ exchanger can be viewed as an innocent bystander manipulated by hyperinsulinemia. Conversely, we could postulate that the metabolic cascade starts with a primary genetic defect in the Na^+-proton exchanger. Last, these two pathogenetic sequences are not mutually exclusive. We could postulate that excessive Na^+-H^+ pump activity is an inherited trait but in itself is not sufficient to cause hypertension. Only in individuals with insulin resistance and secondary hyperinsulinemia will the phenotypic expression (i.e., hypertension) of the $Na^+$$H^+$ exchanger become manifest.

Enhanced growth factor activity. Insulin acting directly or indirectly through the stimulation of growth factors, such as insulinlike growth factor I (IGF-I), also may contribute to the development of hypertension by causing hypertrophy of the vascular wall and narrowing of the lumen [channel within] of the resistance vessels involved in the regulation of systemic blood pressure. The components of vascular hypertrophy include increases in the size and number of myocytes [muscle cells] and in the amount of contractile protein, DNA, and collagen, all of which can be increased by the actions of insulin and IGF-I. Consistent with this, receptors for IGF-I and insulin have been identified on blood vessels. Further support for the growth factor hypothesis comes from the classic experiment of Cruz et al., who demonstrated that chronic insulin infusion into one femoral artery of the dog causes vascular hypertrophy only on the ipsilateral [same] side.

In summary, much evidence exists supporting the hypothesis that hyperinsulinemia may play an important pathogenetic role in the development of hypertension in several insulin-resistant states, including obesity, diabetes mellitus, and essential hypertension. Insulin can elevate the blood pressure via various mechanisms: kidney Na^+ retention; SNS activation; enhanced fluxes of Na^+ and Ca^+ into vascular smooth muscle cells, leading to an increased vascular sensitivity to the vasoconstrictor effect of pressor amines; and proliferation of arteriolar smooth muscle cells.

Insulin Resistance, Hyperinsulinemia, and Hyperlipidemia

The characteristic lipid [fat] profile in an individual with NIDDM includes 1) decreased serum HDL-chol; 2) increased serum very-low-density lipoprotein (VLDL); and 3) less commonly, an increase in LDL-chol. A decrease in HDL-chol and an increase in LDL-chol are well-established risk factors for coronary artery disease (CAD) in both nondiabetic and diabetic subjects. Although less commonly appreciated, evidence is mounting that elevated VLDL levels also are a risk factor for the development of CAD in both nondiabetic and NIDDM subjects.

According to current concepts, LDL is synthesized from hepatic-derived VLDL by the progressive elimination of lipids and apolipoproteins (apoAI and apoAII) [the protein part of the lipoproteins—a combination of lipid and protein] and the accumulation of apoC and apoE. Intermediate-density lipoprotein (IDL) represents an intermediate, which is formed during the conversion of VLDL to LDL, and these IDL particles are particularly atherogenic. From these interconversions, it can be anticipated that factors that enhance VLDL synthesis also will increase the formation of IDL and LDL and predispose to accelerated atherogenesis.

The plasma VLDL concentration is determined by two factors: 1) the rate of VLDL synthesis by the liver and 2) the rate of VLDL removal by peripheral tissues. The former in turn is regulated by the ambient plasma insulin concentration and substrate availability. In obese nondiabetic subjects, individuals with impaired glucose tolerance, and NIDDM patients with mild to moderate fasting hyperglycemia, insulin resistance is universally present. However, this is offset by enhanced pancreatic insulin secretion, and the resultant hyperinsulinemia in turn augments hepatic VLDL synthesis. Note that a close relationship between hyperinsulinemia and hypertriglyceridemia [elevated amounts of triglycerides—a fat compound—in the blood] has also been described in population-based studies in healthy normal-weight subjects. The association between plasma insulin and triglyceride levels has also been demonstrated in normoinsulinemic [normal insulin levels in the blood] individuals. In addition to elevated insulin levels, NIDDM subjects, especially if they are obese, have increased plasma free fatty acid and glucose concentrations, providing an abundant substrate supply to drive VLDL formation. Resistance to the action of insulin on lipoprotein lipase has also been described in obesity and diabetes, and a defect in VLDL removal has been shown to contribute to the hyperlipidemia [elevated amounts of lipids—fats—in the blood] in these disorders.

In summary, there is much evidence that suggests that insulin resistance, working through hyperinsulinemia, enhances hepatic VLDL synthesis and contributes to the elevated plasma triglyceride levels observed in normal-weight healthy subjects, obese nondiabetic subjects, and NIDDM subjects. Resistance to the action of insulin on lipoprotein lipase also contributes to the hypertriglyceridemia in some obese and diabetic people.

Reduced HDL-chol concentration is a well-established risk factor for CAD in nondiabetic and diabetic individuals. Many epidemiological studies have demonstrated an inverse correlation between the plasma insulin and HDL concentration in otherwise healthy subjects. A similar inverse relationship has been demonstrated in obese and NIDDM patients. Golay et al. have provided insight into the mechanism of the reduced HDL levels in NIDDM. With [³H]apoAI (apoAI is the major lipoprotein in HDL), Golay et al. demonstrated that, despite enhanced HDL synthesis, the plasma HDL concentration was significantly reduced in NIDDM versus control subjects. This decrease in plasma HDL was entirely accounted for by an increase in the rate of apoAI/HDL degradation, which exceeded an enhanced rate of apoAI/HDL synthesis. Within both the control and NIDDM groups, the plasma insulin concentration and the plasma HDL concentration (and apoAI clearance rate) were strongly and inversely correlated. Although the precise cellular mechanisms by which insulin regulates HDL metabolism remain to be defined, it is nonetheless clear that hyperinsulinemia is associated with a decline in circulating HDL levels and an increased risk for CAD.

In summary, there is abundant evidence that now implicates hyperinsulinemia with various lipid abnormalities (increased VLDL/IDL/LDL and decreased HDL), which are known risk factors for CAD and other macrovascular complications. Although hyperinsulinemia may be the final common denominator ultimately responsible for the abnormal plasma lipid profile, it is important to recognize that insulin resistance represents the basic underlying metabolic defect.

Insulin Resistance, Hyperinsulinemia, and Atherosclerosis

Epidemiologists interested in atherosclerosis have long recognized that insulin is a major risk factor for the development of CAD and that the effect is independent of blood pressure and plasma lipid levels. A growing body of experimental evidence has accumulated to support this association. The major effects of insulin on arterial tissues are summarized in Table 11.3. The atherosclerotic plaque is characterized by excessive amounts of lipid and collagen, foam macrophages [large cells that "eat" foreign particles], and proliferated smooth muscle cells. All of these constituents are affected by the plasma insulin concentration. In a now classic experiment, Cruz et al. demonstrated that chronic insulin infusion into one femoral artery of the

Table 11.3. Effect of insulin on arterial tissues

Proliferation of smooth muscle cells

Enhanced cholesterol synthesis and low-density lipoprotein-receptor activity

Increased formation and decreased regression of lipid plaques

Stimulation of connective tissue synthesis

Stimulation of growth factors

dog resulted in marked intimal [the inner layer of the blood vessel] and medial [the middle portion] proliferation and the accumulation of cholesterol and fatty acids on the insulin-infused side but was without effect on the contralateral [opposite side] femoral artery. Subsequent studies have shown that adding insulin to cultured smooth muscle cells markedly stimulates their proliferation. Enhanced LDL-receptor activity and increased cholesterol and triglyceride synthesis have been demonstrated in arterial smooth muscle cells, fibroblasts [connective tissue cells], and mononuclear cells both *in vivo* and *in vitro* after the addition of insulin. The effect of insulin to augment lipid synthesis by vascular smooth muscle cells probably results from its stimulatory action on the lipogenic enzymes [enzymes that help make lipids] glucose-6-phosphate dehydrogenase, malic enzyme, and 3-hydroxyacyl-CoA dehydrogenase. In addition to fostering the development of the atherosclerotic plaque, hyperinsulinemia has been shown to inhibit the reabsorption of plaques once formed. Collagen is an integral component of the atherosclerotic lesion, and it is well established that collagen synthesis is augmented by insulin and insulinlike growth factors. Last, not only is insulin itself a growth-promoting substance, but it stimulates various other growth factors, including IGF-I, which cause cells to proliferate and thereby contribute to the atherosclerotic process.

In summary, various different sorts of evidence have implicated insulin, independent of changes in plasma lipid levels or blood pressure, in the pathogenesis of atherosclerosis. Although this relationship was initially promulgated by epidemiological observations, a significant body of experimental data has accumulated to provide the biochemical/cellular basis of this association.

One of the great paradoxes in medicine is the inability of effective antihypertensive therapy to diminish the increased incidence of coronary artery disease in patients with hypertension. Normalizing blood pressure in hypertensive individuals reduces the incidence of stroke, kidney failure, congestive heart failure, and accelerated hypertension but has never been shown to prevent CAD. This paradox may be explained by the failure of antihypertensive therapy to reverse the basic underlying metabolic problem: insulin resistance with its compensatory hyperinsulinemia. In fact, most antihypertensive regimens exacerbate the existing insulin resistance/hyperinsulinemia and promote a more atherogenic plasma lipid profile. This is particularly true of ß-adrenergic antagonists and diuretics (see subsequent discussion).

Which Is the Culprit: Insulin Resistance or Hyperinsulinemia?

An important question that arises from the preceding discussion is whether the abnormalities in blood pressure regulation, plasma lipid profile, and/or susceptibility to atherogenesis observed in obese, diabetic, elderly, and hypertensive individuals are related to the insulin resistance per se or to the compensatory increase in plasma insulin concentration. This is a difficult issue to address, because the two conditions usually go hand in hand. However, the question may be approached indirectly by examining the mechanism(s) responsible for the insulin resistance in these four common clinical disorders. A defect in total-body glucose metabolism could result from an abnormality in glucose oxidation, nonoxidative glucose disposal (glycogen formation), or suppression of hepatic glucose production. If one metabolic abnormality could be shown to be related consistently to the clustering of hypertension, lipid abnormalities, and atherosclerosis, the case for insulin resistance as a primary etiological factor would be strengthened. If, on the other hand, a variety of different metabolic abnormalities are shown to contribute to the defect in insulin action, it becomes more difficult to argue that the clustering of hypertension, hyperlipidemia, and atherosclerosis is due to the insulin resistance per se. Rather, a stronger argument could be made for the pathogenetic role of hyperinsulinemia, which is a consistent feature of all insulin-resistant states. Defects in glucose oxidation, nonoxidative glucose disposal, and suppression of hepatic glucose production all contribute, in varying amounts, to the insulin resistance in obesity, NIDDM, aging, and hypertension. Although certainly not conclusive, these observations favor the primacy of hyperinsulinemia rather than insulin resistance in the pathogenesis of the hyperlipidemia, elevated blood pressure, and accelerated atherogenesis. In support of this, there are several well-established mechanisms by which insulin can lead to hypertension, diminished HDL-chol, elevated VLDL, and atherosclerosis. However, we cannot avoid being impressed by the rather striking decrease in nonoxidative glucose disposal that occurs in individuals with obesity, NIDDM, and essential hypertension. Therefore, it behooves the investigator to gain a more in-depth appreciation of the potential mechanisms by which a defect in glycogen synthesis might be related to an abnormality in blood pressure regulation, lipid metabolism, and atherogenesis.

Insulin Resistance: A Multifaceted Syndrome

From the preceding discussion, it appears that insulin resistance is a multifaceted syndrome that can express itself in many ways, depending on a particular individual's genetic background. Insulin resistance is a common disorder, which occurs with high frequency in the general population. There is a clear-cut age-related decline in the body's sensitivity to insulin. However, within any given age-group, i.e., young, middle aged, and elderly, there is a wide range of insulin sensitivity. For instance, within the young group, the most insulin-sensitive individual uses glucose at a rate that is four times that of the most insulin-resistant person. To compensate for this defect in insulin-mediated glucose metabolism, the ß-cell must augment its secretion of insulin. In a sense, this is an adaptive process in that the hyperinsulinemia prevents the development of glucose intolerance and frank diabetes mellitus. However, in other ways, this adaptive process is maladaptive. In most people, the increase in plasma insulin concentration probably has little or no consequence. However, in genetically predisposed individuals, the hyperinsulinemia may have important clinical ramifications. For instance, in individuals who have simultaneously inherited a gene that limits the ß-cell's ability to augment insulin secretion (i.e., the diabetic gene), the presence of insulin resistance presents a major problem. Because insulin secretion cannot be augmented sufficiently to offset the insulin resistance, the phenotypic expression is that of NIDDM. If, in other individuals, the Na^+-H^+ gene is overexpressed, the simultaneous presence of hyperinsulinemia (i.e., secondary to the insulin resistance) will lead to the intracellular accumulation of sodium, enhanced sensitivity to angiotensin-norepinephrine, and eventually hypertension. Still, in others who have inherited a primary abnormality in lipid metabolism, hyperinsulinemia may interact with this gene to cause a phenotype characterized by high plasma VLDL or decreased HDL levels. Similarly, in individuals who have inherited a gene or set of genes that predispose to atherosclerosis, the simultaneous presence of hyperinsulinemia will manifest itself as CAD. Note that excessive caloric intake and the development of obesity, although an acquired form of insulin resistance, can be viewed in the same light as the inherited form of insulin resistance.

In summary, the gene(s) for insulin resistance is (are) endemic in the general population. However, in most individuals, the phenotypic expression of this gene(s) goes undetected, and rarely is its biochemical counterpart (i.e., hyperinsulinemia) picked up because measurement of the plasma insulin concentration is not routinely performed.

When the insulin-resistance gene coexists with some other gene, i.e., the hypertension gene, the diabetes gene, the hyperlipidemia gene, or the atherogenesis gene, the phenotypic expression assumes the characteristic of the latter. Thus, a "touch" of the hypertension gene may in itself be insufficient to elevate blood pressure. However, in the presence of hyperinsulinemia (which is a compensatory response to the insulin resistance), the expression of the hypertension gene can be amplified, and the phenotypic result is essential hypertension. The same scenario can be postulated for diabetes, hyperlipidemia, and atherosclerosis. This pathogenetic sequence may help explain the common clustering of diabetes, obesity, hypertension, elevated VLDL, decreased HDL, and atherosclerosis in the same individual.

Clinical Implications of Insulin Resistance

Diabeles and hypertension are common clinical disorders that affect about 10 and about 40 percent of the elderly population, respectively. The treatment of both of these disorders involves the choice of medications that have the potential to adversely affect the body's sensitivity to insulin. Exercise and weight loss represent the cornerstones of diabetic management for NIDDM patients. However, these therapeutic interventions are often insufficient to restore normoglycemia, and pharmacological approaches are required. In the United States, sulfonylureas represent the only class of oral agents available for the treatment of NIDDM. Acutely, these drugs improve glucose tolerance by enhancing insulin secretion. Fortunately, their beneficial long-term effects are related to an improvement in insulin sensitivity, and the initially elevated plasma levels usually, but not always, return to pretreatment values. If insulin resistance with its compensatory hyperinsulinemia plays a role in the development of atherosclerosis, hypertension, and abnormal serum lipid profile, it makes sense to develop antidiabetic drugs whose primary mechanism of action is to improve the body's sensitivity to insulin. We also must be concerned about the use of insulin to treat the patient with NIDDM. There are many data to support the concept that hyperglycemia and poor metabolic control play an important role in the development of the chronic microvascular complications (neuropathy, nephropathy, retinopathy) of diabetes mellitus. Therefore, the American Diabetes Association has advocated that physicians strive for the best possible glycemic control without untoward side effects from hypoglycemia. On the other hand, evidence reviewed in the preceding sections of this text suggest that hyperinsulinemia may be deleterious to various organ systems and may lead to macrovascular disease. To place this controversy in perspective, some quantitative considerations are helpful. The normal ß-cell secretes about 30 U insulin/day. To normalize the plasma glucose profile in NIDDM patients, especially if they are obese, more than 100 U insulin/day is required. Thus, the physician is faced with a dilemma. Does he/she aggressively treat the abnormal plasma glucose profile with the aim of achieving normoglycemia if this can only be achieved at the expense of marked hyperinsulinemia? This is a difficult issue to resolve, because the relationship between glycemic control and microvascular complications is difficult to quantitate, whereas the relationship between insulin and macrovascular disease is even more elusive. Obviously, the best approach would be to use drugs that improve glucose tolerance by enhancing tissue sensitivity to insulin, thereby lowering the plasma insulin concentration. Unfortunately, such drugs are not yet available in the U.S.

Treatment of hypertension has been shown to effectively reduce the incidence of stroke, congestive heart failure, kidney insufficiency, and accelerated/malignant hypertension but not the incidence of CAD. It has become apparent that several categories of drugs that have gained widespread use in the treatment of hypertension are associated with worsening glucose tolerance and a more atherogenic plasma lipid profile. In particular, both diuretics and ß-adrenergic antagonists have been shown to cause insulin resistance and worsening glucose tolerance despite an increase in circulating insulin levels. When diuretics and ß-blockers are used in combination, the deleterious effects on insulin resistance, glucose metabolism, and plasma lipid profile are even more pronounced. Of particular concern is the recent observation that the insulin resistance and glucose intolerance persists for many months after discontinuation of diuretics and ß-blocking agents. Because insulin resistance, hyperinsulinemia, impaired glucose tolerance, and hyperlipidemia are all components of the insulin-resistance syndrome, we must be concerned about the atherogenic potential of these antihypertensive drugs, particularly in diabetic patients. Given the choice, it would seem preferable to select antihypertensive medications that are metabolically inert. The closest approximation to such an ideal drug are the Ca^{2+}-channel blockers and the converting enzyme inhibitors. Neither have any known adverse effects on glucose or lipid metabolism, and there is even the suggestion that the converting enzyme inhibitors may enhance insulin sensitivity and improve glucose tolerance.

Summary

Insulin resistance with respect to glucose utilization no longer can be considered an uncommon metabolic disorder. In addition to NIDDM and obesity, insulin resistance has been shown to be a characteristic feature of the normal aging process and essential hypertension. Moreover, within the normal healthy adult population, there is a wide (3- to 4-fold) spectrum of insulin sensitivity. In fact, a small but significant percentage of the normal population is as resistant as individuals with diabetes mellitus or obesity. Nonetheless, glucose tolerance remains unaltered in such individuals, because the pancreatic ß-cells are capable of augmenting their secretion of insulin to precisely offset the insulin action. However, much evidence has begun to accumulate that chronic day-long hyperinsulinemia is associated with the development of hypertension, hyperlipidemia, and atherosclerosis. In a sense, insulin resistance can be viewed as a large iceberg submerged just below the surface of the water. The physician recognizes only the tips of the iceberg—diabetes, obesity, hypertension, hypertriglyceridemia, diminished HDL-chol, and atherosclerosis—which extrude above the surface, and the complete insulin-resistance syndrome may be missed. With the recognition that insulin resistance consists of a cluster of disorders and biochemical abnormalities, it is important for the various subspecialties (diabetes, metabolism, lipidology, hypertension, cardiology) to interact more closely and to focus their attention on defining the mechanism(s) responsible for the defect in insulin-mediated glucose metabolism. Such an understanding may lead to the development of a new class of drugs, "insulin sensitizers." By lowering the elevated plasma insulin concentration, such agents may provide a wide spectrum of beneficial metabolic effects, which not only improve glucose utilization but normalize the plasma lipid profile and decrease the risk for CAD.

Acknowledgements

We thank Rhonda Wolfe and Stella Merla for expert help in preparation of the manuscript.

References

[The original copy of this text contains a list of more than 300 technical references. To consult this list, please refer to: DeFronzo, Ralph A. and Eleuterio Ferrannini. "Insulin Resistance: A Multifaceted

Syndrome Responsible for NIDDM, Obesity, Hypertension, Dyslipidemia, and Atherosclerotic Cardiovascular Disease," *Diabetes Care*, Vo. 14. No. 3, March 1991.]

Chapter 12

Hypoglycemia

What Is Hypoglycemia?

Glucose, a form of sugar, is the body's main fuel. Hypoglycemia, or low blood sugar, occurs when blood levels of glucose drop too low to fuel the body's activity.

Carbohydrates (sugars and starches) are the body's main dietary sources of glucose. During digestion, the glucose is absorbed into the blood stream (hence the term "blood sugar"), which carries it to every cell in the body. Unused glucose is stored in the liver as glycogen.

Hypoglycemia can occur as a complication of diabetes, as a condition in itself, or in association with other disorders.

How Does the Body Control Glucose?

The amount of glucose in the blood is controlled mainly by the hormones insulin and glucagon. Too much or too little of these hormones can cause blood sugar levels to fall too low (hypoglycemia) or rise too high (hyperglycemia). Other hormones that influence blood sugar levels are cortisol, growth hormone, and catecholamines (epinephrine and norepinephrine).

The pancreas, a gland in the upper abdomen, produces insulin and glucagon. The pancreas is dotted with hormone-producing tissue called the islets of Langerhans, which contain alpha and beta cells.

National Institute of Diabetes and Digestive and Kidney Diseases, NIH Pub No. 95–3926, May 1995.

143

When blood sugar rises after a meal, the beta cells release insulin. The insulin helps glucose enter body cells, lowering blood levels of glucose to the normal range. When blood sugar drops too low, the alpha cells secrete glucagon. This signals the liver to release stored glycogen and change it back to glucose, raising blood sugar levels to the normal range. Muscles also store glycogen that can be converted to glucose.

Blood Sugar Range. The normal range for blood sugar is about 60 mg/dl (milligrams of glucose per deciliter of blood) to 120 mg/dl, depending on when a person last ate. In the fasting state, blood sugar can occasionally fall below 60 mg/dl and even to below 50 mg/dl and not indicate a serious abnormality or disease. This can be seen in healthy women, particularly after prolonged fasting. Blood sugar levels below 45 mg/dl are almost always associated with a serious abnormality.

What Are the Symptoms of Hypoglycemia?

A person with hypoglycemia may feel weak, drowsy, confused, hungry, and dizzy. Paleness, headache, irritability, trembling, sweating, rapid heart beat, and a cold, clammy feeling are also signs of low blood sugar. In severe cases, a person can lose consciousness and even lapse into a coma.

The symptoms associated with hypoglycemia are sometimes mistaken for symptoms caused by conditions not related to blood sugar. For example, unusual stress and anxiety can cause excess production of catecholamines, resulting in symptoms similar to those caused by hypoglycemia but having no relation to blood sugar levels.

Hypoglycemia in Diabetes

The most common cause of hypoglycemia is as a complication of diabetes. Diabetes occurs when the body cannot use glucose for fuel because either the pancreas is not able to make enough insulin or the insulin that is available is not effective. As a result, glucose builds up in the blood instead of getting into body cells.

The aim of treatment in diabetes is to lower high blood sugar levels. To do this, people with diabetes may use insulin or oral drugs, depending on the type of diabetes they have or the severity of their condition. Hypoglycemia occurs most often in people who use insulin to lower their blood sugar. All people with insulin-dependent diabetes

(IDDM or Type I) and some people with noninsulin-dependent diabetes (NIDDM or Type II) use insulin. People with Type II diabetes who take oral drugs called sulfonylureas are also vulnerable to low blood sugar episodes.

Conditions that can lead to hypoglycemia in people with diabetes include taking too much medication, missing or delaying a meal, eating too little food for the amount of insulin taken, exercising too strenuously, drinking too much alcohol, or any combination of these factors. People who have diabetes often refer to hypoglycemia as an "insulin reaction."

Managing Hypoglycemia in Diabetes

People with diabetes should consult their health care providers for individual guidelines on target blood sugar ranges that are best for them. The lowest safe blood sugar level for an individual varies, depending on the person's age, medical condition, and ability to sense hypoglycemic symptoms. A target range that is safe for a young adult with no diabetes complications, for example, may be too low for a young child or an older person who may have other medical problems.

Because they are attuned to the symptoms, people with diabetes can usually recognize when their blood sugar levels are dropping too low. They can treat the condition quickly by eating or drinking something with sugar in it such as candy, juice, or non-diet soda. Taking glucose tablets or gels (available in drug stores) is another convenient and quick way to treat hypoglycemia.

People with IDDM are most vulnerable to severe insulin reactions, which can cause loss of consciousness. A few patients with long-standing insulin-dependent diabetes may develop a condition known as hypoglycemia unawareness, in which they have difficulty recognizing the symptoms of low blood sugar. For emergency use in patients with IDDM, physicians often prescribe an injectable form of the hormone glucagon. A glucagon injection (given by another person) quickly eases the symptoms of low blood sugar, releasing a burst of glucose into the blood.

Emergency medical help may be needed if the person does not recover in a few minutes after treatment for hypoglycemia. A person suffering a severe insulin reaction may be admitted to the hospital so that blood sugar can be stabilized.

People with diabetes can reduce or prevent episodes of hypoglycemia by monitoring their blood sugar levels frequently and learning to recognize the symptoms of low blood sugar and the situations that may trigger it. They should consult their health care providers for advice about the best way to treat low blood sugar. Friends and relatives should know about the symptoms of hypoglycemia and how to treat it in case of emergency.

Episodes of hypoglycemia in people with IDDM may become more common now that research has shown that carefully controlled blood sugar helps prevent the complications of diabetes. Keeping blood sugar in a close-to-normal range requires multiple injections of insulin each day or use of an insulin pump, frequent testing of blood glucose, a diet and exercise plan, and guidance from health care professionals.

Other Causes of Hypoglycemia

Hypoglycemia in people who do not have diabetes is far less common than once believed. However, it can occur in some people under certain conditions such as early pregnancy, prolonged fasting, and long periods of strenuous exercise. People on beta blocker medications who exercise are at higher risk of hypoglycemia, and aspirin can induce hypoglycemia in some children. Drinking alcohol can cause blood sugar to drop in some sensitive individuals, and hypoglycemia has been well documented in chronic alcoholics and binge drinkers. Eating unripe ackee fruit from Jamaica is a rare cause of low blood sugar.

Diagnosis

To diagnose hypoglycemia in people who do not have diabetes, the doctor looks for the following three conditions:

- The patient complains of symptoms of hypoglycemia

- Blood glucose levels are measured while the person is experiencing those symptoms and found to be 45 mg/dl or less in a woman or 55 mg/dl or less in a man

- The symptoms are promptly relieved upon ingestion of sugar.

For many years, the oral glucose tolerance test (OGTT) was used to diagnose hypoglycemia. Experts now realize that the OGTT can actually trigger hypoglycemic symptoms in people with no signs of the disorder. For a more accurate diagnosis, experts now recommend that blood sugar be tested at the same time a person is experiencing hypoglycemic symptoms.

The doctor will also check the patient for health conditions such as diabetes, obtain a medication history, and assess the degree and severity of the patient's symptoms. Laboratory tests to measure insulin production and levels of C-peptide (a substance that the pancreas releases into the bloodstream in equal amounts to insulin) may be performed.

Reactive Hypoglycemia

A diagnosis of reactive hypoglycemia is considered only after other possible causes of low blood sugar have been ruled out. Reactive hypoglycemia with no known cause is a condition in which the symptoms of low blood sugar appear 2 to 5 hours after eating foods high in glucose.

Ten to 20 years ago, hypoglycemia was a popular diagnosis. However, studies now show that this condition is actually quite rare. In these studies, most patients who experienced the symptoms of hypoglycemia after eating glucose-rich foods consistently had normal levels of blood sugar—above 60 mg/dl. Some researchers have suggested that some people may be extra sensitive to the body's normal release of the hormone epinephrine after a meal.

People with symptoms of reactive hypoglycemia unrelated to other medical conditions or problems are usually advised to follow a healthy eating plan. The doctor or dietitian may suggest that such a person avoid foods high in carbohydrates; eat small, frequent meals and snacks throughout the day; exercise regularly; and eat a variety of foods, including whole grains, vegetables, and fruits.

Rare Causes of Hypoglycemia

Fasting hypoglycemia occurs when the stomach is empty. It usually develops in the early morning when a person awakens. As with other forms of hypoglycemia, the symptoms include headache, lack of energy, and an inability to concentrate. Fasting hypoglycemia may be caused by a variety of conditions such as hereditary enzyme or hormone deficiencies, liver disease, and insulin-producing tumors.

In hereditary fructose intolerance, a disorder usually seen in children, the body is unable to metabolize the natural sugar fructose. Attacks of hypoglycemia, marked by seizures, vomiting, and unconsciousness, are treated by giving glucose and eliminating fructose from the diet.

Galactosemia, a rare genetic disorder, hampers the body's ability to process the sugar galactose. An infant with this disorder may appear normal at birth, but after a few days or weeks of drinking milk (which contains galactose), the child may begin to vomit, lose weight, and develop cataracts. The liver may fail to release stored glycogen into the blood, triggering hypoglycemia. Removing milk from the diet is the usual treatment.

A deficiency of growth hormone causes increased sensitivity to insulin. This sensitivity occurs because growth hormone opposes the action of insulin on muscle and fat cells. For this reason, children with growth hormone deficiency sometimes suffer from hypoglycemia, which goes away after treatment.

People with insulin-producing tumors, which arise in the islet cells of the pancreas, suffer from severe episodes of hypoglycemia.

To diagnose these tumors, called insulinomas, a doctor will put the patient on a 24- to 72-hour fast while measuring blood levels of glucose, insulin, and proinsulin. High levels of insulin and proinsulin in the presence of low levels of glucose strongly suggest an insulin-producing tumor. These tumors are usually benign and can be surgically removed.

In rare cases, some cancers such as breast cancer and adrenal cancer may cause hypoglycemia through secretion of a hormone called insulin-like growth factor II. The treatment is removal of the tumor, if possible.

Research

The National Institute of Diabetes and Digestive and Kidney Diseases (NIDDK) was established by Congress in 1950 as one of the National Institutes of Health, the research arm of the Public Health Service under the U.S. Department of Health and Human Services.

The NIDDK conducts and supports research in diabetes, glucose metabolism, insulin action, and the hormonal controls of blood sugar. Current studies also focus on fasting hypoglycemia, obesity, and insulin resistance.

Resources on Hypoglycemia

American Diabetes Association (ADA)
National Service Center
1660 Duke Street
Alexandria, VA 22314
(800) 232-3472 or (703) 549-1500

The ADA is a private, voluntary organization that fosters public awareness of diabetes and supports and promotes diabetes research and education. The ADA distributes printed information on many aspects of diabetes, and local affiliates sponsor community programs. Local affiliates, located in every state, are listed in telephone directories or can be located by contacting the national office.

The American Dietetic Association
National Center for Nutrition and Dietetics
216 West Jackson Boulevard
Chicago, IL 60606-6995
(800) 366-1655 or (312) 899-0040

The American Dietetic Association is a professional organization for registered dietitians. It publishes a variety of materials for patient and professional education and supports an information and referral service for the general public.

Juvenile Diabetes Foundation International
120 Wall Street
New York, NY 10005-4001
(212) 785-950; (800) JDF-CURE
(212) 785-9595 Fax

The JDF is a private, voluntary organization that promotes research and public education in diabetes, primarily insulin-dependent diabetes. Local chapters, located across the country, are listed in telephone directories or can be found by contacting the national office.

National Diabetes Information Clearinghouse (NDIC)
One Information Way
Bethesda, MD 20892-3560

The NDIC is a service of NIDDK. The clearinghouse distributes a variety of diabetes-related materials to the public and to health professionals, including a literature search listing publications and articles about hypoglycemia in diabetes.

Additional Readings

Bennion, Lynn J., "Hypoglycemia: A diagnostic challenge," *Clinical Diabetes*, July/August 1985, pp. 85–90.

DCCT Research Group, "Epidemiology of Severe Hypoglycemia in the Diabetes Control and Complications Trial," *The American Journal of Medicine,* vol. 90, April 1991, pp. 450–459.

Field, James B., "Hypoglycemia: Definition, clinical presentations, classifications and laboratory tests," in *Endocrinology and Metabolism Clinics of North America*, vol. 18, no. 1, March 1989.

Foster, Daniel & Rubenstein, Arthur, "Hypoglycemia, insulinoma, and other hormone-secreting tumors of the pancreas" in *Principles of Internal Medicine*. Ed. E. Braunwald et al [K. J. Isselbacher, R. G. Petersdorf, J. D. Wilson, J. B. Martin, & A. S. Fauci] McGraw-Hill Book Company, 1987, pp. 1800–1807.

Metz, Robert J., "Is the problem hypoglycemia?," *Patient Care*, Oct. 15, 1983, pp. 61–89.

Nelson, Roger L., "Oral glucose tolerance test: Indications and limitations," *Mayo Clinic Proceedings,* vol. 63, 1988, pp. 263–269.

Palardy, Jean et al., "Blood glucose measurements during symptomatic episodes in patients with suspected postprandial hypoglycemia," *New England Journal of Medicine*, Nov. 23, 1989, pp. 1421–1425.

Service, F. John, "Hypoglycemic Disorders," *New England Journal of Medicine*, April 27, 1995, pp. 1144–1152.

Service, F. John, "Hypoglycemia," in *Cecil's Textbook of Medicine*. James B. Wyngaarden & Lloyd H. Smith, Jr. (Eds). W. B. Saunders Company, 1988, pp. 1381–1387.

Service, F. John, "Hypoglycemia and the postprandial syndrome," *New England Journal of Medicine*, (Editorial), Nov. 23, 1989, pp. 1472–1474.

National Diabetes Information Clearinghouse

One Information Way
Bethesda, MD 20892-3560

The National Diabetes Information Clearinghouse is a service of the National Institute of Diabetes and Digestive and Kidney Diseases, part of the National Institutes of Health, under the U.S. Public Health Service. The clearinghouse, established in 1978, is designed to increase knowledge and understanding about diabetes among patients and their families, health care professionals, and the public. The clearinghouse answers inquiries; develops, reviews, and distributes publications; and works closely with professional and patient organizations and government agencies to coordinate resources about diabetes.

Publications produced by the clearinghouse are reviewed carefully for scientific accuracy, content, and readability. Materials produced by other sources are also reviewed for scientific accuracy and are used, along with clearinghouse publications, to answer requests.

Chapter 13

Nutritional Recommendations for People with Diabetic Disorders

Nutrition Recommendations and Principles for People with Diabetes Mellitus

Medical nutrition therapy is integral to total diabetes care and management. Although adherence to nutrition and meal planning principles is one of the most challenging aspects of diabetes care, nutrition therapy is an essential component of successful diabetes management.

Achieving nutrition-related goals requires a coordinated team effort that includes the person with diabetes. Because of the complexity of nutrition issues, it is recommended that a registered dietitian, knowledgeable and skilled in implementing current principles and recommendations for diabetes, be a member of the treatment team.

Effective self-management training requires an individualized approach, appropriate for the personal lifestyle and diabetes management goals of the individual with diabetes. Monitoring of glucose and glycated hemoglobin, lipids, blood pressure, and renal status is essential to

This chapter includes "Position Statement: Nutrition Recommendations and Principles for People with Diabetes Mellitus," reprinted with permission from *Diabetes Care*, Volume 17:519-522, 1994, Copyright © 1994 by American Diabetes Association, Inc.; and selected excerpts from: *Diet and Nutrition: Guides, Manuals, Fact Sheets, and Cookbooks for People with Diabetes*, National Diabetes Information Clearinghouse, 1 Information Way, Bethesda, MD 20892-5360; (301) 654-3327. March 1996. Because the American Diabetes Association updated nutritional recommendations in 1994, citations for documents dated before that year have been deleted.

evaluate nutrition-related outcomes. If goals are not met, changes must be made in the overall diabetes care and management plan.

Nutrition assessment is used to determine what the individual with diabetes is able and willing to do. A major consideration is the likelihood of adherence to nutrition recommendations. To facilitate adherence, sensitivity to cultural, ethnic, and financial considerations is of prime importance.

This text reflects scientific nutrition and diabetes knowledge as of 1994. However, there are limited published data for some recommendations and, under these circumstances, recommendations are based on clinical experiences and consensus. This position paper is based on the concurrent technical review paper, which discusses published research and issues that remain unresolved (1).

Goals of Medical Nutrition Therapy

Although the overall goal of nutrition therapy is to assist people with diabetes in making changes in nutrition and exercise habits leading to improved metabolic control, there are additional specific goals:

1. Maintenance of as near-normal blood glucose levels as possible by balancing food intake with insulin (either endogenous or exogenous) or oral glucose-lowering medications and activity levels.

2. Achievement of optimal serum lipid levels.

3. Provision of adequate calories for maintaining or attaining reasonable weights for adults, normal growth and development rates in children and adolescents, increased metabolic needs during pregnancy and lactation, or recovery from catabolic illnesses. Reasonable weight is defined as the weight an individual and health care provider acknowledge as achievable and maintainable, both short- and long-term. This may not be the same as the traditionally defined desirable or ideal body weight.

4. Prevention and treatment of the acute complications of insulin-treated diabetes such as hypoglycemia, short-term illnesses, and exercise-related problems, and of the long-term complications of diabetes such as renal disease, autonomic neuropathy, hypertension, and cardiovascular disease.

5. Improvement of overall health through optimal nutrition. *Dietary Guidelines for Americans* (2) and the *Food Guide*

154

Pyramid (3) summarize and illustrate nutritional guidelines and nutrient needs for all healthy Americans, and can be used by people with diabetes and their family members.

Nutrition Therapy and Type I Diabetes

A meal plan based on the individual's usual food intake should be determined and used as a basis for integrating insulin therapy into the usual eating and exercise patterns. It is recommended that individuals using insulin therapy eat at consistent times synchronized with the time-action of the insulin preparation used. Further, individuals need to monitor blood glucose levels and adjust insulin doses for the amount of food usually eaten. Intensified insulin therapy, such as multiple daily injections or use of an insulin pump, allows considerable flexibility in when and what individuals eat. With intensified therapy, insulin regimens should be integrated with lifestyle and adjusted for deviations from usual eating and exercise habits.

Nutrition Therapy and Type II Diabetes

The emphasis for medical nutrition therapy in type II diabetes should be placed on achieving glucose, lipid, and blood pressure goals. Weight loss and hypocaloric diets usually improve short-term glycemic levels and have the potential to increase long-term metabolic control. However, traditional dietary strategies, and even very-low-calorie diets, have usually not been effective in achieving long-term weight loss; therefore, emphasis should be placed instead on glucose and lipid goals. Although weight loss is desirable, and some individuals are able to lose and maintain weight loss, several additional strategies can be implemented to improve metabolic control. There is no one proven strategy or method that can be uniformly recommended.

An initial strategy is improvement in food choices, as illustrated by *Dietary Guidelines for Americans* and the *Food Guide Pyramid*. A nutritionally adequate meal plan with a reduction of total fat, especially saturated fats, can be employed. Spacing meals (spreading nutrient intake throughout the day) is another strategy that can be adopted. Mild to moderate weight loss (5-10 kg [10-20 pounds]) has been shown to improve diabetes control, even if desirable body weight is not achieved. Weight loss is best attempted by a moderate decrease in calories and an increase in caloric expenditure. Moderate caloric restriction (250-500 calories less than average daily intake) is recommended.

Regular exercise and learning new behaviors and attitudes can help facilitate long-term lifestyle changes. Monitoring blood glucose levels, glycated hemoglobin, lipids, and blood pressure is essential. However, if metabolic control has not improved after employment of better nutrition and regular exercise, an oral glucose-lowering medication or insulin may be needed.

Many individuals with refractory obesity may have limited success with the above strategies. Newer pharmacological agents, i.e., the serotonergic appetite suppressants, as well as gastric reduction surgery (for people with a body mass index >35 kg/m²), may prove to be potentially beneficial to this group. Studies on the long-term efficacy and safety of these methods are, however, unavailable.

Protein

There is limited scientific data upon which to establish firm nutritional recommendations for protein intake for individuals with diabetes. At the present time, there is insufficient evidence to support protein intakes either higher or lower than average protein intake for the general population. For people with diabetes, this translates into about 10-20% of the daily caloric intake from protein. Dietary protein should be derived from both animal and vegetable sources.

With the onset of nephropathy, lower intakes of protein should be considered. A protein intake similar to the adult Recommended Dietary Allowance (0.8 g-kg body wt⁻¹ day⁻¹), about 10% of daily calories, is sufficiently restrictive and is recommended for individuals with evidence of nephropathy.

Total Fat

If dietary protein contributes 10-20% of the total caloric content of the diet, then 80-90% of calories remain to be distributed between dietary fat and carbohydrate. Less than 10% of these calories should be from saturated fats and up to 10% calories from polyunsaturated fats, leaving 60-70% of the total calories from monounsaturated fats and carbohydrates. The distribution of calories from fat and carbohydrate can vary and be individualized based on the nutrition assessment and treatment goals.

The recommended percentage of calories from fat is dependent on desired glucose, lipid, and weight outcomes. For individuals who have normal lipid levels and maintain a reasonable weight (and for normal growth and development in children and adolescents) the *Dietary*

Guidelines for Americans recommendations of 30% or less of the calories from total fat and less than 10% of calories from saturated fat can be implemented.

If obesity and weight loss are the primary issues, a reduction in dietary fat intake is an efficient way to reduce caloric intake and weight, particularly when combined with exercise.

If elevated low-density lipoprotein (LDL) cholesterol is the primary problem, the National Cholesterol Education Program Step II diet guidelines, in which less than 7% of total calories are from saturated fat, up to 30% of the calories are from total fat, and dietary cholesterol is less than 200 mg/day, should be implemented.

If elevated triglycerides and very low density lipoprotein cholesterol are the primary problems, one approach that may be beneficial, other than weight loss and increased physical activity, is a moderate increase in monounsaturated fat intake, with less than 10% of calories each from saturated and polyunsaturated fats, monounsaturated fats up to 20% of calories, and a more moderate intake of carbohydrate. However, in obese individuals the increase in fat intake may perpetuate or aggravate the obesity. In addition, patients with triglyceride levels more than 1,000 mg/dl may require reduction of all types of dietary fat to reduce levels of plasma dietary fat in the form of chylomicrons.

Monitoring glycemic and lipid status and body weight, on any diet, is essential to assess the effectiveness of the nutrition recommendations.

Saturated Fat and Cholesterol

A reduction in saturated fat and cholesterol consumption is an important goal to reduce the risk of cardiovascular disease (CVD). Diabetes is a strong independent risk factor for CVD, over and above the adverse effects of an elevated serum cholesterol. Therefore, less than 10% of the daily calories should be from saturated fats, and dietary cholesterol should be limited to 300 mg or less daily. However, even these recommendation must be incorporated with consideration of an individual's cultural and ethnic background.

Polyunsaturated fats of the omega-3 series are provided naturally in fish and other seafood, and the intake of these foods need not be curtailed in people with diabetes mellitus.

Carbohydrate and Sweeteners

The percentage of calories from carbohydrate will also vary, and is individualized based on the patient's eating habits and glucose and lipid goals. For most of this century, the most widely held belief about the dietary treatment of diabetes has been that "simple" sugars should be avoided and replaced with complex carbohydrates. This belief appears to be based on the assumption that sugars are more rapidly digested and absorbed than are starches and thereby aggravate hyperglycemia to a greater degree. There is, however, very little scientific evidence that supports this assumption. Fruits and milk have been shown to have a lower glycemic response than most starches, and sucrose produces a glycemic response similar to that of bread, rice, and potatoes. Although various starches do have different glycemic responses, from a clinical perspective first priority should be given to the total amount of carbohydrate consumed rather than the source of the carbohydrate.

Sucrose

Scientific evidence has shown that the use of sucrose as part of the meal plan does not impair blood glucose control in individuals with type I or type II diabetes. Sucrose and sucrose-containing foods must be substituted for other carbohydrates and foods and not simply added to the meal plan. In making such substitutions, the nutrient content of concentrated sweets and sucrose-containing foods, as well as the presence of other nutrients frequently ingested with sucrose such as fat, must be considered.

Fructose

Dietary fructose produces a smaller rise in plasma glucose than isocaloric amounts of sucrose and most starchy carbohydrates. In that regard, fructose may offer an advantage as a sweetening agent in the diabetic diet. However, because of potential adverse effects of large amounts of fructose (i.e., double the usual intake [20% of calories]) on serum cholesterol and LDL cholesterol, fructose may have no overall advantage as a sweetening agent in the diabetic diet. Although people with dyslipidemia should avoid consuming large amounts of fructose, there is no reason to recommend that people avoid consumption of fruits and vegetables, in which fructose occurs naturally, or moderate consumption of fructose-sweetened foods.

Other Nutritive Sweeteners

Nutritive sweeteners other than sucrose and fructose include corn sweeteners such as corn syrup, fruit juice or fruit juice concentrate, honey, molasses, dextrose, and maltose. There is no evidence that these sweeteners have any significant advantage or disadvantage over sucrose in terms of improvement in caloric content or glycemic response.

Sorbitol, mannitol, and xylitol are common sugar alcohols (polyols) that produce a lower glycemic response than sucrose and other carbohydrates. Starch hydrolysates are formed by the partial hydrolysis and hydrogenation of edible starches, thus becoming polyols. The exact caloric value of the polyols is difficult to determine. There appear to be no significant advantages of the polyols over other nutritive sweeteners. Excessive amounts of polyols may, however, have a laxative effect.

Nonnutritive Sweeteners

Saccharin, aspartame, and acesulfame K are approved for use by the Food and Drug Administration (FDA) in the United States. The FDA also determines an acceptable daily intake for approved food additives, including nonnutritive sweeteners. Nonnutritive sweeteners approved by the FDA are safe to consume by all people with diabetes.

Fiber

Dietary fiber may be beneficial in treating or preventing several gastrointestinal disorders, including colon cancer, and large amounts of soluble fiber have a beneficial effect on serum lipids. There is no reason to believe that people with diabetes would be more or less amenable to these effects that those without diabetes. Although selected soluble fibers are capable of delaying glucose absorption from the small intestine, the effect of dietary fiber on glycemic control is probably insignificant. Therefore, fiber intake recommendations for people with diabetes are the same as for the general population. Daily consumption of a diet containing 20-35 g dietary fiber from a wide variety of food sources is recommended.

Sodium

People differ greatly in the sensitivity to sodium and its effect of blood pressure. Because it is impractical to asses individual sodium sensitivity, intake recommendations for people with diabetes are the same as for the general population. Some health authorities recommend no more than 3,000 mg/day of sodium for the general population, while other authorities recommend no more than 2,400 mg/day.

For people with mild to moderate hypertension, 2,400 mg or less per day of sodium is recommended.

Alcohol

The same precautions regarding the use of alcohol that apply to the general public also apply to people with diabetes. Under normal circumstances, however, blood glucose levels will not be affected by moderate use of alcohol when diabetes is well controlled. For people using insulin, up to 2 alcoholic beverages (1 alcoholic beverage = 12 oz beer, 5 oz wine, or 1 1/2 oz distilled spirits) can be ingested with and in addition to the usual meal plan.

Special considerations for further modification of alcohol intake include the following. Abstention from alcohol should be advised for people with a history of alcohol abuse or during pregnancy. Alcohol may increase the risk for hypoglycemia in people treated with insulin or sulfonylureas. If alcohol is consumed by such people, it should only be ingested with a meal. Reduction of or abstention from alcohol intake may be advisable for people with diabetes with other medical problems such as pancreatitis, dyslipidemia, or neuropathy. When calories from alcohol need to be calculated as part of the total caloric intake, alcohol is best substituted for fat exchanges or fat calories (1 alcoholic beverage = 2 fat exchanges).

Micronutrients: Vitamins and Minerals

When dietary intake is adequate, there is generally no need for additional vitamin and mineral supplementation for the majority of people with diabetes. Although there are theoretical reasons to supplement with antioxidants, there is little confirmatory evidence at present that such therapy has any benefits.

The only known circumstance in which chromium replacement has any beneficial effect on glycemic control is for people who are chromium deficient as a result of long-term chromium-deficient parenteral nutrition. However, it appears that most people with diabetes are not chromium deficient and, therefore, chromium supplementation has no known benefit.

Similarly, although magnesium deficiency may play a role in insulin resistance, carbohydrate intolerance, and hypertension, the available data suggest that routine evaluation of serum magnesium levels is recommended only in patients at high risk for magnesium deficiency. Levels of magnesium should be repleted only if hypomagnesium can be demonstrated.

Potassium loss may be sufficient to warrant dietary supplementation in patients taking diuretics. Hyperkalemia sufficient to warrant dietary potassium restriction may occur in patients with renal insufficiency or hyporeninemic hypoaldosteronism or in patients taking angiotensin-converting enzyme inhibitors.

Pregnancy

Nutrition recommendations for women with preexisting and gestational diabetes mellitus should be based on a nutrition assessment. Monitoring blood glucose levels, urine ketones, appetite, and weight gain can be a guide to developing and evaluating an appropriate individualized meal plan and to making adjustments to the meal plan throughout pregnancy to ensure desired outcomes.

Summary

A historical perspective of nutrition recommendations is provided in Table 13.1. Today there is no ONE "diabetic" or "ADA" diet. The recommended diet can only be defined as a dietary prescription based on nutrition assessment and treatment goals.

Table 13.1. Historical perspective of nutrition recommendations

	Distribution of Calories		
Year	%Carbohydrate	%Protein	%Fat
Before 1921		Starvation diets	
1921	20	10	70
1950	40	20	40
1971	45	20	35
1986	up to 60	12-20	<30
1994	*	10-20	*.+

*Based on nutritional assessment and treatment goals.
+less than 10% of calories from saturated fats.

Medical nutrition therapy for people with diabetes should be individualized, with consideration given to usual eating habits and other lifestyle factors. Nutrition recommendations are then developed to meet treatment goals and desired outcomes. Monitoring metabolic parameters including blood glucose, glycated hemoglobin, lipids, blood pressure, and body weight, as well as quality of life, is crucial to ensure successful outcomes.

References

1. Franz MJ, Horton ES, Bantle JP, Beebe CA, Brunzell JD, Coulston AM, Henry RR, Hoogwerf BJ, Stacpoole PW: Nutrition principles for the management of diabetes and related complications (Technical review). *Diabetes Care* 17:490-518. 1994

2. U.S. Department of Agriculture, U.S. Department of Health and Human Services: *Nutrition and Your Health: Dietary Guide lines for Americans.* 3rd Ed, Hyattsville, MD. USDA's Human Nutrition Information Service. 1990

3. U.S Department of Agriculture: *The Food Guide Pyramid.* Hyattsville, MD. USDA's Human Nutrition Information Service. 1992

Guides, Manuals, Fact Sheets, and Cookbooks for People with Diabetes

This literature search is from the Diabetes subfile of the Combined Health Information Database (CHID). Each citation contains information about the author, title, and source of the item, as well as a summary of its contents. Depending on the type of material, the citation also may include information about a corporate author, where to obtain the item, and its price. Formats of audiovisuals are provided.

The following codes are used in a literature search:

TI Title
AU Author
CN Corporate Author
SO Source
PD Physical Description
AV Producer/Availability
AB Abstract

With the exception of journal articles, sources for items listed are given after the code AV (Producer/Availability). Please contact the producer listed after the AV code for a copy of the item.

Copies of journal articles are available at most public and medical libraries using the information provided after the SO (Source) code.

CHID is available online through Ovid Online. If you would like references to materials on other topics, you may request a special literature search of CHID from a library that subscribes to Ovid Online, or from the National Diabetes Information Clearinghouse, 1 Information Way, Bethesda, MD 20892-3560; telephone: (301) 654-3327; fax: (301) 907-8906; e-mail: ndic@aerie.com

TI 1200-Calorie Meal Plan.
SO Indianapolis, IN: Eli Lilly and Company. 1995. 5 p.
CN Eli Lilly and Company.
AV Available from Eli Lilly and Company. Lilly Corporate Center, Indianapolis, IN 46285. (800) 545-5979 or (317) 276-2000. PRICE: Single copy free.
AB This brochure presents the exchange list for a 1,200-calorie meal plan, designed for people with diabetes. The recommended exchange list values for this level of caloric intake are noted, along with textual material describing how to use exchange lists, two sample menus, and a blank chart for the reader to fill in a personal meal plan. The brochure unfolds to a 11-inch x 22-inch chart that presents the food exchange lists in seven categories: breads and starches, meat and meat substitutes, vegetables, fruits, milk and milk products, fats, and free foods. General nutritional recommendations and meal planning suggestions for people with diabetes are also included.

TI 1500-Calorie Meal Plan.
SO Indianapolis, IN: Eli Lilly and Company. 1995. 5 p.
CN Eli Lilly and Company.
AV Available from Eli Lilly and Company. Lilly Corporate Center, Indianapolis, IN 46285. (800) 545-5979 or (317) 276-2000. PRICE: Single copy free.
AB This brochure presents the exchange list for a 1,500-calorie meal plan, designed for people with diabetes. The recommended exchange list values for this level of caloric intake are noted, along with textual material describing how to use exchange lists, two sample menus, and a blank chart for the

reader to fill in a personal meal plan. The brochure unfolds to a 11-inch x 22-inch chart that presents the food exchange lists in seven categories: breads and starches, meat and meat substitutes, vegetables, fruits, milk and milk products, fats, and free foods. General nutritional recommendations and meal planning suggestions for people with diabetes are also included.

TI 2000-Calorie Meal Plan.
SO Indianapolis, IN: Eli Lilly and Company. 1995. 5 p.
CN Eli Lilly and Company.
AV Available from Eli Lilly and Company. Lilly Corporate Center, Indianapolis, IN 46285. (800) 545-5979 or (317) 276-2000. PRICE: Single copy free.
AB This preplanned menu sheet is designed to help patients with newly-diagnosed diabetes begin learning about diabetes meal planning. The brochure provides two menus for an 2,000-calorie meal plan as well as a detailed introduction to the exchange list system. One side of the brochure (which unfolds to poster size) lists the seven exchange list categories and notes foods and serving sizes for each category. The opposite side lists the menus as well as some brief introductory material about instituting and following a meal plan. The sheet includes a brief section on including fast foods.

TI 366 Low-Fat Brand-Name Recipes in Minutes!
AU Smith, M.J.
SO Minneapolis, MN: Chronimed Publishing, Inc. 1994. 360 p.
AV Available from Chronimed Publishing, Inc. P.O. Box 47945, Minneapolis, MN 55447-9727. (612) 541-0239. PRICE: $12.95 plus $3 for shipping and handling.
AB This cookbook features low-fat, easy-to-prepare recipes that include brand name foods. The recipes are presented in 13 categories: beverages, appetizers, breads, bread machine breads, salads, soups and stews, main dish salads, casseroles, grain-based side dishes, low- or no-meat entrees, entrees, vegetables, and desserts. Each recipe includes nutritional information that follows the same format as the new food labels. The author also includes tips on reducing the fat in brand name foods, recipe preparation times, and food exchange lists for weight loss and diabetes. An index concludes the cookbook.

TI **Balance Your Food Act: A Food Book for Adults With Diabetes.**

SO Atlanta, GA: Pritchett and Hull Associates, Inc. 1995. 12 p.

CN Pritchett and Hull Associates, Inc.

AV Available from Pritchett and Hull Associates, Inc. 3440 Oakcliff Road NE., Suite 110, Atlanta, GA 30340-3079. (800) 241-4925 or (404) 451-0602. Fax (800) 752-0510 or (404) 454-7130. PRICE: $25 per pack of 20. Item Number 224.

AB This booklet helps people with diabetes balance what they eat with how much and when they eat. Focusing on the role of diet therapy as an important facet of diabetes care, the booklet covers food groups and exchange lists; measuring foods for exact amounts; seasonings and free foods; sweets and desserts that can be worked into a healthy diabetes meal plan; the use of artificial sweeteners; foods labeled 'dietetic'; the role of high fiber foods; cholesterol and saturated fats; and eating at restaurants. The booklet concludes with a list of books and exchange list resources for readers wishing to obtain additional information. Simple line drawings and cartoons illustrate the booklet.

TI **Carbohydrate Counting, Adding Flexibility to Your Food Choices.**

AU Barry, B.; Castle, G.

SO Minneapolis, MN: International Diabetes Center. 1994. 15 p.

AV Available from Chronimed Publishing. P.O. Box 47945, Minneapolis, MN 55447-9727. (800) 848-2793. PRICE: $18.50; plus shipping and handling. ISBN: 1885115067.

AB This booklet outlines the use of carbohydrate counting as a meal planning option for people with diabetes. The authors stress that carbohydrate counting is a great way to add variety to food choices and flexibility to the meal plan. Topics include how to count carbohydrates, carbohydrate counting and exchange lists, flexibility and control, protein and fats, the role of sugar, counting carbohydrates within the meal plan, and using food labels. The booklet uses quizzes throughout the text to test readers' comprehension of the material presented. The brochure concludes with a blank form for readers and/or their dietitians to individualize the amount of carbohydrate recommended.

TI **Complete Step-by-Step Diabetic Cookbook.**

AU Chappell, A.C., ed.

SO Birmingham, AL: Oxmoor House, Inc. 1995. 368 p.

AV Available from Oxmoor House, Inc. P.O. Box 2463, Birmingham, AL 35201. (800) 633-4910. PRICE: $17.95 plus $3.95 shipping. ISBN: 0848714318.

AB This cookbook, designed to help people with diabetes or those who cook for them, features recipes and meal planning techniques for everyone who is concerned about healthy eating. The cookbook includes over 300 recipes, including sugar-free, low-fat recipes developed and tested by registered dietitians at the University of Alabama at Birmingham. The cookbook provides diabetes exchange values for each recipe, along with nutrient values for calories, carbohydrate, protein, fat, fiber, sodium, and cholesterol. The introductory material presents guidelines for smart eating, meal planning, meals away from home, using exchange lists, and using nutritional analyses. Recipes are presented for beverages; breads and cereals; eggs and cheese; fish and shellfish; meats; poultry; rice, pasta, and starchy vegetables; vegetables; salads and salad dressings; sauces and toppings; soups; and desserts. Recipe title and subject indexes are included.

TI Coping with Diabetes: The New Food Label.
AU Kurtzweil, P.
SO *FDA Consumer*. 28(9): 20-25. November 1994.
AV Available from Food and Drug Administration. (HFI-40), 5600 Fishers Lane, Rockville, MD 20857.
AB This article, the third in a series of articles telling readers how to use the new food labels to meet specific dietary needs, concentrates on managing diabetes. Labeling benefits include print size and color, helpful for persons with visual impairment; more complete nutrition information, particularly about saturated fat and cholesterol; how labels can be used by people following various meal plans, including exchange lists; weight loss; serving sizes; calorie and other information; and front label information. The article also lists general dietary guidelines for people with diabetes, as recommended by the American Diabetes Association (ADA). One sidebar presents a nutrient claims guide for individual foods, defining such terms as fat, saturated fat, cholesterol, healthy, calories, light, fiber, sugar-free, and no-added-sugar. One figure depicts a food label, with key information noted. Another figure illustrates three diet planning guides for people with diabetes: the Food Guide Pyramid, Exchange Lists, and carbohydrate counting. 2 figures.

TI **Diabetes and Food Shopping.**
SO Washington, DC: Giant Food, Inc. 1994. 7 p.
CN Giant Food, Inc.
AV Available from Giant Food, Inc. Consumer Affairs Department 597, P.O. Box 1804, Washington, DC 20013. PRICE: Single copy free.
AB This consumer information pamphlet, produced by a major food store, provides basic guidelines for food shopping for people with diabetes. The brochure can help readers understand the basics of diabetes; learn about healthful eating, including the use of meal plans and the Food Guide Pyramid; use the Nutrition Facts label on food packages; learn more about weight control and exercise; and locate other resources about diabetes management. Numerous food labels are reproduced to serve as illustrations for the section on interpreting labels. The pamphlet concludes with an annotated list of organizations, books, cookbooks, and magazines through which readers can obtain more information.

TI **Diabetes and Nutrition: Eating for Health.**
SO Timonium, MD: Milner-Fenwick, Inc. 1994.
CN American Association of Diabetes Educators (AADE).
PD 1/2 in VHS videocassette (12 min 30 sec), color.
AV Available from Milner-Fenwick, Inc. 2125 Greenspring Drive, Timonium, MD 21093. Voice (800) 432-8433 or (410) 252-1700; fax (410) 252-6316. PRICE: $175 Item Number DB-22.
AB This videotape teaches healthy food choices and modified eating habits. The program explains the importance of limiting high fat and sugary foods to best maintain healthy weight, blood glucose levels, and the cardiovascular system. Patients also learn how to work with a dietitian to develop a personal meal plan. The video is available in Spanish and with closed captioning.

TI **Diabetes and the Food Pyramid.**
SO Madison, WI: University of Wisconsin Hospital and Clinics. 1994.
CN University of Wisconsin Hospital and Clinics.
PD 1/2 in VHS or 3/4 in broadcast master videocassette (30 min), color.
AV Available from University of Wisconsin Hospital and Clinics, Department of Outreach Education. Picture of Health, 2870 University Avenue, Suite 206, Madison, WI 53705-3611. (800)

757-4354 or (608) 263-6510. Fax (608) 265-5444. PRICE: $14.95 for VHS, $36.95 for broadcast master, plus $5.75 shipping and handling (as of 1995); discounts available for larger quantities. Item Number 121494A.

AB In this patient education videotape, the viewer is introduced to the new nutritional guidelines for people with diabetes, issued by the American Diabetes Association. Narrated by Ann Martin, a registered dietitian, the program highlights the changes in the new guidelines, focusing on how to incorporate those changes into everyday diabetes management. The program also offers suggestions for quick meals on days when one does not feel like cooking.

TI **Diabetes: Diet.**

SO New York, NY: Nidus Information Services, Inc. 1994. 8 p.

CN Nidus Information Services, Inc.

AV Available from Nidus Information Services, Inc. 175 Fifth Avenue, Suite 2338, New York, NY 10010. (800) 334-9355 or (212) 260-4268. PRICE: $5.95 if mailed first class; $9.95 if faxed. Bulk discounts available.

AB This wellness publication aids readers in understanding current medical knowledge and diabetes. As part of a series of reports, it uses a question-and-answer format to cover various topics, including why people with diabetes require special diets, the general guidelines for a diabetes diet, exchange lists, meal planning or schedules, the use of sodium and alcohol, food labels, and weighing and measuring foods. The document covers behavioral considerations in diabetes management such as blood glucose monitoring, preventing hypoglycemia, and weight control. The document concludes with an annotated list of resource organizations, through which readers can obtain additional information. 11 tables. 6 references.

TI **Diabetes: Nutrition Guidelines Emphasize Personal Touch.**

SO *Mayo Clinic Health Letter*. 12(8): 4-5. August 1994.

CN Mayo Foundation.

AV Available from Mayo Clinic Health Letter. Subscription Services, P.O. Box 53889, Boulder, CO 80322-3889. (800) 333-9037.

AB This brief newsletter article reports on the new set of nutrition guidelines for people with diabetes. The guidelines, recently released by the American Diabetes Association (ADA), underscore the important role of diet in keeping blood glucose levels under control. The new recommendations stress the need for individualizing the diet and developing a meal plan based on the individual's food preferences, health concerns such as weight or blood cholesterol level, and insulin therapy. The article concludes by urging readers to work closely with a registered dietitian and other members of the diabetes care team in planning the diet.

TI Diabetic's Innovative Cookbook: A Positive Approach to Living With Diabetes.
AU Juliano, J.; Young, D.
SO New York, NY: Henry Holt and Company, Inc. 1994. 416 p.
AV Available from Henry Holt and Company, Inc. 115 West 18th Street, New York, NY 10011. (800) 488-5233. PRICE: $25 ISBN: 0805025189.
AB The authors present a positive approach to living well with diabetes. Juliano, himself a physician with diabetes, shares with the reader his 30 years of experience in dealing with the day-to-day challenges of diabetes. He advocates a take-charge attitude toward living well within the confines of a diabetes diet. He also reviews the guidelines for good nutrition and discusses issues such as fiber, fruit and fruit sugar, vegetable and fruit juices, and desserts. In the second part of the book, Young presents more than 145 low-fat, heart-healthy recipes for appetizers, breakfast, broths and soups, sauces and relishes, salads, vegetables and side dishes, rice and pasta, entrees, and desserts. The recipes include exchange list and nutritional information. The book also includes the full American Diabetes Association Exchange Lists, a selected reading list, and subject and recipe indexes.

TI Exchange Lists for Meal Planning.
SO Alexandria, VA: American Diabetes Association. 1995. 33 p.
CN American Diabetes Association. American Dietetic Association.
AV Available from American Diabetes Association. ADA Order Department. P.O. Box 930850, Atlanta, GA 31193. (800) 232-6733. PRICE: $1.20 (members) or $1.50 (nonmembers) for single copy; $30 (members) or $37.50 (nonmembers) for package of 25.
AB This illustrated manual, revised in 1995, provides nutrition guidelines and management tips for people with either insulin-dependent or non-insulin-dependent diabetes. The manual

details food exchanges for each of the following food categories: starches, fruit, milk, other carbohydrates, vegetables,
meat and meat substitutes, fats, free foods, combination foods,
and fast foods. The fat list is broken down into monounsaturated, polyunsaturated, and saturated fats, and high sodium
foods are identified. Tips for deciphering food labels, a glos-
sary, and an index close the manual. The inside back cover is
a chart that can be used to devise a personal meal plan.

TI Fast Food Facts. 4th ed.
AU Franz, M.J.
SO Minneapolis, MN: Chronimed Publishing. 1994. 145 p.
AV Available from Chronimed Publishing. P.O. Box 59032, Minneapolis, MN 55459. (800) 848-2793 or (612) 546-1146. PRICE:
$4.95.
AB This book provides information about nutritional and exchange values for the food served at 15 fast food chains.
Charts offer per serving counts for calories, carbohydrates,
protein, fat, saturated fat, cholesterol, and sodium. The lists
identify menu items containing large amounts of refined
sugar, salt, and fat.

TI Flexibility is Key in New Diabetes Meal Plan.
AU Franz, M.J.
SO *Diabetes in the News.* 14(3): 6-12. June 1995.
AV Available from Diabetes in the News. P.O. Box 4548, South
Bend, IN 46634. (312) 664-9782.
AB This article presents information about the American Diabetes Association's 1994 nutrition guidelines for people with diabetes. The new guidelines stress flexibility, with the goal of
helping patients maintain near-normal blood glucose levels,
achieve optimal blood fat levels, attain a reasonable weight,
prevent complications, and improve overall health through
proper nutrition. The author stresses that the flexibility offered is designed only for people whose diabetes is in good
control and that readers should consult their health care team
for assistance in updating their meal plans. Other topics include specific guidelines in the areas of carbohydrates and
sweeteners, dietary fat, protein, fiber, sodium, and alcohol. A
companion article provides details for patients who want to
incorporate the new guidelines into their everyday program of
diabetes management. 1 table.

TI Flexible Meal Planning with Diabetes.
SO Washington, DC: Sugar Association, Inc. 1994. 4 p.
CN Sugar Association, Inc.
AV Available from Sugar Association, Inc. 1101 15th Street NW,
Suite 600, Washington, DC 20005. (202) 785-1122. PRICE: Up
to 50 copies free.
AB This brochure is designed to help readers with diabetes follow
the new dietary guidelines, which allow the limited use of
sugar in a diabetic diet. The guidelines also address proportions of carbohydrates, fats, and protein in the diet. Topics include weight loss; the use of sugar in moderation; and meal
planning and optimal nutrition. Three meal plans are provided, as are recipes for Chocolate Dunking Biscotti; Black-
berry Tea Bars; Watermelon Ice; and Cinnamon Apple-Nut
Muffins

TI Good Nutrition Counts!: 1200-Calorie Meal Plan.
SO Princeton, NJ: Novo Nordisk Pharmaceuticals, Inc. 7 p.
CN Novo Nordisk Pharmaceuticals, Inc.
AV Available from Novo Nordisk Pharmaceuticals, Inc. 100 Overlook Center Suite 200, Princeton, NJ 08540-7810. (800) 727-
6500. PRICE: Single copy free.
AB This brochure presents the exchange list for a 1,200-calorie
meal plan designed for people with diabetes. The recommended exchange list values for this level of caloric intake are
noted, along with material describing how to use exchange
lists, a suggested meal plan, and a blank chart for the reader
to fill in a personal meal plan. The brochure unfolds to a 17
inch x 17 inch chart that presents the food exchange lists in
seven categories: bread and starch, meat, vegetable, fruit,
milk, fat, and free foods. General nutritional recommendations for people with diabetes are also included.

TI Good Nutrition Counts!: 1500-Calorie Meal Plan.
SO Princeton, NJ: Novo Nordisk Pharmaceuticals, Inc. 7 p.
CN Novo Nordisk Pharmaceuticals, Inc.
AV Available from Novo Nordisk Pharmaceuticals, Inc. 100 Overlook Center, Suite 200, Princeton, NJ 08540-7810. (800) 727-
6500. PRICE: Single copy free.
AB This brochure presents the exchange list for a 1,500-calorie
meal plan designed for people with diabetes. The recommended exchange list values for this level of caloric intake are

noted, along with material describing how to use exchange lists, a suggested meal plan, and a blank chart for the reader to fill in a personal meal plan. The brochure unfolds to a 17 inch x 17 inch chart that presents the food exchange lists in seven categories: bread and starch, meat, vegetable, fruit, milk, fat, and free foods. General nutritional recommendations for people with diabetes are also included.

TI Good Nutrition Counts!: 2000-Calorie Meal Plan.
SO Princeton, NJ: Novo Nordisk Pharmaceuticals, Inc. 7 p.
CN Novo Nordisk Pharmaceuticals, Inc.
AV Available from Novo Nordisk Pharmaceuticals, Inc. 100 Overlook Center, Suite 200, Princeton, NJ 08540-7810. (800) 727-6500. PRICE: Single copy free.
AB This brochure presents the exchange list for a 2,000-calorie meal plan designed for people with diabetes. The recommended exchange list values for this level of caloric intake are noted, along with material describing how to use exchange lists, a suggested meal plan, and a blank chart for the reader to fill in a personal meal plan. The brochure unfolds to a 17 inch x 17 inch chart that presents the food exchange lists in seven categories: bread and starch, meat, vegetables fruit, milk, fat, and free foods. General nutritional recommendations for people with diabetes are also included.

TI Good Nutrition Counts!: 1800-Calorie Meal Plan.
SO Princeton, NJ: Novo Nordisk Pharmaceuticals, Inc. 7 p.
CN Novo Nordisk Pharmaceuticals, Inc.
AV Available from Novo Nordisk Pharmaceuticals, Inc. 100 Overlook Center, Suite 200, Princeton, NJ 08540-7810. (800) 727-6500. PRICE: Single copy free.
AB This brochure presents the exchange list for an 1,800-calorie meal plan designed for people with diabetes. The recommended exchange list values for this level of caloric intake are noted, along with material describing how to use exchange lists, a suggested meal plan, and a blank chart for the reader to fill in a personal meal plan. The brochure unfolds to a 17 inch x 17 inch chart that presents the food exchange lists in seven categories: bread and starch, meat, vegetable, fruit, milk, fat, and free foods. General nutritional recommendations for people with diabetes are also included.

TI **Good Nutrition Counts!: 2200-Calorie Meal Plan.**
SO Princeton, NJ: Novo Nordisk Pharmaceuticals, Inc. 7 p.
CN Novo Nordisk Pharmaceuticals, Inc.
AV Available from Novo Nordisk Pharmaceuticals, Inc. 100 Overlook Center, Suite 200, Princeton, NJ 08540-7810. (800) 727-6500. PRICE: Single copy free.
AB This brochure presents the exchange list for a 2,200-calorie meal plan designed for people with diabetes. The recommended exchange list values for this level of caloric intake are noted, along with material describing how to use exchange lists, a suggested meal plan, and a blank chart for the reader to fill in a personal meal plan. The brochure unfolds to a 17 inch x 17 inch chart that presents the food exchange lists in seven categories: bread and starch, meat, vegetable, fruit, milk, fat, and free foods. General nutritional recommendations for people with diabetes are also included.

TI **Good Nutrition Counts!: 2500-Calorie Meal Plan.**
SO Princeton, NJ: Novo Nordisk Pharmaceuticals, Inc. 7 p.
CN Novo Nordisk Pharmaceuticals, Inc.
AV Available from Novo Nordisk Pharmaceuticals, Inc. 100 Overlook Center, Suite 200, Princeton, NJ 08540-7810. (800) 727-6500. PRICE: Single copy free.
AB This brochure presents the exchange list for a 2,500-calorie meal plan designed for people with diabetes. The recommended exchange list values for this level of caloric intake are noted, along with material describing how to use exchange lists, a suggested meal plan, and a blank chart for the reader to fill in a personal meal plan. The brochure unfolds to a 17 inch x 17 inch chart that presents the food exchange lists in seven categories: bread and starch, meat, vegetable, fruit, milk, fat, and free foods. General nutritional recommendations for people with diabetes are also included.

TI **Love Your Heart Italian Low Cholesterol Cookbook.**
AU Kruppa, C.
SO Chicago, IL: Surrey Books. 1994. 364 p.
AV Available from Surrey Books. 230 East Ohio Street, Suite 120, Chicago, IL 60611. (312) 751-7330 or (800) 326-4430. PRICE: $12.95. ISBN: 0940625814.
AB Emphasizing fresh foods and produce, natural herbs and spices, and low-fat cooking methods, this book presents over

250 Italian recipes. Recipes are presented in 18 categories: condiments; appetizers; omelets; salads and dressings; soups; pasta; pizza; poultry; meat; seafood; vegetables; rice, risotto, and polenta; dinner sauces; breads; biscotti; desserts; sweet sauces; and Italian styles coffees. Nutritional data and diabetic exchanges follow each recipe.

TI Making Sense of Food Exchanges.
AU Dinsmoor, R.S.
SO *Diabetes Self-Management.* 11(4): 44, 46-48. July-August 1994.
AV Available from R.A. Rapaport Publishing, Inc. 150 West 22nd Street, New York, NY 10011. (800) 234-0923.
AB This article presents an introduction to the use of food exchange lists for meal planning for people with diabetes. Topics include defining dietary goals; how and why the exchange lists were created; how to obtain the complete Exchange Lists for Meal Planning from the American Dietetic Association; the six categories on the exchange lists, including starch/bread, meat and meat substitutes, vegetable, fruit, milk, fat, and free foods; the dietitian's role; converting food label information; and hints and tips for successful use of the exchange list system. One sidebar looks at other meal-planning approaches, including the Health Food Choices plan, carbohydrate counting, and the Total Available Glucose (TAG) plan.

TI Meal Planning: Eating Right for People With Diabetes.
SO Evanston, IL: Altschul Group Corporation. 1994.
CN Altschul Group Corporation.
PD 1/2 in VHS videocassette (13 min), color.
AV Available from Altschul Group Corporation. 1560 Sherman Avenue, Suite 100, Evanston, IL 60201. (800) 421-2363 or (708) 328-6700. Fax (708) 328-6706. PRICE: $295 (as of 1995). Order no. 7846.
AB This videotape program is one of a series of six videotapes that present a common sense approach for living with and controlling diabetes mellitus. This program provides a sensible approach to meal planning and good eating for people with diabetes. This approach follows the Department of Agriculture's Food Guide Pyramid recommendations. The program depicts a dietitian leading a workshop on healthy eating, including tips for shopping, family meals, parties, and snacks.

TI **Menu Plan Can Save Time, Money.**
AU Hall, D.
SO *Diabetes in the News*. 14(3): 18-19. June 1995.
AV Available from Diabetes in the News. P.O. Box 4548, South
   Bend, IN 46634. (312) 664-9782.
AB In this article, the author explains to readers how a detailed
   menu plan can save time and money for people with diabetes
   and their families. Topics include how to plan menus in advance; flexibility in food choices; and scheduling in special occasions, including picnics or meals at restaurants. The author
   lists important things to consider, including nutritional goals
   and needs, budget, time and scheduling factors, food preparation skills, family preferences, planning for foods that are in
   season, and variety.

TI **Month of Meals 5: A Menu Planner.**
SO Alexandria, VA: American Diabetes Association. 1994. 70 p.
CN American Diabetes Association.
AV Available from American Diabetes Association. ADA Order
   Center. P.O. Box 930850, Atlanta, GA 31193. (800) 232-6733.
   PRICE: $9.95 for ADA members; $12.50 for nonmembers.
   ISBN: 0945448341. Order Number CMPMOM5.
AB This cookbook, the fifth in the Month of Meals series, offers
   complete vegetarian menus for a month of breakfasts, lunches,
   and dinners, and three calorie levels of snacks. An introduction describes the benefits of a vegetarian diet, the different
   types of vegetarian diets, the six food groups used in the exchange list system, the necessity of eating whole grains, the
   role of micronutrients, and blank forms for individualized
   meal planning. Each page of the cookbook is cut into thirds, so
   readers can mix and match these meatless meals and snacks
   into countless combinations. A recipe index is included.

TI **New Nutritional Guidelines for a New Day in Diabetes
   Care: Most Commonly Asked Diet Questions.**
AU Brackenridge, B.
SO Van Nuys, CA: Prana Publications. 1995. Audiocassette.
PD Audiocassette (60 min).
AV Available from Prana Publications. 5623 Matilija Avenue, Van
   Nuys, CA 91401. (800) 735-7726 or (818) 780-1308. Fax (818)
   786-7359. E-mail prana@earthspirit.org. PRICE: $11.95 plus
   $3.25 shipping and handling (as of 1995). Order Number A12.

AB In this audiocassette program for people with diabetes, Betty Brackenridge, former president of the American Association of Diabetes Educators, explains the American Diabetes Association's 1994 nutritional guidelines. Topics include changes in the guidelines; new guidelines regarding sugar; weight loss and determining appropriate weight levels; and other common concerns.

TI **NutriScore Board for Diabetes: Food Group Version.**
SO LaGrange, IL: Health Promotion Services, Inc. 1995. Food record chart.
CN Health Promotion Services, Inc.
PD Pad of charts (8.5 in x 11 in), 25 sheets per pad.
AV Available from Health Promotion Services, Inc. 339 South Sixth Avenue, LaGrange, IL 60525. (708) 354-0256. Fax (708) 354-0409. PRICE: $4.75 for 1 to 24 pads (Item Number NP1); discounts for larger quantities.
AB This food record chart provides a visual method for people with diabetes to record food intake for a 1-week period of time. Seven food groups are depicted: grains, beans, and starchy vegetables; vegetables; fruit; milk; meat; fat; and sweets. For each food group, the appropriate amounts are noted in words and depicted with graphic symbols; space is provided for each day of the week. The weekly totals space provides a goal for each food group, as well as a place for the user to write down his or her actual total for each food group. The chart is also available in a write-on, wipe-off version and in a version designed for people who do not have diabetes.

TI **Pocket Food Guide.**
SO Toronto, Ontario: Canadian Diabetes Association. 1995. 2 p.
CN Canadian Diabetes Association.
AV Available from Canadian Diabetes Association. 15 Toronto Street, Suite 1001, Toronto, ON, Canada M5C 2E3. PRICE: Free, but $3 (Canadian) shipping and handling. Available only in tablets of 100 tear-off sheets. Recommended for professional use only.
AB This pocket food guide is designed to convey the basic concepts important to the nutritional management of diabetes: what to eat, how much to eat, and when to eat. The guide provides brief information to help people with diabetes understand variety, moderation, and balance as they relate to

eating. The guide includes a tear-off, wallet-sized legend of food symbols that represent food groups, including starch foods, fruits and vegetables, milk, sugars, protein foods, fats and oils, and extras. The tear-off portion also has space to record the name and telephone number of one's dietitian. The guide is available in English or French.

TI **Respect the Gift of Food.**
AU McCarter, M.
SO Albuquerque, NM: Indian Health Service Diabetes Program. 1994. Poster.
CN Indian Health Service Diabetes Program.
PD 1 poster: color.; 36 x 24 in.
AV Available from Indian Health Service Diabetes Program. 5300 Homestead Road NE., Albuquerque, NM 87110. (505) 837-4182. PRICE: Free to Native Americans and to professionals serving them.
AB This poster is one of a group of posters designed to increase Native American awareness of the problem of diabetes and to remind people with diabetes of important aspects of diabetes management. The text of the poster reads, Respect the Gift of Food . . . You can prevent and control diabetes. Eat food low in fat and sugar. The main part of the poster consists of a water-color illustration of Southwestern Native Americans eating at a table laden with healthy foods. The poster is printed on heavy poster paper.

TI **Restaurant Companion: A Guide to Healthier Eating Out. 2nd ed.**
AU Warshaw, H.S.
SO Chicago, IL: Surrey Books. 1995. 360 p.
AV Available from Surrey Books. 230 East Ohio Street, Suite 120, Chicago, IL 60611. (312) 751-7330 or (800) 326-4430. PRICE: $13.95 plus shipping and handling (as of 1995). ISBN: 0940625938.
AB This guide was designed to help people make healthful choices from restaurant menus and, using model meals, shows how to order in a restaurant to keep calories under control and re-duce fat, cholesterol, and sodium intakes. This book strives to show that restaurant food can be good and healthy when or-dered by an informed consumer. It covers European and Asian as well as American cuisines and presents a wide variety of

foods to replace traditional eating patterns. The various sections of the book cover different food styles, including Mexican, Chinese, Italian, Thai, Japanese, Indian, Middle Eastern, vegetarian, and traditional American, as well as seafood, fast food, salad bar, luncheon, breakfast and brunch, airline food, and alcoholic versus nonalcoholic beverages. The book represents a departure from the high-fat, high-cholesterol, high-calorie foods often associated with dining out.

TI **Telling It Like It Is: A Look at The New Food Labels.**
AU Holzmeister, L.A.
SO *Diabetes Self-Management.* 11(2): 40, 42, 44, 46-47. March-April 1994.
AV Available from R.A. Rapaport Publishing, Inc. 150 West 22nd Street, New York, NY 10011. (800) 234-0923.
AB This article gives readers an overview of the new requirements for food labels that went into effect in May 1994. The author notes that the information provided by the new labels shows for the first time how each food fits, nutrient by nutrient, into an overall healthy diet. Topics covered include foods that are exempt from the labeling requirements, terminology and what is included in each section, serving sizes versus food exchanges, daily values and percent daily values, figuring out the sugar entry on the label, and seven health claims and their definitions as per the new regulation. One diagram shows a sample food label with each part described. The article concludes with a list of common food label terms and what they mean.

TI **The 'Can Have' Diet and More!: The Easy Guide to Informed Exercise and Food Choices.**
AU Stein, P.M.; Winn, N.J.
SO Olathe, KS: NCES, Inc. (Nutritional Counseling and Education Services). 1995. 140p.
AV Available from NCES. 1904 East 123rd Street, Olathe, KS 66061. (800) 445-5653. Fax (800) 251-9349. PRICE: $8.95 (as of 1995). ISBN: 0962096512.
AB This book helps readers adopt a healthy lifestyle and healthy eating habits without resorting to a strict diet. Sixteen chapters cover dieting and weight loss; the benefits of exercise; exercising safely; dietary fats and learning about fats in the diet; controlling blood cholesterol; sodium and limiting sodium

in the diet; planning a diet for people with diabetes; reading food labels; food values; and altering recipes for lower fat content. The chapter on food values lists serving size, grams of fat, calories, and milligrams of sodium for generic foods including bread and cereal products, fruits and fruit juices, vegetables, dairy products, protein foods, fats, oils and salad dressings, desserts and sweets, frozen foods, canned foods, and other prepared foods. The chapter lists the same nutrient values for 29 franchised restaurants, including fast food restaurants and "sit down" restaurants such as Country Kitchen, Olive Garden, and Pizza Hut. 10 references.

TI **You'll Face Many Challenges When You Switch to a Flexible Meal Plan.**
AU Blocker, A.K.
SO *Diabetes in the News.* 14(3): 14-17. June 1995.
AV Available from Diabetes in the News. P.O. Box 4548, South Bend, IN 46634. (312) 664-9782.
AB In this article, the author familiarizes readers with the details of using a flexible meal plan as part of a diabetes management program. Topics include designing the meal plan, working with a dietitian, calculating carbohydrates, monitoring blood glucose levels and adjusting food intake accordingly, working with the diabetes health care team, determining appropriate exercise levels, and maintaining the flexible meal planning approach. The article includes a chart that summarizes the exchange values and carbohydrate levels of common snack foods.

Chapter 14

The Role of Exercise Combined with Diet in Metabolic Control

In 1988 Reaven[1] called it 'Syndrome X,' and in 1989 Kaplan[2] called it 'the deadly quartet', while Foster[3] suggested that it is 'a secret killer.' They were all referring to the aggregation of coronary heart disease (CHD) risk factors including obesity, hypertension [high blood pressure], hypertriglyceridemia [high levels of tryglycerides—a fatty substance—in the blood], depressed high density lipoprotein (HDL) cholesterol and glucose intolerance or hyperinsulinemia [excess insulin secreted by the pancreas]. The aggregation of all these risk factors would greatly increase the risk for CHD. In 1990, Landin et al.[4] reported that individuals with this combination of risk factors were also likely to have elevated levels of fibrinogen [a coagulation factor] and tissue plasminogen activator inhibitor [involved in clot formation]. More recently, it has been reported that the definition of the syndrome should be expanded to include small, dense low density lipoprotein (LDL) particles.[5-7] As the list grows, the risk for CHD obviously increases greatly. This syndrome is now well recognized, and is usually referred to as the 'insulin resistance syndrome' or simply the 'metabolic syndrome'.

The exact rate of occurrence of this syndrome is not known, but it is suspected to be quite common. It has been estimated that 25 to 35%

Barnard, R. James and Stephen J. Wen. "Exercise and Diet in the Prevention and Control of the Metabolic Syndrome," *Sports Medicine*, 18(4):218-228, 1994; reprinted with permission. Bracketed comments have been added to help explain technical terms to the lay reader.

of the populations in Western, industrialized societies have at least several aspects of the metabolic syndrome.[8-9] Ferrannini et al.[9] found that only 36% of a studied population were free of all 6 measures that they had characterized as making up the syndrome: obesity, hypertension, hypertriglyceridemia, glucose intolerance, hypercholesterolemia [high cholesterol] and non-insulin-dependent diabetes mellitus (NIDDM). Large proportions of the studied population, ranging from 17% for the obese to a high of 56% for hypertensives, also had 3 or more of the other metabolic syndrome characteristics. The syndrome has also been found in a high percentage of obese, young adults aged 18 to 26 years.[10]

The purpose of this review is to investigate the underlying mechanisms of the syndrome, and to see how exercise and diet might prevent or control the metabolic syndrome.

Cause of the Metabolic Syndrome

The traditional view has been that obesity is the underlying factor responsible for the metabolic syndrome.[2] However, more recently it has been suggested[7] that insulin resistance is the underlying factor, and that once an individual develops insulin resistance they will then develop the other characteristics of the syndrome if they have the genetic predisposition. Haffner et al.[11] reported that baseline insulin levels, independent of bodyweight or body fat distribution, were predictors of subsequent development of metabolic disorders. This does not mean that obesity is not important in the development of the syndrome. In 1947, Vague[12] observed that women with upper body or android obesity were far more likely to develop diabetes and atherosclerosis than women with lower body or gynoid obesity. Many studies have reported that upper body obesity, as determined by the waist-to-hip ratio, computed tomography or similar measures, correlates more strongly with the metabolic factors than do total weight or body mass index.[13-16] In a review of the literature, Després et al.[13] concluded that the risk for cardiovascular disease in gluteal-femoral-obese individuals is only moderately elevated from that of the nonobese, whereas cardiovascular-disease risk increases in trunk-abdominal-obese individuals, and is highest in individuals with deep abdominal fat. The degree of insulin resistance and the accumulation of metabolic risk factors also increase with the different types of obesity.

Precisely how or why upper body fat and, especially, deep abdominal fat are related to the metabolic syndrome is unknown. Björntrop[14] has proposed that deep abdominal or portal adipose tissue plays an important role in the metabolic syndrome by releasing free fatty acids (FFAs) into the portal circulation which then go directly to the liver. The lipid mobilizing capacity of portal adipose tissue is pronounced in men and in abdominally obese women, because of an abundance of ß-adrenergic receptors and little a-adrenergic inhibition [adrenergic refers to the actions or characteristics of the adrenal gland hormones epinephrine and norepinephrine]. The high level of portal FFAs induces the liver to secrete triglyceride-rich, very low density lipoproteins (VLDLs). The high portal FFA concentration also decreases the ability of the liver to clear insulin, which results in the hyperinsulinemia that is indicative of the metabolic syndrome.

We would agree with Björntrop[14] regarding the release of fatty acids from deep abdominal fat stores; however, we do not feel that elevated portal FFAs are the true mediator of the syndrome. It is our belief that the combination of physical inactivity with the typical high-fat, refined-sugar diet currently consumed by most people in the industrialized nations is the major underlying cause of the metabolic syndrome in genetically susceptible individuals, as outlined in Figure 14.1. With an animal model, it was found that feeding the animals a diet in which 40% of the calories were obtained from fat and 40% from sucrose resulted in skeletal muscle insulin resistance and hyperinsulinemia to maintain normal glycemia.[17, 18] These changes occurred in 10 weeks, without any change in bodyweight or whole body fat. Others[19, 20] have also reported that feeding rats a diet high in fat and/or sucrose leads to insulin resistance within a few weeks. In addition to skeletal muscle insulin resistance, these diets can also lead to insulin resistance in the liver.[21]

Further support for the suggestion that abdominal fat is not the real underlying factor for the metabolic syndrome comes from intervention studies, which have shown that most of the metabolic factors (including hyperinsulinemia, hypertriglyceridemia and hypertension) can be significantly reduced with little or no change in bodyweight.[22] The belief that diet is the major underlying factor comes from a long term (2-year) feeding study where rats were raised on either a very-low-fat, high-complex-carbohydrate (LFCC) diet or a high-fat, sucrose (HFS) diet.[23] After 2 years, the HFS rats were obese, hyperinsulinemic, hypertensive and hypertriglyceridemic, and had enhanced clotting (Table 14.1).

Interestingly, much of the excess body fat in the HFS rats was observed to be in the abdominal cavity. All of the rats were obese, and there was significant aggregation of other risk factors. However, not all of the HFS rats exhibited all of the other characteristics of the

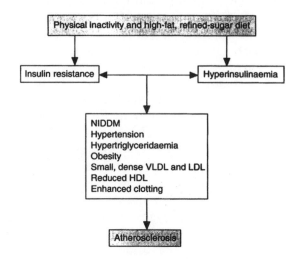

Figure 14.1. *Proposed scheme for the development of insulin resistance leading to non-insulin-dependent diabetes mellitus (NIDDM) and the metabolic syndrome, the eventual outcome being the development of atherosclerosis and its clinical sequalae. Abbreviations: HDL = high density lipoproteins; LDL = low density lipoproteins; VLDL = very low density lipoproteins.*

Table 14.1. Effects of diet on female Fischer rats. Rats were raised for 2 years on a low-fat, complex-carbohydrate (LFCC) or a high-fat, sucrose (HFS) diet[23]

Parameter	LFCC	HFS[a]
Bodyweight (g)	223±3	287±6
Body fat (%)	15±1	38±1
Fasting insulin (pmol/L)	98±10	439±118
Systolic blood pressure (mm Hg)	123±3	140±3
Fasting triglycerides (mmol/L)	0.4±0.07	1.1±0.2
Clot viscoelasticity (cP)	51±5	77±7

[a] $p < 0.05$

metabolic syndrome even though they were from an inbred strain. In the LFCC group, only 1 rat had a slightly elevated insulin level and 1 a slightly elevated triglyceride level. Thus, if genetics are involved, as suggested by DeFronzo and Ferrannini,[7] they must only predispose the organism, and once insulin resistance develops the other characteristics of the syndrome will follow but seem to be exacerbated by abdominal obesity. However, it may be that those individuals with a genetic predisposition for central obesity also have a genetic predisposition for the other characteristics of the metabolic syndrome. In addition to the animal data showing the importance of diet, studies on groups such as the Australian Aborigines, the American Pima Indians and other similar populations have found a very high incidence of insulin resistance and some aspects of the metabolic syndrome since these societies have adopted a Western diet and lifestyle.[24] However, all of the characteristics are not always observed, a further indication of a genetic involvement.

While most individuals in the highly industrialized societies are inactive and consume a high-fat, refined-sugar diet, stress associated with this lifestyle might also contribute to the metabolic syndrome.[25, 26] Stress is associated with the release of hormones, especially glucocorticoids, that antagonise [act in opposition to] the actions of insulin. Stress-induced release of glucocorticoids and FFAs may lead to insulin resistance.

Thus, it appears that lifestyle is the major underlying factor in the metabolic syndrome. Once an organism develops insulin resistance and hyperinsulinemia, other characteristics of the syndrome will follow in genetically susceptible individuals or animals. Insulin has been shown to induce hepatic [in the liver] production of triglycerides and VLDLs.[27-30] This effect of insulin would be exacerbated by a high-fat diet as well as by the direct release of FFAs from abdominal fat tissue into the portal circulation. This excessive production of triglyceride by the liver is also associated with the production of highly atherogenic [causes hardening of the arteries], small, dense lipoproteins if the individual is consuming the typical Western high-fat, high-cholesterol diet.[31] However, if the diet is very low in fat but high in carbohydrate, the triglycerides are packaged into large, less dense VLDL which may be less atherogenic.[32]

In addition to increased production of triglyceride and VLDL, insulin resistance is associated with reduced clearance of chylomicrons [a substance in the blood that transports fats and cholesterol] and triglyceride-rich remnants.[33-36] This abnormal clearance of triglyceride is due to a reduction in lipoprotein lipase activity. The reduced clearance of VLDL is also, in part, responsible for the low levels of HDL cholesterol characteristic of the metabolic syndrome.[1, 2, 7, 13, 36] Increased catabolism [breaking a compound down into simpler compounds] of HDL apoprotein A-1 and apoprotein A-11, which is associated with central obesity, also reduces HDL cholesterol.

Numerous studies have reported a correlation between insulin resistance, hyperinsulinemia and hypertension.[36, 37] The exact mechanisms responsible for the elevated blood pressure are not known but may involve increased sodium reabsorption, increased sympathetic nervous system activity, altered cellular cation [an ion with a positive electrical charge] exchange or smooth muscle cell proliferation.[36]

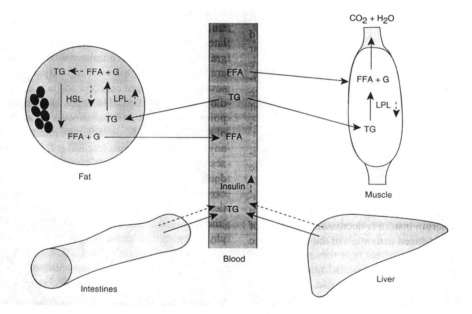

Figure 14.2. *Proposed scheme for the development of obesity as a result of consuming a high-fat, refined-sugar diet. The dietary-induced hyperinsulinemia would result in: (i) increased triglyceride formation in the liver; (ii) reduced skeletal muscle lipoprotein lipase activity; (iii) enhanced fat cell lipoprotein lipase activity; and (iv) depressed fat cell hormone-sensitive lipase activity. Abbreviations: FFA = free fatty acids; G = glucose; HSL = hormone-sensitive lipase; LPL = lipoprotein lipase; TG = triglycerides.*

186

The metabolic syndrome is also associated with changes in the hemostatic [stops blood flow] system, and is thought to be a major factor responsible for myocardial infarction.[4, 38] Increased levels of fibrinogen and plasminogen activator inhibitor-1 (PAI-1) have been documented. The mechanisms linking these changes with the metabolic syndrome are unknown. However, it has been reported that high levels of insulin and lipoprotein abnormalities affect PAI-1 synthesis by both endothelial cells [found in the lining of blood vessels, lymph vessels, and the heart] and hepatocytes [a type of cell found in the liver] in culture.[39-41]

In our view, obesity is the result of physical inactivity combined with a high-fat, refined-sugar diet which causes insulin resistance and hyperinsulinemia. Those who are genetically predisposed to central obesity (most men and some women) deposit fat in that particular region, and this may then exacerbate the syndrome. Obesity may result from overconsumption of calories due to the high caloric density of fatty foods. However, obesity may develop as a result of the insulin resistance and hyperinsulinemia without consuming excess calories, as outlined in Figure 14.2. It has been demonstrated that skeletal muscle lipoprotein lipase activity is related to insulin sensitivity.[42, 43] Conversely, hyperinsulinemia has been shown to stimulate lipoprotein lipase [a substance that helps create free fatty acids] while inhibiting hormone-sensitive lipase [an enzyme involved in fat metabolism] in fat cells.[44, 45] These changes in lipase activity resulting from hyperinsulinemia would favor fat storage in adipocytes as opposed to fat metabolism by muscle.

In conclusion, the bulk of evidence indicates that insulin resistance and hyperinsulinemia are the factors responsible for the other characteristics of the metabolic syndrome, including hypertriglyceridemia, hypertension, obesity, small dense lipoproteins, and enhanced clotting. The true underlying factor is the high-fat, refined-sugar diet consumed by individuals in most industrialized nations. It has been shown that, when rats are placed on a high-fat and/or refined-sugar diet, skeletal muscle insulin resistance develops within a few weeks.[17-20] Since skeletal muscle is the most important target tissue for insulin action, removing up to 75% of the glucose during hyperinsulinemia, resistance in muscle would be a major factor responsible for hyperinsulinemia and the metabolic syndrome. Exactly how a high-fat, refined-sugar diet induces skeletal muscle insulin resistance is not known.

Studies have reported no change in the number of insulin receptors or insulin-responsive glucose transporters (GLUT-4).[46, 47] Boyd et al.[48] studied insulin receptor tyrosine kinase in rats fed a high-fat, sucrose diet and reported no change. Iwanishi and Kobayashi,[49] however, reported a decrease in insulin receptor autophosphorylation and tyrosine kinase activity in high-fat-fed rats. A decrease in insulin receptor tyrosine kinase has also been reported in skeletal muscle insulin receptors from patients with NIDDM, an insulin-resistant condition.[50]

Controlling the Metabolic Syndrome

Assuming that insulin resistance and resultant hyperinsulinemia are the physiological factors responsible for the other aspects of the metabolic syndrome, it would seem imperative to control these factors. Both diet and exercise can play important roles in controlling or preventing insulin resistance. Anderson et al.[51] concluded that high-complex-carbohydrate, high-fiber diets are effective for improving metabolic control in NIDDM or other insulin-resistant states. Using isotope-tracer and insulin-clamp studies, Fukagawa et al.[52] reported that when healthy adults were switched from the typical Western high-fat, refined-sugar diet to a high-complex-carbohydrate, high-fiber diet, peripheral insulin sensitivity was significantly increased. Thus, the available data indicate that diet is an important factor in the production of insulin resistance, and can also be an important factor in controlling or reversing insulin resistance.

Exercise can also play an important role in controlling or preventing insulin resistance. A single bout of exercise has a well known insulin-like effect, dramatically increasing skeletal muscle glucose transport.[46, 53] This effect is observed at a time when serum insulin is decreased as a result of the exercise-induced activation of the sympathetic nervous system. The effect lasts for several hours, and does not involve the insulin signaling pathway. Following the initial response, there is another response which involves increased insulin sensitivity and may last up to 24 hours after the completion of exercise.[46] This response to a single bout of exercise has been observed in insulin-resistant states, including the obese Zucker rat[54] as well as NIDDM and obese patients.[55, 56]

If a single bout of exercise increases insulin sensitivity, it would be assumed that repeated bouts of exercise, resulting in a state of training, would also increase insulin sensitivity. Numerous studies in normal, healthy humans and animals have reported an increase in insulin sensitivity following exercise training.[46, 57] Exercise training has also been shown to increase insulin sensitivity in the insulin-resistant, obese Zucker rat[58, 59] and in diet-induced insulin-resistant rats.[18, 60] Exercise training has also been effective in treating some, but not all, patients with NIDDM. Exercise has been shown to improve the diabetic state in young NIDDM patients but is less effective in older patients.[61] The intensity of exercise appears to be important.

Rogers et al.[62] reported that 1 week of intensive exercise training improved oral glucose tolerance before any significant changes in bodyweight or maximal oxygen uptake (VO_{2max}) were observed. The fact that exercise has not been shown to be effective in controlling NIDDM in many studies, especially in older individuals, may be related to the frequency and intensity of training programs. Many older individuals with NIDDM are limited in their exercise capacity, due to being severely overweight or having orthopedic or cardiovascular problems. However, Després et al.[63] pointed out that insulin sensitivity as well as plasma lipids can be modified by exercise without any increase in cardiorespiratory fitness as assessed by VO_{2max}. They suggest that brisk walking done on a regular basis probably represents the best exercise prescription for the metabolic complications of abdominal obesity. They suggest the term 'metabolic fitness' to describe these important physiological changes resulting from low-level exercise. Several epidemiological studies have reported that exercise plays an important role in reducing the risk for NIDDM.[64-66] However, those who exercise regularly might also have a healthier diet.

Since exercise has been shown to control insulin resistance and reduce insulin levels, it should affect the metabolic syndrome if our model is indeed correct.[46, 57-59] Després et al.[67] studied the effects of a short term (22 days) intensive exercise program in male twins. Significant reductions were reported for plasma insulin, body fat and plasma triglycerides while HDL cholesterol levels significantly increased. There was no significant change in the ratio of trunk to extremity skinfold fat. Furthermore, the change in trunk fat was unrelated to the significant changes in insulin, triglycerides or HDL cholesterol. There were differences in the amount of change observed between groups of twins, but within pairs of twins the changes were similar, which would suggest a hereditary influence.

This same group of investigators studied the effects of intensive (90 minutes, 4 to 5 times/week) training in obese women.[63, 68] After 6 months there was no significant change in body composition, but there were significant changes in insulin and lipids levels in those women who initially had elevated waist-to-hip ratios. In a longer training study (14 months) with obese women, Després et al.[69] did find reductions in abdominal fat and greater changes in insulin and lipids levels. It was concluded that changes in insulin and lipids are not correlated with changes in VO_{2max}. Insulin and lipid changes can also be observed without changes in body composition, but the changes are greater when accompanied by reductions in abdominal fat.[63]

Lampman et al.[70-72] conducted several 9- to 10-week training studies on men with insulin resistance and hypertriglyceridemia. They concluded that moderate activity, without any weight change, did not improve the metabolic syndrome characteristics of insulin resistance and lipid metabolism. However, with more intensive training but still no change in bodyweight, improvements were seen in insulin sensitivity and serum triglycerides; small but nonsignificant increases were also observed for HDL cholesterol.

While there are not many studies looking at the effects of exercise training on the metabolic syndrome *per se*, numerous studies have examined the response of individual characteristics of the metabolic syndrome, including insulin sensitivity, triglycerides, HDL cholesterol and hypertension.[73] All of these aspects of the metabolic syndrome respond positively to exercise training. Acute exercise has a positive effect to reduce blood clotting, but there is no substantial evidence indicating that exercise training has any significant influence on the clotting system.[73]

Thus, the available data clearly indicate that regular aerobic exercise can play an important role in helping to control insulin resistance and the other characteristics of the metabolic syndrome.

The one area that has not been extensively investigated is the effect of exercise or training on lipoprotein particle size. Since small dense LDL particles have been associated with elevated levels of triglyceride, it is assumed that exercise should result in larger, less dense particles, as exercise is highly effective in reducing serum triglycerides. Two studies have examined the effects of a single prolonged bout of exercise on LDL particles. Baumstark et al.[74] reported a reduction in LDL triglyceride content and a change in LDL density, which were correlated with the change in serum triglycerides. Lamon-Fava et al.[75] reported an increase in LDL particle size in 7 men following a triathlon. The changes were correlated with a change in serum triglycerides. This same group compared LDL particle size in a group of women distance runners with a that of a group of age-matched controls.[76] The eumenorrheaic [with normal menstruation] female runners had greater LDL particle sizes than did the controls, but those of the amenorrheaic [with absence of menstruation] runners were not significantly different from the controls.

Williams et al.[77] found similar results in male long-distance runners. There were fewer small dense LDL particles as well as lower triglycerides in the distance runners. The differences observed between the distance runners and sedentary controls may have been due to different dietary habits. Williams et al.[78] also examined the effects of a 1-year exercise training program and found no significant changes in small or large LDL particles when the exercisers were compared with controls. The lack of change may have been because the study participants were relatively healthy at the start of the study with low lipid levels, only experienced a 7.5 ml/kg/min increase in VO_{2max} and had no changes in LDL or VLDL levels. In another study,[79] where VLDL was significantly reduced, they did find a small increase in LDL particle size after 1 year.

Switching from the typical Western high-fat, refined-sugar diet to a low-fat, high-complex-carbohydrate diet has been shown to increase insulin sensitivity. The effects of diet on other aspects of the metabolic syndrome have not been studied extensively, and, especially in the case of triglycerides, what studies there are have been very controversial. In a review article, Anderson et al.[51] reported that high-fiber diets reduced triglycerides in 6 of 7 studies; however, the overall reduction was not significant. More recently, several studies[80-83] have reported an increase in triglycerides with high-carbohydrate diets; these data agree with those of our rat study.[23] However, Ullman et al.[84] reported that when study participants were slowly switched to a low-fat, high complex-carbohydrate diet, hypertriglyceridemia did not develop. However, when dietary carbohydrate was suddenly increased, hypertriglyceridemia was observed.

Thus, the data indicate that, if the diet contains a large amount of refined or simple carbohydrate, hypertriglyceridemia will develop. If the diet contains a large amount of complex-carbohydrate, high-fiber foods, especially if gradually introduced, hypertriglyceridemia will not develop. Even if triglycerides do increase on high-carbohydrate diets, LDL cholesterol is dramatically reduced and the lipoprotein particles formed (VLDL and LDL) are large, less dense particles thought to be much less atherogenic.[32]

One well-documented effect of a high-carbohydrate, low-fat diet is a reduction in HDL cholesterol, which is due to a reduction in apoprotein-A synthesis as well as to an increase in catabolism by the liver.[85] However, Brinton et al.[85] state that it is inappropriate to assume that a low-fat, high-carbohydrate diet-induced decrease in HDL cholesterol carries the same risk of atherosclerosis as does a low HDL cholesterol level found in people on a typical Western high-fat diet where the risk for atherosclerosis is increased. Societies that habitually consume low-fat, high-complex-carbohydrate diets have low HDL-cholesterol levels but also very low rates of atherosclerosis.[32, 84]

High-complex-carbohydrate, high-fiber diets can play an important role in controlling high blood pressure. This was emphasized long before the relationship between insulin resistance and hypertension was discovered. Most individuals in nonindustrialized societies, who exist on high-complex-carbohydrate diets, maintain low blood pressure throughout their lives, and hypertension is almost nonexistent.[86] Wright et al.[87] compared dietary fiber intake and blood pressure in 94 healthy individuals, and found a significant negative correlation. When dietary fiber was increased, blood pressure decreased. Anderson[88] examined blood pressure responses in diabetic patients treated with a high-complex-carbohydrate, high-fiber diet without restricting salt. Not only was the dose of insulin required to control diabetes drastically reduced, but blood pressure was also reduced in normotensive as well as in hypertensive individuals. Thus, these data further support the important relationship between serum insulin and blood pressure.

Reducing fat in the diet down to 25% of total calories has been shown to significantly reduce platelet aggregation and increase fibrinolytic activity.[89, 90] In both human and animal studies, saturated fat has been shown to adversely affect whole blood clotting and platelet aggregation, while polyunsaturated fat seems to improve these parameters.[89] Steele and Rainwater[91] reported a significant increase in platelet survival time in hyperlipidemic patients treated with diet or drugs to reduce lipids. ?-3 Fatty acids obtained through supplements or from a diet high in fish also reduces platelet aggregation and thromboxane formation.[92-94]

We have investigated the effects on the metabolic syndrome of the Pritikin high-complex-carbohydrate diet combined with aerobic exercise. In a study specifically addressing the metabolic syndrome, insulin, triglyceride, blood pressure and body mass index changes were observed over a 3-week period.[22] Of the 13 participants with NIDDM, 5 initially had all 4 factors elevated, while in the insulin-resistant group 10 of 29 individuals had all 4 factors elevated. At the end of the program, only 1 of the study participants with NIDDM and 2 of the insulin-resistant individuals still had all 4 factors elevated. For both groups, there were significant reductions in fasting insulin levels (Figure 14.3). The large reduction of insulin in the NIDDM group was partly due to the discontinuation of insulin injections in 2 of 6 participants and of oral hypoglycemic agents in 4 of 5 participants. The reduction in the insulin-resistant group primarily reflected a change in insulin sensitivity. Serum triglycerides were significantly reduced in both groups, with the biggest decrease observed in the NIDDM group which also had the biggest drop in insulin (Figure 14.4). Systolic blood pressure was reduced from 143 ± 9mm Hg to 132 ± 6mm Hg in the NIDDM group and from 130 ± 4mm Hg to 125 ± 5mm Hg in the insulin-resistant group. Diastolic pressure was reduced from 83 ± 3mm Hg to 71 ± 3mm Hg for the NIDDM group, and from 84 ± 3mm Hg to 78 ± 2mm Hg for the insulin-resistant group. In addition, 4 of 10 individuals in the NIDDM group and 1 of 10 in the insulin resistant group discontinued antihypertensive drugs. Body mass index was significantly reduced in both groups; however, most of the study participants were still overweight or obese at the end of the study (Figure 14.5), further indicating that obesity is not the under-lying cause of the metabolic syndrome.

The changes in triglycerides and blood pressure observed in this study[22] of the metabolic syndrome are similar to changes reported in other studies of this lifestyle modification program. In a large popu-lation (4587) of men and women, triglycerides were reduced by 38 and 23% respectively.[95] In a 5-year follow-up study of 64 cardiac patients and a 2- to 3-year follow-up of 69 NIDDM patients, we found that a

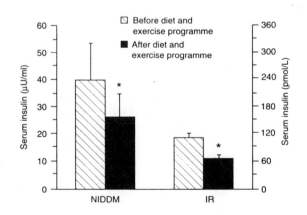

Figure 14.3. Effects of a high-complex-carbohydrate diet combined with daily aerobic exercise on fasting insulin in non-insulin-dependent diabetes mellitus (NIDDM) patients and insulin resistant (IR) individuals.[22] * p < 0.05.

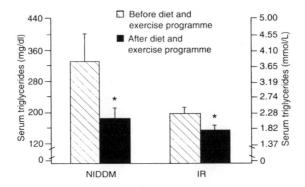

Figure 14.4. *Effects of a high complex-carbohydrate diet combined with daily aerobic exercise on serum triglycerides in non-insulin-dependent diabetes mellitus (NIDDM) patients and insulin resistant (IR) individuals.[22] * p < 0.05.*

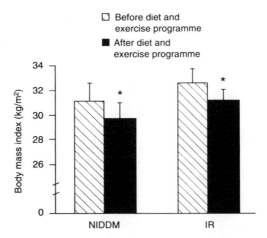

Figure 14.5. *Effects of a high-complex-carbohydrate diet combined with daily aerobic exercise on body mass index in non-insulin-dependent diabetes mellitus (NIDDM) patients and insulin resistant (IR) individuals.[22] * p < 0.05.*

majority were maintaining the reduced levels of triglycerides.[96, 97] Improvements in blood pressure with significant reductions in the use antihypertensive drugs were reported for 268 patients.[98] These improvements in blood pressure were still observed at 4 years of follow-up for most individuals.

In 2 small studies, the effects of the Pritikin diet and exercise program on blood clotting factors were examined.[99] Platelet aggregation was studied in platelet-rich plasma with collagen and with adenosine diphosphate stimulation. In both cases, platelet aggregation and thromboxane formation were significantly reduced. Two of the clotting factors included in the metabolic syndrome, tPAI and fibrinogen, were also examined.[100] Fibrinogen was lower at the conclusion of the study, but not statistically significant; however, tPAI was significantly reduced.

Conclusions

The available data suggest that the metabolic syndrome is a result of a genetic predisposition and the typical sedentary lifestyle combined with a high-fat, refined-sugar diet consumed by most Western societies. Diet appears to be a major factor and can even induce the syndrome in laboratory animals. Since diet and inactivity seem to be important in the etiology of the syndrome, it is not surprising to find that regular aerobic exercise, especially when combined with a very low-fat, high-complex-carbohydrate diet, can reverse the syndrome. Since the syndrome is made up of many factors shown to be independent risk factors for coronary heart disease, it must be playing an important role in the etiology of the number one killer in Western societies.

Acknowledgements

R. James Barnard is supported by NIH Grant AG 075299.

References

1. Reaven GM. Role of insulin resistance in human disease. *Diabetes* 1988; 37:1595-607

2. Kaplan NM. The deadly quartet: upper-body obesity, glucose intolerance, hypertriglyceridemia, and hypertension. *Arch Intern Med* 1989; 149:1514-20

3. Foster DW. Insulin resistance—a secret killer? *N Engl J Med* 1989; 320:733-4

4. Landin K, Tengborn L, Smith U. Elevated fibrinogen and plasminogen activator inhibitor (PAI-1) in hypertension are related to metabolic risk factors for cardiovascular disease. *J Intern Med* 1990; 227:273-8

5. Barakat HA, Carpenter JW, McLendon VD, et al. Influence of obesity, impaired glucose tolerance, and NIDDM on LDL structure and composition. *Diabetes* 1990; 39:1527-33

6. Reaven GM, Chen Y-DI, Jeppesen J, et al. Insulin resistance and hyperinsulinemia in individuals with small, dense, low density lipoprotein particles. *J Clin Invest* 1993; 92:141-6

7. DeFronzo RA, Ferrannini E. Insulin resistance: a multifaceted syndrome responsible for NIDDM, obesity, hypertension, dyslipidemia, and atherosclerotic cardiovascular disease. *Diabetes Care* 1991; 14:173-94

8. Rupp H. Insulin resistance, hyperinsulinemia, and cardiovascular disease: the need for novel dietary prevention strategies. *Basic Res Cardiol* 1992; 87:99-105

9. Ferrannini E, Haffner SM, Mitchell BD. et al. Hyperinsulinemia: the key feature of a cardiovascular and metabolic syndrome. *Diabetiologia* 1991; 34:416-22

10. Srinivasan SR, Bao W, Berenson GS. Coexistence of increased levels of adiposity, insulin, and blood pressure in a young adult cohort with elevated very-low-density lipoprotein cholesterol: the Bogalusa Heart Study. *Metabolism* 1993; 42:170-6

11. Haffner SM, Valdez RA, Hazuda HP, et al. Prospective analysis of the insulin-resistance syndrome (Syndrome X). *Diabetes* 1992; 41:715-22

12. Vague J. La différenciation sexuelle, facteur déterminant des formes de l'obésité. *Presse Med* 1947; 30:339-40

13. Després J-P, Moorjani S, Lupien PJ, et al. Regional distribution of body fat, plasma lipoproteins, and cardiovascular disease. *Arteriosclerosis* 1990; 10:497-511

14. Björntorp P. 'Portal' adipose tissue as a generator of risk factors for cardiovascular disease and diabetes. *Arteriosclerosis* 1990; 10:495-6

15. Kissebah AH, Peiris AN. Biology of regional body fat distribution: relationship to non-insulin-dependent diabetes mellitus. *Diabetes Metab Rev* 1989; 5:83-109

16. Bouchard C, Bray GA, Hubbard VS. Basic and clinical aspects of regional fat distribution. *Am J Clin Nutr* 1990; 52:946-50

17. Grimditch GK, Barnard RJ, Sternlicht E. et al. Effect of diet on insulin binding and glucose transport in rat sarcolemmal vesicles. *Am J Physiol* 1987; 252:E420-E425

18. Grimditch GK, Barnard RJ, Hendrick L, et al. Effects of diet and exercise training on peripheral insulin sensitivity. *Am J Clin Nutr* 1988; 48: 38-43

19. Storlien LH, Pan DA, Kirketos AD, et al. High fat diet-induced insulin resistance. Lessons and implications from animal studies. *Ann NY Acad Sci* 1993; 683:82-90

20. Vrána A, Kazdová L, Dobesová Z, et al. Triglyceridemia, glucoregulation, and blood pressure in various rat strains. Effects of dietary carbohydrates. *Ann NY Acad Sci* 1993; 683:57-9

21. Davidson MB, Garvey D. Studies on mechanisms of hepatic insulin resistance in cafeteria-fed rats. *Am J Physiol* 1993 264:E18-E23

22. Barnard RJ, Ugianskis EJ, Martin DA, et al. Role of diet and exercise in the management of hyperinsulinemia and associated atherosclerotic risk factors. *Am J Cardiol* 1992; 69:440-4

23. Barnard RJ, Faria DJ, Menges JE, et al. Effects of a high-fat, sucrose diet on serum insulin and related atherosclerotic risk factors in rats. *Atherosclerosis* 1993; 100:229-36

24. O'Dea K. Diabetes in Australian Aborigines: impact of the western diet and life style. *J Intern Med* 1992; 232:103-17

25. Brindley DN, Rolland Y. Possible connections between stress, diabetes, obesity, hypertension and altered lipoprotein metabolism that may result in atherosclerosis. *Clin Sci* 1989; 77:453-61

26. Mårin P, Björntorp P. Endocine-metabolic pattern and adipose tissue distribution. *Hormone Res* 1993; 39 Suppl. 3:81-5

27. Salans LB, Reaven GM. Effect of insulin pretreatment on glucose and lipid metabolism of liver slices from normal rats. *Proc Soc Exp Biol Med* 1966, 122:1208-13.

28. Olefsky JM, Farquhar JW, Reaven GM. Reappraisal of the role of insulin in hypertriglyceridemia. *Am J Med* 1974; 57:551-60

29. Tobey TA, Greenfield M, Kraemer F, et al. Relationship between insulin resistance, insulin secretion, very low density lipoprotein kinetics, and plasma triglyceride levels in normotriglyceridemic man. *Metabolism* 1981; 30:165-71

30. Reaven GM, Risser TR, Chen Y-DI, et al. Characterization of a model of dietary-induced hypertriglyceridemia in young, nonobese rats. *J Lipid Res* 1979; 20:371-8

31. McNamara JR, Jenner JL, Li Z, et al. Change in LDL panicle size is associated with change in plasma triglyceride concentration. *Arterioscler Thromb* 1992; 12:1284-90

32. Stacpoole PW, Von Bergmann K, Kilgore LL, et al. Nutritional regulation of cholesterol synthesis and apolipoprotein B kinetics: studies in patients with familial hypercholesterolemia and normal subjects treated with a high carbohydrate, low fat diet. *J Lipid Res* 1991; 32:1837-40

33. Taskinen MR. Lipoprotein lipase in diabetes. *Diabetes Metab Rev* 1987; 3:551-70

34. Brunzell JD, Porte Jr D, Bierman EL. Abnormal lipoprotein mediated plasma triglyceride removal in untreated diabetes mellitus associated with hypertriglyceridemia. *Metabolism* 1979; 28:901-7

35. Ooi TC, Simo IE, Yakichuk JA. Delayed clearance of postprandial chylomicrons and their remnants in the hypoalphalipoproteinemia and mild hypertriglyceridemia syndrome. *Arterioscler Thromb* 1992; 12:1184-90

36. DeFronzo RA. Insulin resistance, hyperinsulinemia, and coronary artery disease: a complex metabolic web. *J Cardiovasc Pharmacol* 1992; 20 Suppl. II:S1-S16

37. Gans ROB, Donker AJM. Insulin and blood pressure regulation. *J Intern Med* 1991; 229 Suppl. 2:49-64

38. Juhan-Vague I, Thompson SG, Jespersen J. Involvement of the hemostatic system in the insulin resistance syndrome: a study of 1500 patients with angina pectoris. *Arterioscler Thromb* 1993; 13:1865-73

39. Alessi MC, Juhan-Vague I, Kooistra T, et al. Insulin stimulates the synthesis of plasminogen activator inhibitor 1 by the human hepatocellular cell line Hep G2. *Thromb Haemost* 1988; 60:491-4

40. Stiko-Rahm A, Wiman B, Hamsten A, et al. Secretion of plasminogen activator inhibitor 1 from cultured human umbilical vein endothelial cells is induced by very low density lipoprotein. *Arteriosclerosis* 1990; 10:1067-73

41. Latron Y, Chautan M, Anfosso E, et al. Stimulating effect of oxidized-low-density lipoproteins on plasminogen activator inhibitor I synthesis by endothelial cells. *Arterioscler Thromb* 1991:11:1821-9

42. Pollare T, Vessby B, Lithell H. Lipoprotein lipase activity in skeletal muscle is related to insulin sensitivity. *Arterioscler Thromb* 1991; 11:1192-203

43. Kiens B, Lithell H, Mikines KJ, et al. Effects of insulin and exercise on muscle lipoprotein lipase activity in man and its relation to insulin action. *J Clin Invest* 1989; 84:1124-9

44. Farese RV, Yost TJ, Eckel RH. Tissue-specific regulation of lipoprotein lipase activity by insulin/glucose in normal weight humans. *Metabolism* 1991; 40:214-16

45. Ong JM, Kirchegessner TG, Schatz MC, et al. Insulin increases the synthetic rate and messenger RNA level of lipoprotein lipase in isolated rat adipocytes. *J Biol Chem* 1988; 263: 12933-8

46. Barnard RJ, Youngren JE. Regulation of glucose transport in skeletal muscle. *FASEB J* 1992; 6:3238-44.

47. Fryer LG, Kruszynska YT. Insulin resistance in high fat fed rats. Role of glucose transporters, membrane lipids, and triglyceride stores. *Ann NY Acad Sci* 1993; 683:91-7

48. Boyd JJ, Contreras I, Kern M, et al. Effect of a high-fat-sucrose diet on in vivo insulin receptor kinase activation. *Am J Physiol* 1990; 259:E111-E116

49. Iwanishi M, Kobayashi M. Effect of pioglitazone on insulin receptors of skeletal muscles from high-fat-fed rats. *Metabolism* 1993; 42:1017-21

50. Scheck SH, Barnard RJ, Lawani LO, et al. Effects of NIDDM on the glucose transport system in human skeletal muscle. *Diabetes Res* 1991; 16:111-9

51. Anderson JW, Gustafson NJ, Bryant CA, et al. Dietary fiber and diabetes: a comprehensive review and practical application. *J Am Diet Assoc* 1987; 87:1189-97

52. Fukagawa NK, Anderson JW, Hogeman G, et al. High-carbo-hydrate, high-fiber diets increase peripheral insulin sensitivity in healthy young and old adults. *Am J Clin Nutr* 1990; 52:524-8

53. Ivy JL. The insulin-like effect of muscle contraction. *Exercise Sport Sci Rev* 1987; 15:29-51

54. Brozinick JT, Etgen GJ, Yaspelkis BB, et al. Contraction activated glucose uptake is normal in insulin-resistant muscle of the obese Zucker rat. *J Appl Physiol* 1992; 73:382-8

55. Devlin JT, Hirshman M, Horton ED, et al. Enhanced peripheral and splanchnic insulin sensitivity in NIDDM men after a single bout of exercise. *Diabetes* 1987; 36:434-9

56. Burstein R, Epstein Y, Shapiro Y, et al. Effect of an acute bout of exercise on glucose disposal in human obesity. *J Appl Physiol* 1990; 69:299-304

57. Mikines KJ. The influence of physical activity and inactivity on insulin action and secretion in man. *Acta Physiol Scand* 1992; 146 Suppl. 609:1-43

58. Ivy JL, Brozinick JR, Torgan CE, et al. Skeletal muscle glucose transport in obese Zucker rats after exercise training. *J Appl Physiol* 1989; 66:2635-41

59. Willems MET, Brozinick JT, Torgan CE, et al. Muscle glucose uptake of obese Zucker rats trained at two different intensities. *J Appl Physiol* 1991; 70:36-42

60. Kraegen EW, Storlien LH, Jenkins AB, et al. Chronic exercise compensates for insulin resistance induced by a high fat diet in rats. *Am J Physiol* 1989; 256:E242-E249

61. Wallberg-Henricksson H. Exercise and diabetes mellitus. *Exer Spon Sci Rev* 1992; 20:339-68

62. Rogers MA, Yamamoto C, King DS, et al. Improvement in glucose tolerance after 1 week of exercise in patients with NIDDM. *Diabetes Care* 1988; 11:613-8

63. Després J-P, Prud'Homme D, Tremblay A, et al. Contribution of low intensity exercise training to treatment of abdominal obesity. In: Guy-Grand B, Ricquier D, Lafontan M, et al., editors. *Importance of 'metabolic fitness' in obesity in Europe 91.* London: John Libby, 1992:177-81

64. Helmrich SP, Ragland DR, Leung RW, et al. Physical activity and reduced occurrence of non-insulin-dependent diabetes mellitus. *N Engl J Med* 1991; 325:147-52

65. Manson JE, Rimm EB, Stampfer MJ, et al. Physical activity and incidence of non-insulin-dependent diabetes mellitus in women. *Lancet* 1991; 338:774-8

66. Manson JE, Nathan DM, Krolewski AS, et al. A prospective study of exercise and incidence of diabetes among US male physicians. *JAMA* 1992; 268:63-7

67. Després J-P, Moorjani S, Tremblay A, et al. Heredity and changes in plasma lipids and lipoproteins after short-term exercise training in men. *Arteriosclerosis* 1988; 8:402-9

68. Després J-P, Trembley A, Nadaeu A, et al. Physical training and changes in regional adipose tissue distribution. *Acta Med Scand* 1988; Suppl. 723:205-12

69. Després J-P, Pouliot MC, Moorjani S, et al. Loss of abdominal fat and metabolic response to training in obese women. *Am J Physiol* 1991; 261:E159-E167

70. Lampman RM, Santinga JT, Bassett DR, et al. Effectiveness of unsupervised and supervised high intensity physical training in normalizing serum lipids in men with type IV hyperlipoproteinemia. *Circulation* 1978; 57:172-80

71. Lampman RM, Santinga JT, Savage PJ, et al. Effect of exercise training on glucose tolerance, in vivo insulin sensitivity, lipid and lipoprotein concentrations in middle-aged men with mild hypertriglyceridemia. *Metabolism* 1985; 34:205-11

72. Lampman RM, Schteingart DE, Santinga JT, et al. The influence of physical training on glucose tolerance, insulin sensitivity, and lipid and lipoprotein concentrations in middle-aged

hypertriglyceridemic, carbohydrate intolerant men. *Diabetologia* 1987; 30:380-5

73. Bouchard C, Shephard RJ, Stephens T. *Physical activity, fitness and health. International proceedings and consensus statement.* Champaign: Human Kinetics Publishers, 1994:417-683

74. Baumstark MU, Frey I, Berg A. Acute and delayed effects of prolonged exercise on serum lipoproteins II. Concentration and composition of low density lipoprotein subfractions and very low-density lipoproteins. *Europ J Appl Physiol* 1993; 66:526-30

75. Lamon-Fava S, McNamara JR, Farber HW, et al. Acute changes in lipid lipoprotein, apolipoprotein, and low-density lipoprotein particle size after an endurance triathlon. *Metabolism* 1989; 38:921-5

76. Lamon-Fava S, Fischer EC, Nelson ME, et al. Effect of exercise and menstrual cycle status on plasma lipids, low density lipoprotein particle size, and apolipoproteins. *J Clin Endocrinol Metab* 1989; 68:17-21

77. Williams PT, Krauss RM, Wood PD, et al. Lipoprotein subfractions of runners and sedentary men. *Metabolism* 1986, 35:45-52

78. Williams PT, Krauss RM, Vranizan KM, et al. Changes in lipoprotein subfractions during diet-induced weight loss in moderately overweight men. *Circulation* 1990; 81:1293-1304

79. Williams PT, Krauss RM, Vranizan KM, et al. Effects of exercise-induced weight loss on low density lipoprotein subfractions in healthy men. *Arteriosclerosis* 1989; 9:623-32

80. Coulston AM, Hollenbeck CB, Swislock ALM. Deleterious metabolic effects of high-carbohydrate, sucrose-containing diets in patients with non-insulin dependent diabetes mellitus. *Am J Med* 1987; 82:213-20

81. Coulston AM, Hollenbeck CB, Suislocki ALM, et al. Persistence of hypertriglyceridemic effect of low-fat, high-carbohydrate diets in NIDDM patients. *Diabetes Care* 1989; 12:94-101

82. Rivellese AA, Giacco R, Genovese S, et al. Effects of changing amount of carbohydrate in diet on plasma lipoproteins and apoproteins in type II patients. *Diabetes Care* 1990; 13:446-8

83. Fuh MMT, Lee MMS, Jeng CY, et al. Effect of low fat-high carbohydrate diet in hypertensive patients with non-insulin-dependent diabetes mellitus. *Am J Hypertens* 1990; 3:527-32

84. Ullman D, Connor WE, Hatcher LF, et al. Will a high-carbohydrate, low-fat diet lower plasma lipids and lipoproteins without producing hypertriglyceridemia? *Arterioscler Thromb* 1991; 11:1059-67

85. Brinton EA, Eisenberg S, Breslow JL. A low-fat diet decreases high density lipoprotein (HDL) cholesterol levels by decreasing HDL apoprotein transport rates. *J Clin Invest* 1990; 85:144-51

86. Trowell H. Hypertension, obesity, diabetes mellitus and coronary heart disease. In: Trowell HC, Burkitt DP editors. *Western diseases: their emergence and prevention*. London: Edward Arnold, 1981:3-32

87. Wright A, Burstyn PE Gibney MJ. Dietary fiber and blood pressure. *BMJ* 1979; 2:1541-3

88. Anderson JW. Plant fiber and blood pressure. *Ann Intern Med* 1983; 98:842-6

89. Iacono JM, Binder RA, Marshall MW, et al. Decreased susceptibility to thrombin and collagen platelet aggregation in man fed a low fat diet. *Haemostasis* 1974; 3:306-18

90. Marckmann P, Sandström B, Jespersen J. Favorable long-term effect of a low-fat/high-fiber diet on human blood coagulation and fibrinolysis. *Arterioscler Thromb* 1993; 13:505-11

91. Steele E, Rainwater J. Effect of dietary and pharmacologic alteration of serum lipids on platelet survival time. *Circulation* 1978; 58:365-7

92. Goodnight SHJ, Harris WS, Connor WE. The effects of dietary W3 fatty acids on platelet composition and function in men: a prospective controlled study. *Blood* 1981; 58;880-5

93. Siess W, Roth P, Scherer B, et al. Platelet membrane fatty acids platelet aggregation and thromboxane formation during a mackerel diet. *Lancet* 1980; I:441-4

94. Dyerberg J, Bang HO. Haemostatic function and polyunsaturated fatty acids in Eskimos. *Lancet* 1979; II:433-5

95. Barnard RJ. Effects of life-style modification on serum lipids. *Arch Intern Med* 1991; 151:1389-94

96. Barnard RJ, Guzy PM, Rosenberg JM, et al. Effects of an intensive exercise and nutrition program on patients with coronary artery disease: five-year follow-up. *J Cardiac Rehab* 1983; 3:183-90

97. Barnard RJ, Massey MR, Cherny S, et al. Long-term use of a high-complex-carbohydrate, high-fiber diet and exercise in the treatment of NIDDM patients. *Diabetes Care* 1983; 6:268-73

98. Barnard RJ, Zifferblatt SM, Rosenberg IM, et al. Effects of a high-complex-carbohydrate diet and daily walking on blood pressure and medication status of hypertensive patients. *J Cardiac Rehab* 1983; 3:839-46

99. Barnard RJ, Hall JA, Chaudhari A, et al. Effects of a low-fat low-cholesterol diet on serum lipids, platelet aggregation and thromboxane formation. *Prostaglandins Leukotrienes Med* 1987; 26:241-52

100. Mehrabian M, Peter JB, Barnard RJ, et al. Dietary regulation of fibrinolytic factors. *Atherosclerosis* 1990; 84:25-32

Correspondence and reprints: Dr. R. James Barnard, Department of Physiological Science, UCLA 2322 Life Sciences Bldg, 405 Hilgard Avenue, Los Angeles, CA 90024-1527 USA

by R. James Barnard and Stephen J. Wen
Department of Physiological Science,
University of California
Los Angeles, California, USA

Chapter 15

Determining When Anti-Diabetic Medication Is Necessary

Diet. Exercise. Been there? Done that? Still have blood glucose levels that aren't quite what you'd like? Then it may be time for diabetes pills.

Docs call diabetes pills "oral agents." Oral agents are an addition to—not a substitute for—a good diet and exercise. You and your doctor should consider oral agents when, despite your best efforts at losing excess weight, getting regular exercise, and eating a healthy diet,

- your blood glucose levels before breakfast are over 140 mg/dl
- your blood glucose levels before bedtime are over 160 mg/dl, or
- your HbA1C is over 8 percent (2 points over the upper limit of normal).

You could also use insulin to get better glucose control, but your doctor will probably want to try oral agents first, unless your blood glucose levels are extremely high. In particular, oral agents are preferred if you're obese, because you would need large doses of insulin, and insulin treatment tends to promote weight gain even more than certain oral agents do. The older you are, the greater the chance that an oral agent will be the first medication prescribed for diabetes care. That's because they cause fewer low blood glucose reactions than insulin, and because pills are easier to take.

"Pill Time," by Robert Sherwin; reprinted with permission from *Diabetes Forecast*. Copyright © 1996 American Diabetes Association.

There are three classes of oral agents for diabetes control:

Sulfonylureas (sul-fa-nil-YUR-ee-ahs). Most diabetes pills are sulfonylureas, which have been available in the United States for 40 years. They lower blood glucose mainly by stimulating the pancreas to produce more insulin. For these pills to work, your pancreas must still be making insulin. These pills don't work for people with type I diabetes, whose bodies don't make any insulin.

Most sulfonylureas are broken down by your liver and excreted by your kidneys. If you have liver or kidney problems, there are some sulfonylureas that you shouldn't use because the drug won't be eliminated from your body properly.

Sulfonylureas may make your blood glucose level drop too low (under 70 mg/dl). This is called hypoglycemia. It can happen if, for example, you skip meals or drink too much alcohol.

You may gain some weight when you start taking sulfonylureas, but probably not as much as you might if you used insulin.

People who are allergic to sulfa drugs should be cautious about using sulfonylureas.

Biguanides (by-GWAN-ides). The biguanide metformin has been used by people with diabetes worldwide for almost 40 years. It's been on the market in the United States for a year.

Metformin lowers blood glucose mainly by keeping your liver from releasing too much glucose. In contrast to sulfonylureas, metformin doesn't raise insulin levels. so under ordinary circumstances, it doesn't cause hypoglycemia. Another advantage: Some people find that they lose a little weight when they start taking metformin.

Alpha-Glucosidase Inhibitor (al-fa glu-KAH-sid-ase). Acarbose (AK-erbose) is an alpha-glucosidase inhibitor that went on the market earlier this year [1996]. It interferes with carbohydrate digestion. When taken with meals, it keeps blood glucose from rising so quickly after meals. It may also prove useful for people who have type I diabetes, when they use it with their usual insulin doses.

Which Drug?

You and your doctor will consider many things in deciding which oral agent you should take.

Do you have kidney problems? The sulfonylurea tolbutamide is broken down completely by the liver. No active drug reaches the kidneys. Therefore, tolbutamide may be a good choice for you.

In addition, tolbutamide is less likely to cause hypoglycemia than other sulfonylureas, because it doesn't hang around in the body a long time. But tolbutamide needs to be taken two or three times a day. If your reaction is "Three times a day?! Forget it!", tolbutamide might not be your best choice.

Have you had hypoglycemia when taking a sulfonylurea? Then you may want to give metformin a shot. Metformin doesn't cause hypoglycemia.

Do you have a high triglyceride level? Metformin may help lower your triglycerides while it helps you control your blood glucose.

Do you have a serious weight problem? You may be less likely to gain weight if you take metformin than if you take a sulfonylurea.

Although metformin has many good points, it's not the drug for everyone. If you have kidney disease, you shouldn't take metformin. People with kidney disease are at risk of developing a serious condition called lactic acidosis if they take metformin.

Is your main problem high glucose after meals? Acarbose can blunt these changes and is relatively safe.

What other medications do you take? Some of these may interact with certain diabetes pills. These interactions may make one or the other drug less effective, or lead to side effects. Tell your doctor all the other drugs you take. Don't forget alcohol and any over-the-counter medications. To give an example, large doses of aspirin can affect the way sulfonylureas work.

Is cost an issue? If your medical condition allows you the pick of any of the drugs, you might want to consider price. All but one of the sulfonylureas are available as generics, which often cost much less than the brand-named version.

The Choice Is Made

You and your doctor have decided which pill you're going to try. Now what?

Ask your doctor or pharmacist what side effects are possible and what you should do about them. For example, some people complain about a metallic taste when they first start taking metformin. Metformin and acarbose may cause nausea or diarrhea. Side effects of sulfonylureas include nausea and vomiting.

If you think a drug is causing side effects, or you've read about side effects that concern you, don't simply stop taking the drug. Consult your doctor or pharmacist.

Table 15.1. Oral Agents

Sulfonylurias

- Generic Name: tolbutamide
- Available as Generic: yes
- Brand Name: Orinase
- Short, Intermediate or Long Acting? Short
- How Often Do I Need to Take It? 2 or 3 times a day
- Comments: May be a good choice if you have kidney problems. Doesn't last long in the body, so the risk of hypoglycemia is lower than with some of the other sulfonylureas. Not a good choice if you often forget to take pills.

- Generic Name: tolazamide
- Available as Generic: yes
- Brand Name: Tolinase
- Short, Intermediate or Long Acting? Intermediate
- How Often Do I Need to Take It? 1 or 2 times a day

- Generic Name: glyburide
- Available as Generic: yes
- Brand Names: DiaBeta, Micronase, Glynase PresTab
- Short, Intermediate or Long Acting? Intermediate
- How Often Do I Need to Take It? 1 or 2 times a day
- Comments: Intermediate-acting, but effects may last entire day. Glynase PresTab is new and more readily absorbed than the other preparations.

- Generic Name: acetohexamide
- Available as Generic: yes
- Brand Name: Dymelor
- Short, Intermediate or Long Acting? Intermediate
- How Often Do I Need to Take It? 1 or 2 times a day

- Generic Name: glipizide
- Available as Generic: yes
- Brand Names: Glucotrol, Glucotrol XL
- Short, Intermediate or Long Acting? Intermediate and long-acting formulas
- How Often Do I Need to Take It? 1 or 2 times a day
- Comments: Appears to be more effective when taken before meals.

- Generic Name: chlorpropamide
- Available as Generic: yes
- Brand Name: Diabinese
- Short, Intermediate or Long Acting? Long
- How Often Do I Need to Take It? Once a day
- Comments: With this sulfonylurea in particular: If you drink alcohol, you may bet a tingling in your neck and arms, red eyes, and flushed face. Hypoglycemia is more of a problem, as this drug is eliminated by the kidneys slowly; therefore may not be a good choice for the elderly or people with kidney disease.

- Generic Name: glimepiride
- Available as Generic: no
- Brand Name: Amaryl
- Short, Intermediate or Long Acting? Long
- How Often Do I Need to Take It? Once a day
- Comments: Approved for marketing in the U.S. in December 1995. The company expects it to be available in April [1996].

Biguanide

- Generic Name: metformin
- Available as Generic: no
- Brand Name: Glucophage
- Short, Intermediate or Long Acting? Intermediate
- How Often Do I Need to Take It? 2 or 3 times a day
- Comments: Under usual circumstances, doesn't cause hypoglycemia. Doesn't promote weight gain. May cause low B_{12} levels. Need to build up dose slowly and take with meals to minimize gastrointestinal side effects. In very rare cases, especially if kidney disease is present, can produce lactic acidosis, a serious complication. Can be used alone or with a sulfonylurea.

Alpha-Glucosidase Inhibitor

- Generic Name: acarbose
- Available as Generic: no
- Brand Name: Precose
- Short, Intermediate or Long Acting? Short
- How Often Do I Need to Take It? 3 times a day, with meals
- Comments: Doesn't cause hypoglycemia or weight gain. Side effects include gas, bloating, and diarrhea. Causes no serious side effects. May cause rise in liver function tests.

If you are going to take a sulfonylurea, ask your doctor or diabetes educator to explain the symptoms and treatment for hypoglycemia, and then tell your family. (See the section titled "Hypoglycemia" below.)

After you start taking your new diabetes pills, it may be helpful for you to test your blood glucose levels daily or every few days. This will show how well your body is responding to this new medication.

Keep records of your blood glucose tests. Your doctor may want you to call in with the results after you've been on the medication for one to two weeks. He or she will raise the dose if necessary. It's important to get to the right dose as quickly as possible. You aren't looking just for relief of the symptoms of high blood glucose but rather good blood glucose control.

Two May Work

If you get up to the maximum recommended dose of an oral agent and still don't have good control, switching to another drug probably won't work. Instead, your doctor may advise using two different medications. This is called combination therapy. Common combinations are a sulfonylurea plus metformin or a sulfonylurea plus acarbose. An oral agent plus insulin might also be used.

No matter which drug your doctor prescribes for you, make sure you take it as prescribed. Also, continue to watch your diet and get regular exercise. These will all help you get blood glucose levels that are near normal, which will help you avoid diabetic complications.

When Pills Don't Work

You use an oral agent and get good blood glucose control for several years. Then it seems the drug isn't working anymore, or not working as well. Your blood glucose levels start creeping up.

Clause: You aren't following your "diet."

Solution: See a dietitian. Dietitians aren't the diet police. A dietitian can help you work out a meal plan that will work with your lifestyle yet still helps you get good control of your blood glucose levels.

Cause: Your diabetes has progressed.

Solution: Try a combination of two different oral agents or use insulin to get good control.

Cause: You've gained weight.

Solution: Lose some of your excess weight. You don't have to get down to your "ideal" weight. Losing just 5 or 10 pounds may be enough to allow your usual diabetes pill to work for you again.

Cause: Your body is suddenly under a lot of stress, for example, you have a heart attack or a major infection.

Solution: Your doctor will switch you to insulin. You may be able to switch back to your usual oral agent after you recover.

Special Case: You get pregnant, or you're planning to.

Solution: Go on insulin. Diabetes pills aren't recommended for pregnant women.

Hypoglycemia

Sulfonylureas may make your blood glucose level drop too low—below 70 mg/dl. This is called hypoglycemia. Some symptoms of hypoglycemia are feeling shaky, confused, or hungry.

If you have symptoms of low blood glucose, you should test your blood glucose level. If it's below 70 mg/dl, or if you can't test your blood, you should eat or drink 15 grams of carbohydrate. Examples:

- 1 cup of skim milk,
- 1/2 can of nondiet soda, or
- 3 teaspoons of sugar.

For more information, see *Forecast*, "Low Blood Glucose Reactions: A Review of the Basics," August 1995, pp. 28-29.

—by Robert Sherwin

Robert Sherwin, MD, is C.N.H. Long Professor of Medicine and director of the Diabetes Endocrinology Research Center at Yale School of Medicine, New Haven. Conn. He is past-president of the ADA Connecticut Affiliate and is now on its board of directors.

Part Three

Adrenal Gland Disorders

Chapter 16

Cushing's Syndrome: The Facts You Need to Know

Cushing's syndrome is a hormonal disorder caused by prolonged exposure of the body's tissues to high levels of the hormone cortisol. Sometimes called "hypercortisolism," it is relatively rare and most commonly affects adults aged 20 to 50. An estimated 10 to 15 of every million people are affected each year.

The Facts You Need to Know

Cushing's Syndrome is a disease caused by an excess of cortisol production or by excessive use of cortisol or other similar steroid (glucocorticoid) hormones.

Cortisol is a normal hormone produced in the outer portion, or cortex, of the adrenal glands, located above each kidney. The normal function of cortisol is to help the body respond to stress and change. It mobilizes nutrients, modifies the body's response to inflammation, stimulates the liver to raise the blood sugar, and it helps control the amount of water in the body. Another adrenal cortex hormone, aldosterone, regulates salt and water levels which affect blood volume and blood pressure. Small amounts of androgens (male hormones) are also normally produced in the adrenal cortex. Cortisol production is regulated

This chapter includes text from "Cushing's Syndrome: The Facts You Need to Know," written by Paul Margulies, M.D., Medical Director, NADF, Clinical Associate Professor of Medicine, Cornell University Medical College for the National Adrenal Diseases Foundation, 505 Northern Boulevard, Great Neck, New York 11021 (516) 487-4992; reprinted with permission.

by adrenocorticotrophic hormone (ACTH), made in the pituitary gland, which is located just below the brain.

When too much cortisol is produced in the adrenal glands, or an excess is taken in treating other diseases, significant changes occur in all of the tissues and organs of the body. All of these effects together are called Cushing's syndrome.

Cushing's disease is the name given to a type of Cushing's syndrome caused by too much ACTH production in the pituitary. Dr. Harvey Cushing first described a woman with signs and symptoms of this disease in 1912, and in 1932 he was able to link the adrenal overproduction of cortisol to an abnormality in the pituitary.

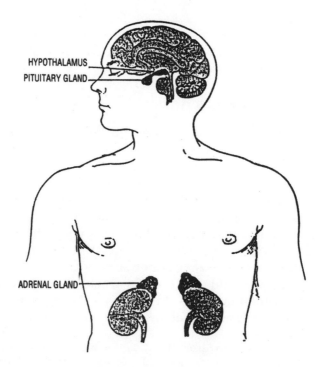

Figure 16.1. *Location of glands important in the development of Cushing's Syndrome.*

What Causes Cushing's Syndrome?

When cortisol or other glucocorticoid hormones (such as hydrocortisone, prednisone, methylprednisolone or dexamethasone) are taken in excess of the normal daily requirement for a prolonged period of time, it causes Cushing's syndrome. This "iatrogenic" (caused by the treatment) form is unfortunately a necessary side effect when high doses of these steroid hormones must be used to treat certain life-threatening illnesses, such as asthma, rheumatoid arthritis, systemic lupus, inflammatory bowel disease, some allergies, and others.

Spontaneous overproduction of cortisol in the adrenals is divided into two groups—those due to an excess of ACTH and those that are independent of ACTH. A pituitary tumor producing too much ACTH, stimulating the adrenals to grow (hyperplasia) and to produce too much cortisol is the most common type, and this is called Cushing's disease. It is the cause of 70% of spontaneous Cushing's syndrome. ACTH can also be produced outside the pituitary in a benign or malignant tumor in the lung, thymus gland, pancreas, or other organ. This is called "ectopic" ACTH production.

When the source of excess cortisol production is a tumor of the adrenal gland itself, then it is not dependent on ACTH. The tumor makes cortisol on its own, and the other adrenal gland shrinks because ACTH production is suppressed. Adrenal cortex tumors can be benign (an adenoma), or malignant (a carcinoma) and are usually found on only one side. A very rare type is caused by multiple benign adenomas on both sides.

Although almost all types of spontaneous Cushing's syndrome are ultimately caused by one type of tumor or another, little is known about what makes these tumors occur. There does not appear to be any specific genetic, immune, or environmental factor.

How Common Is Cushing's Syndrome?

Iatrogenic. Cushing's syndrome from taking steroid medication is extremely common because of the widespread use of these medicines in treating many illnesses.

Spontaneous. Cushing's syndrome and Cushing's disease can occur in children and adults. Pituitary Cushing's disease generally occurs after puberty with equal frequency in boys and girls. In adults, it has a greater frequency in women than men, with most found a age 25 to 45. The total incidence is about 5 to 25 cases per million people

217

per year. Ectopic ACTH as a cause of Cushing's syndrome is more common because of the high rate of lung cancer (about 660 per million per year), but it often goes unrecognized. The incidence increases with age.

Adrenal tumors are relatively rare, and cause Cushing's syndrome in only 2 people per million per year for both adenomas and carcinomas. Both are also 4 to 5 times more common in women than men.

What Are the Symptoms and Signs of Cushing's Syndrome?

Cortisol excess produces significant and serious changes in the appearance and health of affected individuals. Depending on the cause and duration of the Cushing's syndrome, some people may have more dramatic changes, some might look more masculinized, some may have more blood pressure or weight changes.

General physical features include a tendency to gain weight, especially on the abdomen, face (moon face), neck and upper back (buffalo hump), thinning and weakness of the muscles of the upper arms and upper legs; thinning of the skin, with easy bruising and pink or purple stretch marks (striae) on the abdomen, thighs, breasts and shoulders; increased acne, facial hair growth, and scalp hair loss in women; sometimes a ruddy complexion on the face and neck; often a skin darkening (acanthosis) on the neck. Children will show obesity and poor growth in height.

On physical examination, a physician will notice these changes and will also usually find high blood pressure and evidence of muscle weakness in the upper arms and legs, and sometimes some enlargement of the clitoris in females.

Symptoms usually include fatigue, weakness, depression, mood swings, increased thirst and urination, and lack of menstrual periods in women.

Common findings on routine laboratory tests in people with Cushing's syndrome include a higher white blood count, a high blood sugar (often into the diabetic range), and a low serum potassium. These will often reinforce a physician's suspicion about Cushing's syndrome. Ectopic Cushing's syndrome tends to present with less impressive classic features, but more dramatic hypertension and loss of potassium, sometimes in the setting of weight loss from the underlying cancer.

If untreated, Cushing's syndrome will cause continued weakening of the muscles, fatigue, poor skin healing, weakening of the bones of the spine (osteoporosis), and increased susceptibility to some infections including pneumonia and TB.

How Is Cushing's Syndrome Diagnosed?

Most people who appear to have some of the classic physical features of Cushing's syndrome (cushingoid appearance) do not actually have the disease. After iatrogenic Cushing's is excluded, other causes of this appearance can be: polycystic ovary syndrome (androgen excess from the ovaries), ovarian tumors, congenital adrenal hyperplasia, ordinary obesity, excessive alcohol consumption, or just a family tendency to have a round face and abdomen with high blood pressure and high blood sugar.

Because Cushing's syndrome is a rare but serious disorder, it is very important to carefully exclude (rule out) other disorders and then separate the different types, leading eventually to a specific cause that can be treated. This process of testing and excluding usually takes days to weeks and requires a lot of patience and cooperation by the person being tested.

After the initial history, physical exam and routine blood tests, the first step is to prove cortisol excess with specific blood and 24 hour urine tests for cortisol. Inappropriate cortisol production will then be evaluated by doing a dexamethasone suppression test. Dexamethasone (steroid) pills are given by mouth, then blood and urine are collected for cortisol and other adrenal hormones. A screening test might be done initially with an overnight test, but if it is abnormal, usually a 4 day test divided into low and high dose dexamethasone is needed. To separate ACTH dependent from independent types, a blood test for ACTH in the morning is done. Blood and urine tests for adrenal androgens are useful. Testing with other drugs, such as, metyrapone and CRH (corticotropin releasing hormone) may also be needed.

Once all of the blood and urine results are analyzed, they will establish whether some type of Cushing's syndrome is present, and should indicate whether the disease is ACTH dependent (pituitary or ectopic) or independent (an adrenal tumor). Localizing techniques such as CT or MRI are then used to find the tumor. Often a pituitary tumor is tiny and hard to find, so a special test of the release of ACTH from both sides of the pituitary (petrosal sinus sampling) might be needed. Small tumors producing ectopic ACTH are also sometimes difficult to localize and require repeated scans and x-rays.

How Is Cushing's Syndrome Treated?

If the Cushing's syndrome is a side effect of taking high doses of steroid hormones (iatrogenic), withdrawing these medicines will allow the body to go back to normal. The ability to taper or stop the steroids, however, depends on the type of disease being treated and the pattern of response. Sometimes, steroids cannot be totally stopped or may be reduced only to a limited degree because the illness being treated would worsen. In that case, some degree of persistent Cushing's syndrome would remain as an unwanted side effect. Treatment of the effects of steroid excess would include management of high blood sugar with diet and medications, replacement of potassium, treatment of high blood pressure, early treatment of any infections, adequate calcium intake, and appropriate adjustments in steroid doses at times of acute illness, surgery or injury.

Cushing's disease is best treated with the surgical removal of the pituitary tumor, usually with a technique called transsphenoidal resection (behind the nose) by a neurosurgeon. Occasionally, the entire pituitary gland will need to be removed or injured in order to cure the Cushing's disease, leaving the person with a deficiency of ACTH and the other pituitary hormones. This can be treated by giving replacement hormones for cortisol, thyroid and gonadal (sex) hormones. Fertility can be restored with special hormonal therapies. If the pituitary tumor cannot be removed, radiation therapy to the pituitary can be used, but the improvement in the Cushing's syndrome is much slower. Before transsphenoidal surgery became available, the surgical removal of both adrenal glands was common, but this always produced adrenal insufficiency and sometimes caused large ACTH producing pituitary tumors to grow (called Nelson's syndrome). That is why pituitary surgery rather than adrenal surgery is usually preferred for Cushing's disease.

Ectopic ACTH producing tumors are usually malignant (cancer). Removing this cancer or treating it with radiation or chemotherapy may help in improving the Cushing's syndrome. If the tumor is benign, or it can be completely removed, surgery may be a cure. Most of the time, reduction of the cortisol production from the adrenals with medications such as metyrapone, aminoglutethimide or ketoconazole is useful while the ACTH- producing tumor is treated.

Adrenal adenomas are always treated by surgically removing the tumor with either an abdominal or side (flank) incision. The other adrenal is left in, and will grow back to normal size or function. After the surgery, replacement steroid hormones are given and slowly tapered over a few months as the remaining adrenal responds to the normal ACTH production from the pituitary.

Adrenal carcinomas (cancer) can be cured if removed early. Unfortunately, they are usually discovered after they have already spread beyond the adrenal gland and are then not curable. Chemotherapy including o, p'DDD and other medicines are often used to try to control the tumor but do not cure it. The excess cortisol production can be controlled with o, p'DDD or other medications like those mentioned for ectopic ACTH production: metyrapone, aminoglutethimide and ketoconazole. These medicines can be used to treat any form of inoperable or incurable Cushing's syndrome, including Cushing's disease, but they can have serious side effects and require very careful monitoring and balancing with steroid hormone replacement therapies. Surgical cure of the primary cause of the Cushing's syndrome is always the best, if possible.

How Normal Is a Cushing's Patient's Life?

The symptoms, disabilities, and life-style of a person with Cushing's syndrome depend on the degree of cortisol excess, the duration of the disease, the basic health of the person, but especially the type and curability of the Cushing's syndrome. If it is cured, all of the features of the disease can resolve, but this may take as long as 2 to 18 months. During that time, most people get annoyed and frustrated by the slow improvements in physical changes and the combination of Cushing's and adrenal insufficiency signs and symptoms (dizziness, weakness, nausea, loss of appetite) as replacement steroid hormones are tapered and adrenal hormone production slowly improves toward normal. Frequent calls and visits to physicians are necessary.

If the Cushing's syndrome is incurable, or if iatrogenic Cushing's syndrome must remain, these individuals will have to cope with persistent fatigue, muscle weakness, abdominal and facial weight gain, depression, mood swings, and all the other signs and symptoms mentioned earlier. Regular visits to a physician for examinations, blood tests, and treatments of infections and complications will be necessary and are often viewed as a severe burden.

Why Consult an Endocrinologist?

Iatrogenic Cushing's syndrome is generally managed by the physician prescribing the steroid hormones for the primary illness, such as asthma, arthritis or inflammatory bowel disease. Sometimes physicians are able to decrease steroid doses by using other drugs in the treatment of these diseases.

All of the types of spontaneous Cushing's syndrome should be carefully evaluated by an endocrinologist (a specialist in hormonal disease) who has the knowledge and experience in choosing the correct diagnostic studies and evaluating the results. Finding the correct diagnosis often requires prolonged testing and even repetition of tests. Quick shortcuts can be misleading. Referrals for surgery or radiation should be coordinated by the endocrinologist, who will also be directly involved in managing the patient afterwards.

Chapter 17

Cushing's Syndrome: Tests, Treatments, and Research

Tests

Diagnosis of Cushing's Syndrome is based on a review of the patient's medical history, physical examination and laboratory tests. Often x-ray exams of the adrenal or pituitary glands are useful for locating tumors. These tests help to determine if excess levels of cortisol are present and why.

24-Hour Urinary Free Cortisol Level

This is the most specific diagnostic test. The patient's urine is collected over a 24-hour period and tested for the amount of cortisol. Levels higher than 50-100 micrograms a day for an adult suggest Cushing's syndrome. The normal upper limit varies in different laboratories, depending on which measurement technique is used.

Once Cushing's syndrome has been diagnosed, other tests are used to find the exact location of the abnormality that leads to excess cortisol production. The choice of test depends, in part, on the preference of the endocrinologist or the center where the test is performed.

Dexamethasone Suppression Test

This test helps to distinguish patients with excess production of ACTH due to pituitary adenomas from those with ectopic ACTH-producing

This chapter includes text from "Cushing's Syndrome," NIH Pub. No. 96-3007, June 1996; and "Cushing's Syndrome Specialists," National Institute of Diabetes and Digestive and Kidney Diseases (NIDDK).

tumors. Patients are given dexamethasone, a synthetic glucocorticoid, by mouth every 6 hours for 4 days. For the first 2 days, low doses of dexamethasone are given, and for the last 2 days, higher doses are given. Twenty-four hour urine collections are made before dexamethasone is administered and on each day of the test. Since cortisol and other glucocorticoids signal the pituitary to lower secretion of ACTH, the normal response after taking dexamethasone is a drop in blood and urine cortisol levels. Different responses of cortisol to dexamethasone are obtained depending on whether the cause of Cushing's syndrome is a pituitary adenoma or an ectopic ACTH-producing tumor.

The dexamethasone suppression test can produce false-positive results in patients with depression, alcohol abuse, high estrogen levels, acute illness, and stress. Conversely, drugs such as phenytoin and phenobarbital may cause false-negative results in response to dexamethasone suppression. For this reason, patients are usually advised by their physicians to stop taking these drugs at least one week before the test.

CRH Stimulation Test

This test helps to distinguish between patients with pituitary adenomas and those with ectopic ACTH syndrome or cortisol-secreting adrenal tumors. Patients are given an injection of CRH, the corticotropin-releasing hormone which causes the pituitary to secrete ACTH. Patients with pituitary adenomas usually experience a rise in blood levels of ACTH and cortisol. This response is rarely seen in patients with ectopic ACTH syndrome and practically never in patients with cortisol-secreting adrenal tumors.

Direct Visualization of the Endocrine Glands (Radiologic Imaging)

Imaging tests reveal the size and shape of the pituitary and adrenal glands and help determine if a tumor is present. The most common are the CT (computerized tomography) scan and MRI (magnetic resonance imaging). A CT scan produces a series of x-ray pictures giving a cross-sectional image of a body part. MRI also produces images of the internal organs of the body but without exposing the patient to ionizing radiation.

Imaging procedures are used to find a tumor after a diagnosis has been established. Imaging is not used to make the diagnosis of Cushing's syndrome because benign tumors, sometimes called "incidentalomas," are commonly found in the pituitary and adrenal glands.

These tumors do not produce hormones detrimental to health and are not removed unless blood tests show they are a cause of symptoms or they are unusually large. Conversely, pituitary tumors are not detected by imaging in almost 50 percent of patients who ultimately require pituitary surgery for Cushing's syndrome.

Petrosal Sinus Sampling

This test is not always required, but in many cases, it is the best way to separate pituitary from ectopic causes of Cushing's syndrome. Samples of blood are drawn from the petrosal sinuses, veins which drain the pituitary, by introducing catheters through a vein in the upper thigh/groin region, with local anesthesia and mild sedation. X-rays are used to confirm the correct position of the catheters. Often CRH, the hormone which causes the pituitary to secrete ACTH, is given during this test to improve diagnostic accuracy. Levels of ACTH in the petrosal sinuses are measured and compared with ACTH levels in a forearm vein. ACTH levels higher in the petrosal sinuses than in the forearm vein indicate the presence of a pituitary adenoma; similar levels suggest ectopic ACTH syndrome.

The Dexamethasone-CRH Test

Some individuals have high cortisol levels, but do not develop the progressive effects of Cushing's syndrome, such as muscle weakness, fractures and thinning of the skin. These individuals may have Pseudo Cushing's syndrome, which was originally described in people who were depressed or drank excess alcohol, but is now known to be more common. Pseudo Cushing's does not have the same long-term effects on health as Cushing's syndrome and does not require treatment directed at the endocrine glands. Although observation over months to years will distinguish Pseudo Cushing's from Cushing's, the dexamethasone-CRH test was developed to distinguish between the conditions rapidly, so that Cushing's patients can receive prompt treatment. This test combines the dexamethasone suppression and the CRH stimulation tests. Elevations of cortisol during this test suggest Cushing's syndrome.

Some patients may have sustained high cortisol levels without the effects of Cushing's syndrome. These high cortisol levels may be compensating for the body's resistance to cortisol's effects. This rare syndrome of cortisol resistance is a genetic condition that causes hypertension and chronic androgen excess.

Sometimes other conditions may be associated with many of the symptoms of Cushing's syndrome. These include polycystic ovarian syndrome, which may cause menstrual disturbances, weight gain from adolescence, excess hair growth and sometimes impaired insulin action and diabetes. Commonly, weight gain, high blood pressure and abnormal levels of cholesterol and triglycerides in the blood are associated with resistance to insulin action and diabetes; this has been described as the "Metabolic Syndrome-X." Patients with these disorders do not have abnormally elevated cortisol levels.

How Is Cushing's Syndrome Treated?

Treatment depends on the specific reason for cortisol excess and may include surgery, radiation, chemotherapy or the use of cortisol-inhibiting drugs. If the cause is long-term use of glucocorticoid hormones to treat another disorder, the doctor will gradually reduce the dosage to the lowest dose adequate for control of that disorder. Once control is established, the daily dose of glucocorticoid hormones may be doubled and given on alternate days to lessen side effects.

Pituitary Adenomas. Several therapies are available to treat the ACTH-secreting pituitary adenomas of Cushing's disease. The most widely used treatment is surgical removal of the tumor, known as transsphenoidal adenomectomy. Using a special microscope and very fine instruments, the surgeon approaches the pituitary gland through a nostril or an opening made below the upper lip. Because this is an extremely delicate procedure, patients are often referred to centers specializing in this type of surgery. The success, or cure, rate of this procedure is over 80 percent when performed by a surgeon with extensive experience. If surgery fails, or only produces a temporary cure, surgery can be repeated, often with good results. After curative pituitary surgery, the production of ACTH drops two levels below normal. This is a natural, but temporary, drop in ACTH production, and patients are given a synthetic form of cortisol (such as hydrocortisone or prednisone). Most patients can stop this replacement therapy in less than a year.

For patients in whom transsphenoidal surgery has failed or who are not suitable candidates for surgery, radiotherapy is another possible treatment. Radiation to the pituitary gland is given over a 6-week period, with improvement occurring in 40 to 50 percent of adults and up to 80 percent of children. It may take several months or years before patients feel better from radiation treatment alone. However, the combination of radiation and the drug mitotane (Lysodren®) can help speed recovery. Mitotane suppresses cortisol production and lowers plasma and urine hormone levels. Treatment with mitotane alone can be successful in 30 to 40 percent of patients. Other drugs used alone or in combination to control the production of excess cortisol are aminoglutethimide, metyrapone, trilostane and ketoconazole. Each has its own side effects that doctors consider when prescribing therapy for individual patients.

Ectopic ACTH Syndrome. To cure the overproduction of cortisol caused by ectopic ACTH syndrome, it is necessary to eliminate all of the cancerous tissue that is secreting ACTH. The choice of cancer treatment—surgery, radiotherapy, chemotherapy, immunotherapy, or a combination of these treatments—depends on the type of cancer and how far it has spread. Since ACTH-secreting tumors (for example, small cell lung cancer) may be very small or widespread at the time of diagnosis, cortisol-inhibiting drugs, like mitotane, are an important part of treatment. In some cases, if pituitary surgery is not successful, surgical removal of the adrenal glands (bilateral adrenalectomy) may take the place of drug therapy.

Adrenal Tumors. Surgery is the mainstay of treatment for benign as well as cancerous tumors of the adrenal glands. In Primary Pigmented Micronodular Adrenal Disease and the familial Carney's complex, surgical removal of the adrenal glands is required.

What Research Is Being Done on Cushing's Syndrome?

The National Institutes of Health (NIH) is the biomedical research component of the Federal Government. It is one of the health agencies of the Public Health Service, which is part of the U.S. Department of Health and Human Services. Several components of the NIH conduct and support research on Cushing's syndrome and other disorders of the endocrine system, including the National Institute of Diabetes and Digestive and Kidney Diseases (NIDDK), the National Institute of Child Health and Human Development (NICHD), the National Institute of Neurological Disorders and Stroke (NINDS), and the National Cancer Institute (NCI).

NIH-supported scientists are conducting intensive research into the normal and abnormal function of the major endocrine glands and the many hormones of the endocrine system. Identification of the corticotropin releasing hormone (CRH), which instructs the pituitary gland to release ACTH, enabled researchers to develop the CRH stimulation test, which is increasingly being used to identify the cause of Cushing's syndrome.

Improved techniques for measuring ACTH permit distinction of ACTH-dependent forms of Cushing's syndrome from adrenal tumors. NIH studies have shown that petrosal sinus sampling is a very accurate test to diagnose the cause of Cushing's syndrome in those who have excess ACTH production. The recently described dexamethasone suppression-CRH test is able to differentiate most cases of Cushing's from Pseudo Cushing's.

As a result of this research, doctors are much better able to diagnose Cushing's syndrome and distinguish among the causes of this disorder. Since accurate diagnosis is still a problem for some patients, new tests are under study to further refine the diagnostic process.

Many studies are underway to understand the causes of formation of benign endocrine tumors, such as those which cause most cases of Cushing's syndrome. In a few pituitary adenomas, specific gene defects have been identified and may provide important clues to understanding tumor formation. Endocrine factors may also play a role. There is increasing evidence that tumor formation is a multi-step process. Understanding the basis of Cushing's syndrome will yield new approaches to therapy.

NIH supports research related to Cushing's syndrome at medical centers throughout the United States. Scientists are also treating patients with Cushing's syndrome at the NIH Warren Grant Magnuson Clinical Center in Bethesda, Maryland. Physicians who are interested in referring a patient may contact Dr. George P. Chrousos, Developmental Endocrinology Branch, NICHD, Building 10, Room 10N262, Bethesda, Maryland 20892, telephone (301) 496-4686.

Where Can I Find More Information?

The following materials can be found in medical libraries, many college and university libraries, and through interlibrary loan in most public libraries.

Cooper, Paul R. "Contemporary Diagnosis and Management of Pituitary Adenomas," Park Ridge, Illinois: American Association of Neurological Surgeons, 1991.

DeGroot, Leslie J., ed., *et al*. "Cushing's Syndrome," *Endocrinology*. Vol. 2, Philadelphia: W. B. Saunders Company, 1995. 1741–1769.

Isselbacher, Kurt J., ed., *et al*. "Cushing's Syndrome Etiology," *Harrison's Principles of Internal Medicine*. Vol. 2, No. 13, New York: McGraw-Hill Book Company, 1994. 1960–1965.

Wilson, Jean D., ed, *et al*. "Hyperfunction: Glucocorticoids: Hypercortisolism (Cushing's syndrome)," *Williams Textbook of Endocrinology*, No. 8, Philadelphia: W.B. Saunders, 1992; 536–562.

Conn, R.B., Gomez, T., Chrousos, G.P., "Current Diagnosis," No. 8, Philadelphia: W.B. Saunders 1991, 868–872.

NCI Research Report: Cancer of the Lung. Prepared by the Office of Cancer Communications, National Cancer Institute, NIH Publication No. 93–526.

What Other Resources Are Available?

Cushing's Support and Research Foundation, Inc.
65 East India Row 22B
Boston, Massachusetts 02110
(617) 723-3824 or (617) 723-3674
Louise L. Pace, Founder and President

National Adrenal Diseases Foundation
505 Northern Boulevard
Great Neck, NY 11021
(516) 487-4992

Pituitary Tumor Network Association
16350 Ventura Blvd. #231
Encino, CA 91436
(805) 499-997; (805) 499-1523 Fax

Cushing's Syndrome Specialists

Dr. Andy Hoffman
Department of Endocrinology
Stanford University Hospital
Trailer 1A, #111
3801 Miranda
Palo Alto, **California** 94304
(415) 858-3920

Dr. Richard Horton
Section on Endocrinology
University of Southern California
School of Medicine
2250 Alchzar Street
Los Angeles, **California** 90033
(213) 226-4635

Dr. Schlomo Melmed
Division of Endocrinology
Cedars-Sinai Hospital
8700 Beverly Boulevard, B131
Los Angeles, **California** 90048
(310) 855-4691

Dr. Blake Tyrell
University of California, San Francisco
Metabolic Research Building, Room 114
Health Sciences West
San Francisco, **California** 94143
(415) 476-1364

Dr. Martin Weiss
Department of Neurosurgery
University of Southern California
School of Medicine
2250 Alchzar Street
Los Angeles, **California** 90033
(213) 524-3030

Dr. Charles Wilson
Department of Neurosurgery
University of California, San Francisco
School of Medicine
San Francisco, **California** 94143
(415) 476-1087

Dr. Chester Ridgway
University of Colorado
School of Medicine, B141
4200 East Ninth Avenue
Denver, **Colorado** 80262
(303) 270-8443

Dr. Richard Robbins
Department of Neuroendocrinology
Yale University
Tompkins 5
P.O. Box 3333
New Haven, **Connecticut** 06510
(203) 785-5564

Dr. Ace Lipson
2141 K Street, N.W.
Washington, **D.C.** 20037
(202) 296-3443

Dr. Lawrence Fishman
Department of Medicine (D-26)
University of Miami
School of Medicine
P.O. Box 016760
Miami, **Florida** 33101
(305) 324-3195

Dr. Julio Pita
3659 S. Miami Avenue
#6008
Miami, **Florida** 33133
(305) 854-5432

Dr. George Tindall
Department of Neurosurgery
Medical College of Georgia
1327 Clifton Road
Atlanta, **Georgia** 30322
(404) 321-0111

Dr. John VanGilder
Department of Neurosurgery
University of Iowa
C-42, Building GH
Iowa City, **Iowa** 52242
(319) 356-2772

Dr. Janet Schlechte
Clinical Research
University of Iowa
Room 157, MRF
Iowa City, **Iowa** 52242
(319) 335-8652

Dr. Mark Molitch
Endocrinology Center
Northwestern University
Medical Center
303 E. Chicago Avenue
Chicago, **Illinois** 60611
(312) 908-8023

Dr. Ann Klibanski
Neuro-Endocrine Clinic
Massachusetts General Hospital
15 Parkman
Boston, **Massachusetts** 02114
(617) 726-3872

Dr. Beverly Biller
Neuro-Endocrine Clinic
Massachusetts General Hospital
15 Parkman
Boston, **Massachusetts** 02114
(617) 726-3872

Dr. Nicholas Zervas
Department of Endocrinology
Massachusetts General Hospital
15 Parkman
Boston, **Massachusetts** 02114
(617) 726-8581

Dr. David Schteingart
Department of Endocrinology
University of Michigan
1500 Medical Center
Ann Arbor, **Michigan** 48109
(734) 936-5035

Dr. William Daughaday
Metabolic Division
Washington University
Box 8127
660 S. Euclid
St. Louis, **Missouri** 63110
(314) 362-6914

Dr. David Kleinberg
VA Medical Center
408 First Avenue
Room 16042 West
New York, **New York** 10010
(212) 340-6772

Dr. Harold Carlson
VA Medical Center
Northport, **New York** 11768
(516) 261-4400

Dr. Calman Post
Department of Neurosurgery
Columbia University
710 W. 168th Street
New York, **New York** 10032
(212) 305-5491

Dr. William Malarkey
University of Ohio
School of Medicine
Room N1106, Doan Hall
410 W. 10th Street
Columbus, **Ohio** 43210
(614) 293-8775

Dr. Larry Frohmon
Department of Endocrinology
University of Cincinnati
231 Bethesda
ML 547
Cincinnati, **Ohio** 45267
(513) 558-4444

Dr. Warren Selman
Department of Endocrinology
Case Western Reserve University
2074 Abington Road
Cleveland, **Ohio** 44106
(216) 368-1104

Dr. Lynn Loriaux
Department of Endocrinology
Oregon Health Sciences University
3181 S.W. Sam Jackson Blvd.
L607
Portland, **Oregon** 97201-3098
(503) 494-8459

Dr. Peter Snyder
Department of Endocrinology
University of Pennsylvania
611 Clinical Research
422 Currie Blvd.
Philadelphia, **Pennsylvania** 19104
(215) 662-2300

Dr. David Orth
Department of Endocrinology
Vanderbilt University
Room AA-4206
Nashville, **Tennessee** 37232
(615) 322-6199

Dr. James Griffin
Internal Medicine
University of Texas
5323 Harry Hines Blvd.
Dallas, **Texas** 75235
(214) 688-3494

Dr. Samuel Marynick
3707 Gaston Avenue
Suite 325
Dallas, **Texas** 75246
(214) 828-2444

Dr. Glen Cunningham
Department of Endocrinology
Baylor College of Medicine
1 Baylor Plaza
Houston, **Texas** 77030
(713) 795-7470

Dr. Bob Grossman
Department of Endocrinology
Baylor College of Medicine
1 Baylor Plaza
Houston, **Texas** 77030
(713) 798-4696

Dr. William Odell
Department of Endocrinology
University of Utah
50 N. Medical Center
Salt Lake City, **Utah** 84132
(801) 581-7459

Dr. Edward Laws
Department of Neurosurgery
University of Virginia
Box 212
Charlottesville, **Virginia** 22908
(804) 924-2650

Dr. Mary Lee Vance
Department of Endocrinology
University of Virginia
Box 511
Charlottesville, **Virginia** 22908
(804) 924-5929

Dr. John Jane
Department of Endocrinology
University of Virginia
Box 511
Charlottesville, **Virginia** 22908
(804) 924-5929

Chapter 18

Addison's Disease

Addison's disease is a rare endocrine, or hormonal disorder that affects about 1 in 100,000 people. It occurs in all age groups and afflicts men and women equally. The disease is characterized by weight loss, muscle weakness, fatigue, low blood pressure, and sometimes darkening of the skin in both exposed and nonexposed parts of the body.

Addison's disease occurs when the adrenal glands do not produce enough of the hormone cortisol and in some cases, the hormone aldosterone. For this reason, the disease is sometimes called chronic adrenal insufficiency, or hypocortisolism.

Cortisol is normally produced by the adrenal glands, located just above the kidneys. It belongs to a class of hormones called glucocorticoids, which affect almost every organ and tissue in the body. Scientists think that cortisol has possibly hundreds of effects in the body. Cortisol's most important job is to help the body respond to stress. Among its other vital tasks, cortisol:

- helps maintain blood pressure and cardiovascular function;
- helps slow the immune system's inflammatory response;
- helps balance the effects of insulin in breaking down sugar for energy; and
- helps regulate the metabolism of proteins, carbohydrates, and fats.

NIH Publication No. 90–3054, November 1989.

Because cortisol is so vital to health, the amount of cortisol produced by the adrenals is precisely balanced. Like many other hormones, cortisol is regulated by the brain's hypothalamus and the pituitary gland, a bean-sized organ at the base of the brain. First, the hypothalamus sends "releasing hormones" to the pituitary gland. The pituitary responds by secreting other hormones that regulate growth, thyroid and adrenal function, and sex hormones such as estrogen and testosterone. One of the pituitary's main functions is to secrete ACTH (adrenocorticotropin), a hormone that stimulates the adrenal glands. When the adrenals receive the pituitary's signal in the form of ACTH, they respond by producing cortisol. Completing the cycle, cortisol then signals the pituitary to lower secretion of ACTH.

Aldosterone belongs to a class of hormones called mineralocorticoids, also produced by the adrenal glands. It helps maintain blood pressure and water and salt balance in the body by helping the kidney retain sodium and excrete potassium. When aldosterone production falls too low, the kidneys are not able to regulate salt and water balance, causing blood volume and blood pressure to drop.

Causes

Failure to produce adequate levels of cortisol, or adrenal insufficiency, can occur for different reasons. The problem may be due to a disorder of the adrenal glands themselves (primary adrenal insufficiency) or to inadequate secretion of ACTH by the pituitary gland (secondary adrenal insufficiency).

Primary Adrenal Insufficiency

Most cases of Addison's disease are caused by the gradual destruction of the adrenal cortex, the outer layer of the adrenal glands, by the body's own immune system. About 70 percent of reported cases of Addison's disease are due to autoimmune disorders, in which the immune system makes antibodies that attack the body's own tissues or organs and slowly destroy them. Adrenal insufficiency occurs when at least 90 percent of the adrenal cortex has been destroyed. As a result, often both glucocorticoid and mineralocorticoid hormones are lacking. Sometimes only the adrenal gland is affected, as in idiopathic adrenal insufficiency; sometimes other glands also are affected, as in the polyendocrine deficiency syndrome.

The polyendocrine deficiency syndrome is classified into two separate forms, referred to as type I and type II. Type I occurs in children, and adrenal insufficiency may be accompanied by underactive parathyroid glands, slow sexual development, pernicious anemia, chronic candida infections, chronic active hepatitis, and, in very rare cases, hair loss. Type II, often called Schmidt's syndrome, usually afflicts young adults. Features of type II may include an underactive thyroid gland, slow sexual development, and diabetes mellitus. About 10 percent of patients with type II have vitiligo, or loss of pigment, on areas of the skin. Scientists think that the polyendocrine deficiency syndrome is inherited because frequently more than one family member tends to have one or more endocrine deficiencies.

Tuberculosis (TB) accounts for about 20 percent of cases of primary adrenal insufficiency in developed countries. When adrenal insufficiency was first identified by Dr. Thomas Addison in 1849, TB was found at autopsy in 70 to 90 percent of cases. As the treatment for TB improved, however, the incidence of adrenal insufficiency due to TB of the adrenal glands has greatly decreased.

Less common causes of primary adrenal insufficiency are chronic infections, mainly fungal infections; cancer cells spreading from other parts of the body to the adrenal glands; amyloidosis; and surgical removal of the adrenal glands. Each of these causes is discussed in more detail below.

Secondary Adrenal Insufficiency

This form of Addison's disease can be traced to a lack of ACTH, which causes a drop in the adrenal glands' production of cortisol but not aldosterone. A temporary form of secondary adrenal insufficiency may occur when a person who has been receiving a glucocorticoid hormone such as prednisone for a long time abruptly stops or interrupts taking the medication. Glucocorticoid hormones, which are often used to treat inflammatory illnesses like rheumatoid arthritis, asthma, or ulcerative colitis, block the release of both corticotropin-releasing hormone (CRH) and ACTH. Normally, CRH instructs the pituitary gland to release ACTH. If CRH levels drop, the pituitary is not stimulated to release ACTH, and the adrenals then fail to secrete sufficient levels of cortisol.

Another cause of secondary adrenal insufficiency is the surgical removal of benign, or noncancerous, ACTH-producing tumors of the pituitary gland (Cushing's disease). In this case, the source of ACTH is suddenly removed, and replacement hormone must be taken until normal ACTH and cortisol production resumes. Less commonly, adrenal insufficiency occurs when the pituitary gland either decreases in size or stops producing ACTH. This can result from tumors or infections of the area, loss of blood flow to the pituitary, radiation for the treatment of pituitary tumors, or surgical removal of parts of the hypothalamus or the pituitary gland during neurosurgery of these areas.

Symptoms

The symptoms of adrenal insufficiency usually begin gradually. Chronic, worsening fatigue and muscle weakness, loss of appetite, and weight loss are characteristic of the disease. Nausea, vomiting, and diarrhea occur in about 50 percent of cases. Blood pressure is low and falls further when standing, causing dizziness or fainting. Skin changes also are common in Addison's disease, with areas of hyperpigmentation, or dark tanning, covering exposed and nonexposed parts of the body. This darkening of the skin is most visible on scars; skin folds; pressure points such as the elbows, knees, knuckles, and toes; lips; and mucous membranes.

Addison's disease can cause irritability and depression. Because of salt loss, craving of salty foods also is common. Hypoglycemia, or low blood sugar, is more severe in children than in adults. In women, menstrual periods may become irregular or stop.

Because the symptoms progress slowly, they are usually ignored until a stressful event like an illness or an accident causes them to become worse. This is called an addisonian crisis, or acute adrenal insufficiency. In most patients, symptoms are severe enough to seek medical treatment before a crisis occurs. However, in about 25 percent of patients, symptoms first appear during an addisonian crisis.

Symptoms of an addisonian crisis include sudden penetrating pain in the lower back, abdomen, or legs; severe vomiting and diarrhea, followed by dehydration; low blood pressure; and loss of consciousness. Left untreated, an addisonian crisis can be fatal.

Diagnosis

In its early stages, adrenal insufficiency can be difficult to diagnose. A review of a patient's medical history based on the symptoms, especially the dark tanning of the skin, will lead a doctor to suspect Addison's disease.

A diagnosis of Addison's disease is made by biochemical laboratory tests. The aim of these tests is first to determine whether there are insufficient levels of cortisol and then to establish the cause. X-ray exams of the adrenal and pituitary glands also are useful in helping to establish the cause.

ACTH Stimulation Test

This is the most specific test for diagnosing Addison's disease. In this test, blood and/or urine cortisol levels are measured before and after a synthetic form of ACTH is given by injection. In the so called short, or rapid, ACTH test, cortisol measurement in blood is repeated 30 to 60 minutes after an intravenous ACTH injection. The normal response after an injection of ACTH is a rise in blood and urine cortisol levels. Patients with either form of adrenal insufficiency respond poorly or do not respond at all.

When the response to the short ACTH test is abnormal, a "long" ACTH stimulation test is required to determine the cause of adrenal insufficiency. In this test, synthetic ACTH is injected either intravenously or intramuscularly over a 48- to 72-hour period, and blood and/or urine cortisol are measured the day before and during the 2 to 3 days of the injection. Patients with primary adrenal insufficiency do not produce cortisol during the 48- to 72-hour period; however, patients with secondary adrenal insufficiency have adequate responses to the test on the second or third day.

In patients suspected of having an addisonian crisis, the doctor must begin treatment with injections of salt, fluids, and glucocorticoid hormones immediately. Although a reliable diagnosis is not possible while the patient is being treated, measurement of blood ACTH and cortisol during the crisis and before glucocorticoids are given is sufficient to make the diagnosis. Once the crisis is controlled and medication has been stopped, the doctor will delay further testing for up to 1 month to obtain an accurate diagnosis.

Insulin-Induced Hypoglycemia Test

A reliable test to determine how the hypothalamus and pituitary and adrenal glands respond to stress is the insulin-induced hypoglycemia test. In this test, blood is drawn to measure the blood glucose and cortisol levels, followed by an injection of fast-acting insulin. Blood glucose and cortisol levels are measured again at 30, 45, and 90 minutes after the insulin injection. The normal response is for blood glucose levels to fall and cortisol levels to rise.

Other Tests

Once a diagnosis of primary adrenal insufficiency has been made, x-ray exams of the abdomen may be taken to see if the adrenals have any signs of calcium deposits. Calcium deposits may indicate TB. A tuberculin skin test also may be used.

If secondary adrenal insufficiency is the cause, doctors may use different imaging tools to reveal the size and shape of the pituitary gland. The most common is the CT scan, which produces a series of x-ray pictures giving a cross-sectional image of a body part. The function of the pituitary and its ability to produce other hormones also are tested.

Treatment

Treatment of Addison's disease involves replacing, or substituting, the hormones that the adrenal glands are not making. Cortisol is replaced orally with hydrocortisone tablets, a synthetic glucocorticoid, taken once or twice a day. If aldosterone is also deficient, it is replaced with oral doses of a mineralocorticoid, called fludrocortisone acetate (Florinef®), which is taken once a day. Patients receiving aldosterone replacement therapy are usually advised by a doctor to increase their salt intake. Because patients with secondary adrenal insufficiency normally maintain aldosterone production, they do not require aldosterone replacement therapy. The doses of each of these medications are adjusted to meet the needs of individual patients.

During an addisonian crisis, low blood pressure, low blood sugar, and high levels of potassium can be life threatening. Standard therapy involves intravenous injections of hydrocortisone, saline (salt water), and dextrose (sugar). This treatment usually brings rapid improvement. When the patient can take fluids and medications by mouth, the amount of hydrocortisone is decreased until a maintenance dose is achieved. If aldosterone is deficient, maintenance therapy also includes oral doses of fludrocortisone acetate.

Special Problems

Surgery

Patients with chronic adrenal insufficiency who need surgery with general anesthesia are treated with injections of hydrocortisone and saline. Injections begin on the evening before surgery and continue until the patient is fully awake and able to take medication by mouth. The dosage is adjusted until the maintenance dosage given before surgery is reached.

Pregnancy

Women with primary adrenal insufficiency who become pregnant are treated with standard replacement therapy. If nausea and vomiting in early pregnancy interfere with oral medication, injections of the hormone may be necessary. During delivery, treatment is similar to that of patients needing surgery; following delivery, the dose is gradually tapered and the usual maintenance doses of hydrocortisone and fludrocortisone acetate by mouth are not reached until about 10 days after childbirth.

Patient Education

A person who has adrenal insufficiency should always carry identification stating his or her condition in case of an emergency. The card should alert emergency personnel about the need to inject 100 mg of cortisol if its bearer is found severely injured or unable to answer questions. The card should also include the doctor's name and telephone number and the name and telephone number of the nearest relative to be notified. When traveling, it is important to have a needle, syringe, and an injectable form of cortisol for emergencies. A person with Addison's disease also should know how to increase medication during periods of stress or mild upper respiratory infections. Immediate medical attention is needed when severe infections or vomiting or diarrhea occur. These conditions can precipitate an addisonian crisis. A patient who is vomiting may require injections of hydrocortisone.

It is very helpful for persons with medical problems to wear a descriptive warning bracelet or neck chain to alert emergency personnel. Bracelets and neck chains can be obtained from:

Medic Alert Foundation International
2323 Colorado
Turlock, California 95381
(209) 668-3333

Suggested Reading

The following materials can be found in medical libraries, many college and university libraries, and through interlibrary loan in most public libraries.

Wingert, Terence D. and Mulrow, Patrick J., "Chronic Adrenal Insufficiency," in *Current Diagnosis*, edited by Rex B. Conn. Philadelphia, W.B. Saunders Company, 1985, pp 860–863.

Bravo, Emmanuel L., "Adrenocortical Insufficiency," in *Conn's Current Therapy*, edited by Robert E. Rakel. Philadelphia, W.B. Saunders Company, 1987, pp 493–495.

Bondy, Philip K., "Disorders of the Adrenal Cortex," in *Williams Textbook of Endocrinology*, seventh edition, edited by Jean D. Wilson and Daniel W. Foster. Philadelphia, R.B. Saunders Company, 1985, pp 844–858.

Loriaux, D. Lynn and Cutler, Gordon B., "Diseases of the Adrenal Glands," in *Clinical Endocrinology*, edited by Peter O. Kohler. New York, John Wiley & Sons, 1986, pp 208–215.

Williams, Gordon H. and Dluhy, Robert G., "Diseases of the Adrenal Cortex," in *Harrison's Principles of Internal Medicine*, 11th edition, edited by Eugene Braunwald, Kurt J. Isselbacher, Robert G. Petersdorf, Jean D. Wilson, Joseph B. Martin, and Anthony S. Fauci. New York, McGraw-Hill Book Company, 1987, pp 1769–1772.

Baxter, John D. and Tyrrell, I. Blake, "The Adrenal Cortex," in *Endocrinology and Metabolism*, second edition, edited by Philip Felig, John D. Baxter, Arthur E. Broadus, and Lawrence A. Frohman. New York, McGraw-Hill Book Company, 1987, pp 581–599.

Other Resources

National Adrenal Disease Foundation
505 Northern Boulevard, Suite 200
Great Neck, New York 11021
(516) 487-4992

—by Eileen K. Corrigan

Eileen K. Corrigan is affiliated with NIDDK's Office of Health Research Reports.

Chapter 19

Congenital Adrenal Hyperplasia (CAH)

What is CAH?

Congenital adrenal hyperplasia (CAH) is caused by the deficiency of an enzyme that is necessary for the production of the essential steroid hormone, cortisol, in the outer portion of the adrenal gland (adrenal cortex). Cortisol is one of the hormones important in regulating the body's response to stress. Another hormone, aldosterone, essential for regulating salt and water balance, is also produced by this portion of the adrenal gland.

The most common type of CAH is caused by 21-hydroxylase deficiency (21OHD), which disrupts adrenal production of both cortisol and aldosterone. In an effort to counteract deficiency of these hormones, the adrenal enlarges, hence the term "adrenal hyperplasia." As it enlarges, only small amounts of cortisol and aldosterone are produced, and hormone production is shifted toward sex steroids, particularly androgens (male hormones). People severely affected with this disease are unable to respond to stress, cannot properly conserve salt and water, and may become dehydrated and go into shock. The excess androgens produce early signs of sexual development which are especially evident in affected female fetuses who have male-like external genitalia. There is also a mild form of this disease, often referred to as

"Congenital Adrenal Hyperplasia: The Facts You Need to Know," written by Phyllis W. Speiser, MD, for the National Adrenal Diseases Foundation, Inc., 505 Northern Boulevard, Great Neck, NY 11021, (516) 487-4992; reprinted with permission.

245

nonclassic 21-hydroxylase deficiency. This type is quite common, although the physical signs are subtle compared with the classic form of 210HD, and it is diagnosed sometime after infancy, often not until adulthood. There are also several other enzyme deficiencies that can cause rarer forms of classic and nonclassic CAH.

What Causes CAH?

Congenital adrenal hyperplasia 210HD is caused by the inheritance of two defective genes for the 210H enzyme. One defective gene is inherited from the father and one from the mother. In such recessively inherited diseases, there is a 1/4 (25%) risk at each conception that carrier parents will each give the defect to a child. On the other hand, 3/4 (75%) of all children will be healthy. Carriers of the defective gene do not show any signs of disease, but may be detected by hormonal blood tests, or more accurately by genetic tests. There are a few cases in which "new" mutations (defects in the gene's message) are found, and in such situations one or both parents may not be a carrier.

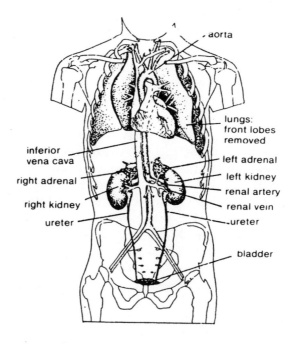

Figure 19.1. Location of the Adrenal Glands.

How Common Is CAH?

Newborn screening studies indicate that the classic form of the disease is found in 1 in every 14,000 live-born infants. This number varies in different parts of the world, but generally holds true for most ethnic groups in Europe, Japan and the U.S. In isolated populations such as the Yupik Eskimos of western Alaska, and on the island of La Reunion in the Indian Ocean, the disease is found in 1 in 400 to 1 in 700 live births.

The nonclassic form of the disease is found in about 1 in 100 people, but again, is higher in select ethnic groups. This is especially true in Jews of Eastern European (Ashkenazi) descent, with approximately 1 in 30 affected. In this milder form of 21OHD many affected individuals never come to medical attention. They may have no visible signs of male hormone excess, and certainly no life-threatening illness.

As stated above, carriers of the gene defect have no symptoms. About 1 in 60 in the entire population carry a classic 21OHD gene defect, and about 1 in 6 carry the nonclassic gene defect.

Less common forms of CAH are defects in the 11ß- hydroxylase, 17a-hydroxylase/17,20-lyases and 3ß-hydroxysteroid dehydrogenase (3ßHSD) enzymes. Since these together comprise only 5-10% of all cases of CAH and are never routinely screened for in the newborns precise statistics regarding population frequencies are unavailable.

What Are the Symptoms of CAH?

For patients affected with the severe disease, the hormonal imbalance begins in prenatal life. Female fetuses develop masculinized external genitals (the clitoris may look like a penis), although they have normal internal reproductive organs. The abnormal appearance of external genitalia in females is a sign that usually brings these infants to prompt medical attention. If the disease is not promptly recognized and treated, both males and females may suffer an "adrenal crisis" due to insufficient cortisol and aldosterone production. Patients who are in crisis must get immediate medical attention, including intravenous fluid, salt and hydrocortisone.

Patients with a mild or nonclassic form of 21OHD have an early onset of sexual development and rapid growth in childhood. In adolescent girls, unwanted facial and body hair and irregular menstrual periods are possible signs of an adrenal hormone imbalance. Severe acne can be a problem in either males or females with the condition.

Although both severely and mildly affected patients can be fertile, some have reproductive difficulties. These are usually treatable.

How Is CAH Diagnosed?

There are several approaches to diagnosing this condition. First, a thorough history and physical examination should be performed by an endocrinologist, who will also inquire in detail about the family history.

Next, blood and urine tests may be obtained to measure adrenal hormones. The most sensitive and specific way to measure these hormones is with an adrenal challenge or stimulation test. Such a test takes one hour to perform and can be done without specific preparation in the office. A blood sample is taken in the early morning, an injection is given of a synthetic form of the normal pituitary hormone ACTH (Adrenal Cortical Tropic Hormone), and one hour later, a second sample of blood is drawn to remeasure the adrenal gland's response to this challenge. If 21-hydroxylase is lacking, some hormones will be elevated (such as progesterone and 17-hydroxyprogesterone, 17OHP), and others will be comparatively low (such as cortisol). Specific published guidelines allow the endocrinologist to decide if the results make the diagnosis.

Often, other blood and urine tests are also obtained to measure additional hormones to exclude conditions which may look like CAH. Sometimes ultrasound and computerized tomography (CAT scan), are done to assess the adrenal size.

Although genetic testing is not usually a first choice test to diagnose patients with the disease, it can be helpful in certain cases if the hormonal tests are inconclusive. However, it is now more common to perform genetic testing for prenatal diagnosis in families where an affected child is already diagnosed. Any such family should be offered genetic counseling with advice regarding patient treatment and diagnosis.

How Is CAH Treated?

Classic congenital adrenal hyperplasia is treated by the administration of hydrocortisone in children. This is usually given in two or three daily doses. Adolescents and adults usually take a longer acting, more potent steroid such as prednisone or dexamethasone. Salt-wasters (those that lack the hormone to retain sodium) also take a drug which replaces aldosterone's effect (Florinef) and/or extra salt tablets. Young patients see the endocrinologist several times yearly to adjust dose and monitor growth. Parents are taught to administer injections of hydrocortisone at home in case of emergency. If a child is unable to take oral fluids or medication, and he/she does not improve following injection of hydrocortisone at home, treatment with intravenous fluid and hydrocortisone is advised under medical supervision. This occurrence is uncommon for most patients.

Girls may require genital surgery to reduce the enlarged clitoris and to separate the urinary opening from the vagina. This procedure should be done by an experienced urologist or gynecologic surgeon.

Psychological consultation is advised for CAH patients, particularly girls, before puberty.

It is recommended that therapy be continuous in all classic patients, even after growth is completed. Females affected with nonclassic 21OHD are usually treated in childhood through the reproductive years. Males with nonclassic 21OHD who have completed their growth most often do not require treatment. If the treatment goal is to suppress adrenal androgens (male hormones), encourage normal growth, and regularize the menstrual cycle, hydrocortisone, prednisone, or dexamethasone (all glucocorticosteroids) are used. Some endocrinologists and gynecologists believe that when relief from hirsutism (excessive facial and body hair) is desired, drugs other than glucocorticoids are more effective. These include spironolactone, which partially blocks androgen action, and oral contraceptives, which suppress any ovarian contribution to androgen production. These drugs may be used individually, or in combination.

Related Diseases

The signs and symptoms found in CAH patients can be associated with several other diseases, but these can be differentiated from CAH by specific hormone measurements. For example, adrenal insufficiency can be caused by Addison's disease, a disease that destroys the adrenal glands. In male infants the listlessness, failure to thrive, and vomiting that are seen with CAH may be mistaken for other illnesses such as intestinal obstruction, kidney disease, or even milk allergy. Abnormal genital appearance may be caused by other rarer genetic conditions. Salt-wasting can be caused by non-hormonal intestinal, kidney, or skin losses, often due to infectious disease.

How Normal Is a CAH Patient's Life?

As long as the proper dose of replacement medication is taken every day, a CAH patient can have a normal, crisis-free life. There are no specific physical or occupational restrictions. Routine care includes regular physician visits, avoidance of dehydration, and the use of extra medication during illness. Pregnancy is possible, but will require extra hormonal monitoring. Prenatal diagnosis is available to parents of affected children. If the fetus proves to be an affected female, severe genital abnormalities can be prevented by treating the pregnant mother with dexamethasone from the first trimester until birth. Every CAH patient should wear an identification bracelet or necklace stating that he or she has the disease, to insure proper emergency treatment. An identification card outlining treatment is also suggested. Today, people with CAH should have a normal life expectancy.

Why Consult an Endocrinologist?

Endocrinologists are specialists in hormonal diseases, including CAH. Because of the relative rarity of this disease, an endocrinologist will have more experience in properly diagnosing and treating CAH than most general physicians.

—by Phyllis W. Speiser, MD

Phyllis W. Speiser, MD is Chief, Division of Pediatric Endocrinology and Metabolism at North Shore University Hospital and Associate Professor of Pediatrics at Cornell University Medical College. The text was edited by Paul Margulies, MD, Medical Director, N.A.D.F. Clinical Associate Professor of Medicine, Cornell University Medical College.

Part Four

Pituitary and Growth Disorders

Chapter 20

Assessing Pituitary Function

The Pituitary Gland and Its Role

The human body is composed of a variety of specialized tissues which must function in an integrated fashion. This integrated control is accomplished by way of two major systems of communication among tissues: the brain and nervous system and the endocrine system. The nervous system conveys electrochemical signals to and from the brain and the body tissues. The endocrine system composed of a series of endocrine glands, releases chemical signals called hormones which act by way of hormone receptors in responsive tissues. The nervous system largely coordinates and directs movement of the body and its interactions with the environment. The endocrine system regulates body metabolism.

The pituitary gland is a unique endocrine gland which serves to link these important communication systems. It resides in a thimble-sized pocket of bone at the base of the brain. It functions as an endocrine transducer system in that it transduces (or converts) nervous into hormonal signals and provides the brain with a direct pathway to influence endocrine gland function. The hypothalamus at the base of the brain contains nerve cells which produce small protein molecules which are transported in small blood vessels to the pituitary gland where they act to regulate production of one or more of the

"The Laboratory Assessment of Pituitary Gland Function," *The Pituitary Patient Resource Guide*, First Edition, ©1995 by the Pituitary Tumor Network Association and Delbert A. Fisher, MD; reprinted with permission.

anterior pituitary hormones. The anterior pituitary hormones, in turn, regulate body metabolism directly or by controlling the activity of other endocrine glands. The anterior gland hormones and their functions include:

- **Growth Hormone (GH)**—Regulates growth in children and has effects on protein sugar and fat metabolism

- **Prolactin (PRL)**—Involved in regulation of breast milk production

- **Gonadotropins**—Regulates the sex glands, including the testes in males and ovaries in females. Two gonadotropins are involved: luteinizing hormone (LH) and follicle stimulating hormone (FSH)

- **Thyroid Stimulating Hormone (TSH)**—Regulates function of the thyroid gland

- **Adrenocorticotropic Hormone (ACTH)**—Regulates function of the adrenal gland

A posterior pituitary gland composed of nerve fibers from the hypothalamus produce other small protein molecules, the Posterior Pituitary Hormones. These include:

- **Vasopressin (VP)**—Also called antidiuretic hormone (ADH) modulates water excretion by the kidney to maintain body fluid volume and composition

- **Oxytocin (OT)**—In females OT stimulates uterine muscle contractions and is involved in labor and delivery; it also stimulates breast milk secretion during breast feeding. OT has no important role in males

The pituitary gland has been referred to as the "master" (endocrine) gland because its hormones are regulatory for a number of the important endocrine glands. These glands, sometimes referred to as "target glands" include:

The Sex Glands, or Gonads. The testes in males produce the male hormone testosterone when stimulated by LH. Both LH and FSH in males regulate sperm production. In females, FSH stimulates growth of ovarian follicles, estrogen production and maturation of the female eggs or ova. LH in females regulates progesterone production which is important for growth of the egg in the uterus after it is released from the follicle and fertilized by a sperm.

The Thyroid Gland. This gland at the front and base of the neck is stimulated by TSH to produce the thyroid hormone thyroxine (T4) a small iodine-containing hormone. Thyroxine, in turn, is converted to the active hormone triiodothyronine (T3) by removal of one of the 4 thyroxine iodine atoms. T3 acts on various body tissues to regulate the level of energy production (metabolic rate). It is also critical for normal childhood growth.

The Adrenal Cortical Glands. These paired glands lie just above the kidneys. When stimulated by pituitary ACTH, they produce the hormones cortisol, aldosterone, and several androgens. Cortisol is required for normal body metabolism and adrenaline and noradrenaline is critical for the body's response to stress. Aldosterone helps regulate body fluid volume and blood pressure by regulating salt (sodium) excretion by the kidney. The adrenal adrogens are weak testosterone-like molecules of limited significance unless secreted in excess in females.

The Role of the Laboratory in the Diagnosis and Management of Pituitary Dividers

During the past three decades, we have witnessed the development of highly sensitive and specific immunoassay methods for the direct measurement of all of the pituitary and target organ hormones in blood. These include those listed in Table 20.1.

Physicians now have the ability to directly measure the levels of these hormones to assess the level of activity of the pituitary and target endocrine glands. An important characteristic of pituitary-target organ interaction is "feedback regulation." The target organ hormone levels in blood circulate or feed back to the pituitary gland and influence the rate of production of the pituitary hormone. For instance, TSH stimulates the thyroid gland to produce thyroxine. The circulating blood levels of thyroxine inhibit or reduce pituitary TSH production such that the blood thyroxine levels are maintained within a narrow normal range. Damage to the thyroid gland reduces thyroxine levels with the result that pituitary TSH production is increased and blood levels of TSH are increased. Such feedback control also is operative for the GH, IGF-I, LH-progesterone or testosterone, FSH-estrogen, and ACTH-cortisol systems. Thus simultaneous measurements of the pituitary and target endocrine gland hormones allows an assessment of feedback regulation and proper pituitary target organ interaction.

Pituitary tumors usually involve specific anterior pituitary cell types and this may produce excess amounts of one of the pituitary hormones. Acromegaly is due to excess GH secretion; Cushing's Disease is due to excess ACTH secretion; other less common tumors secrete TSH or LH/FSH. In these cases, the tumors are "autonomous" or self-controlled so that feedback regulation is abolished and the

Table 20.1. Pituitary and Target Organ Hormones

Pituitary Hormone	Target Hormone
GH	Insulin-Like Growth Factor I (IGF-I) produced in liver
	IGF Binding Proteins produced by liver: IGF-BP2, IGF-BP3
PRL	No target hormone, but PRL suppresses LH, FSH and gonadal function
LH	Testosterone
	Progesterone
FSH	Estrogen
TSH	Thyroxine
	Triiodothyronine
ACTH	Cortisol
	Aldosterone
	Adrenal Androgens
VP	No target hormones
	Can measure urine concentration
OT	No target hormones

excessive, continuous stimulation of the target gland results in the classic signs of the target organ hormone excess. (Acromegaly = IGF-I excess; Cushing's Disease = cortisol excess; Hyperthyroidism = thyroxine excess.)

Many pituitary tumors involve cells which have lost hormone producing capacity. These tumors enlarge and destroy function of other pituitary cells with the result that target organ deficiencies may occur. Even the specific hormone secreting tumors may damage other pituitary cells if they grow large enough. Moreover, damage to functioning pituitary cells may [occur during] the process of treatment of pituitary tumors by surgery or radiation. Pituitary tumors involving posterior pituitary hormones have not been described, but tumors in the area of the hypothalamus can alter production of VP and alter the ability to regulate water (and urine) excretion. Large anterior pituitary tumors sometimes can do this.

It is believed that at least some pituitary tumors are due to the chronic overproduction of the specific hypothalamic regulatory factors (or hormones) which stimulate their respective pituitary cell types. The hypothalamic hormones and the pituitary cell types they stimulate include those listed in Table 20.2.

Table 20.2. Hypothalamic Hormones and Pituitary Cell Types

Hypothalamic Hormone	Pituitary Cell Type
Growth Hormone Releasing Hormone (GHRH)	GH
Corticotrophin Releasing Hormone (CRH)	ACTH
Thyrotropin Releasing Hormone (TRH)	TSH
Gonadotropin Releasing Hormone (GnRH)	LH/FSH

The hypothalamic releasing hormone levels also can be measured in blood. However, in normal circumstances their circulating levels are low because they are not secreted into circulating blood (only into pituitary system blood). However, tissues in various parts of the body are capable of producing small amounts of the hypothalamic hormones, and on occasion excessive amounts can be produced by tumors in the abdomen or chest. Such "ectopic" production of GRH or CRH has been a rare cause of Acromegaly or Cushing's Disease. This can be detected by measurement of these hormones in peripheral blood.

Finally, it is important to recognize that a pituitary tumor or pituitary dysfunction is not usually cured. Long term surveillance and management are essential. Thus, the physician and the patient must depend heavily on the laboratory for initial diagnostic assessment of the pituitary and target hormone activity and for ongoing surveillance of disease activity and treatment management. Many of the hormone measurements are available only in specialized laboratories and some tests require special handling of the specimens and special timing of their collection. Additionally, the physician may conduct scheduled stimulation or suppression tests to assess the responsiveness of the pituitary or target glands or the function of the feedback control systems.

The physician will maintain records of these test results, but it is also important that patients maintain an ongoing record of therapy and test results. Such records may be very important during travel; accidents may occur and the physician records may not be readily available. Having records available in the event of a move or job change may avoid problems. It is also helpful to know the laboratory source of your test results so that recent data can be retrieved in the event of travel or accident.

— by Delbert A. Fisher, MD., President,
Academic Associates Corning Nichols Institute,
San Juan Capistrano, California

Chapter 21

Patterns of Growth

Introduction

"How tall will my 2-year-old be when he grows up?"

"Doctor, my 12-year-old daughter is already 5 feet, 10 inches tall. Is there anything I can do to keep her from growing over 6 feet tall?"

"My child has a cartilage problem and is very short. Will my other children also be short?"

These are questions often asked by parents when the growth of a child seems unusual. What determines how a child grows? How is height inherited? How does one recognize a growth problem? How are growth problems treated? Children may ask parents why they are not as tail as their playmates; parents ask doctors, and doctors ask endocrine (hormone) specialists and geneticists.

This chapter will explain normal and abnormal patterns of growth and answer some of the questions about growth that parents find puzzling.

Normal Growth

Let's discuss the process of normal growth before we talk about its variations and abnormalities. While we all start out about the same

Patterns of Growth ©1976, 1993 Human Growth Foundation, 777 Leesburg Pike, Falls Church, VA 22043; reprinted by permission of Human Growth Foundation, (800) 451-6434.

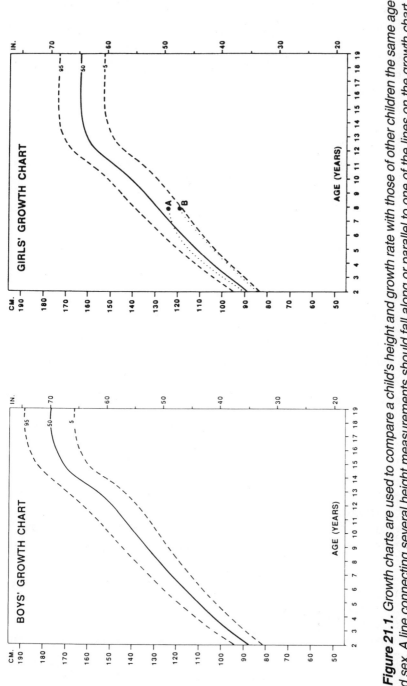

Figure 21.1. *Growth charts are used to compare a child's height and growth rate with those of other children the same age and sex. A line connecting several height measurements should fall along or parallel to one of the lines on the growth chart. On the girl's growth chart, Girl A is more likely to have a growth problem that Girl B because her growth rate has slowed over the past 2 years. Although Girl B is shorter than 95% of girls her age, she is growing at a steady, normal rate.*

size at birth, some of us end up tall and some end up short. Most of us wind up with about the same build as our parents—the characteristics a child inherits will reflect those of the parents.

A baby is about 20 inches long at birth (give or take an inch) and will grow another 10 inches over the first year to reach about 30 inches by 1 year of age. During the second year of life, growth is half this fast, so at 2 years of age, the child will be about 35 inches tall. From 2 years until about 12 years of age, the child will grow at a steady rate of 2 to 2½ inches a year. The growth spurt that goes along with adolescence begins at about age 11 in girls and 13 in boys. This pubertal growth spurt usually lasts 2 years and is accompanied by sexual development. Growth ceases between 16 and 18 years of age, when the growing ends of the bones fuse. A person's adult height is determined by many factors, including the heights of his or her parents, the age at which puberty begins and the length and vigor of the pubertal growth spurt. An x-ray of the hand or knee allows the doctor to assess the maturity of the bones (bone age) and estimate how much growth potential remains.

Normal But Unusual Growth Patterns

Variations from the usual pattern of growth may occur and still be within the range of normal. Some children are taller than expected at a given age, and some are shorter. Parents are more often concerned when their children are shorter than their age-mates than when they are taller, although most short children fall within the normal range of height.

Many children are short because they have inherited shortness from their parents. Even though the American population is taller than in previous generations, there will always be healthy individuals whose height will be in the low part of the normal range. This is called familial short stature.

A common variant of the usual growth pattern occurs when a child is shorter than average for most of his or her life, then is late entering puberty. This condition is called constitutional growth delay with delayed adolescence or delayed maturation. More boys than girls seek medical attention for this condition, although it is not known whether it is really more common in boys. These children generally are the shortest among their age-mates. A 10-year-old child with this condition may be about the size of a 7-year-old; their bone age and growth potential will also be more like that of a 7-year-old. Typical children with constitutional growth delay have been behind their age-mates

261

in height since very early in childhood, but have continued to grow at a slow normal rate. They will enter puberty 2, 3 or even 4 years later than other children their age, but will have a normal growth spurt and end up about as tall as their parents. It is not unusual for this type of growth pattern to run in families—often a father remembers that he didn't have his growth spurt or begin shaving until much later than other boys his age or a mother remembers being late starting her periods.

This type of growth delay may create stress for a child. Nature's timetable can be speeded up by giving a low dose of sex hormone (testosterone or estrogen), although there is a small risk that this will speed up closure of the growth plates, resulting in a slightly shorter adult height. Studies are being done to determine the physical and psychological effects of growth hormone treatment in children with severe constitutional growth delay; the results of these studies are not yet known.

A second type of normal, but unusual, growth pattern is that of the very tall girl. It comes as no surprise to very tall parents that their children grow rapidly and are taller than other children. Some girls feel uncomfortable being 5 or 6 inches taller than their friends. This is an individual matter; some girls feel it is an advantage and enjoy their tallness, while others slouch and try to hide it. Adult height can be predicted on the basis of a bone age x-ray and height measurement. If a height prediction made before age 12 indicates that a girl will be very tall, she can be treated with a high dose of female hormones. These hormones will push the girl into puberty and speed up closure of the growth plates of the bones, so that the girl will end up shorter than she would have been otherwise. These hormones may have undesirable side effects, however, and doctors disagree about the safety and effectiveness of this treatment.

Abnormal Growth Patterns

Poor Nutrition and Systemic Diseases

There are many diseases and disorders that can cause short stature and growth failure. Nutritional deficiencies will cause poor growth eventually—a balanced diet with adequate calories and protein is essential for growth. There are a number of intestinal disorders which may lead to poor absorption of food. Failure to absorb nutrients and energy from food then leads to growth failure. Children with these conditions may have complaints that involve the stomach or intestines (bowels) and may have bowel movements that are unusual in pattern, appearance and odor. Treatment of these conditions often involves a special diet. Normal growth usually resumes after the condition has been treated.

Diseases of the kidneys, lungs and heart may lead to growth failure as a result of inadequate intake of nutrients or buildup of waste products and undesirable substances in the body. Children with diabetes, or "high sugar," may grow slowly, particularly when their blood sugar is not kept near the normal range.

Any disease that is severe, untreated or poorly controlled can have an adverse effect on growth. Severe stress or emotional trauma can also cause growth failure.

Bone Disorders

One form of extreme short stature is caused by abnormal formation and growth of cartilage and bone. Children with a skeletal dysplasia, or chondrodystrophy, are short and have abnormal body proportions; intelligence is normal. Some chondrodystrophies are inherited, others are not. The underlying causes of most of these skeletal dysplasias are not known, although researchers are working to identify the genetic and biochemical mechanisms that are involved. The chances of parents having a second child with the same problem cannot be estimated until the specific type of skeletal dysplasia is identified from physical examination and bone x-rays. The Human Growth Foundation (HGF) booklet, "Achondroplasia," provides more information about a common form of this group of bone disorders. [Information on how to contact the HGF is given at the end of this chapter.]

Children who will be very short as adults and adults with short stature may benefit from social contact with others having similar growth problems and with short adults who are living full and happy lives. The Little People of America is an organization that provides opportunities for such contact. More information can be obtained by writing to LPA, P.O. Box 9897, Washington, DC 20016.

Intrauterine Growth Retardation

Some infants are small at birth. When pregnancy ends earlier than usual, the baby is premature. These babies are small, but usually are normal size given their gestational age (length of time in the womb). However, some infants are shorter and weigh less than they should at birth. In other words, they had a chance to grow in the womb, but

263

did not reach the length and weight they should have for their gestational age. This failure to grow normally in the womb is called intrauterine growth retardation.

This condition may result from a problem with the placenta, the organ in the mother's womb that supplies nutrients and oxygen to the baby. A viral infection, such as German Measles, during pregnancy may affect the placenta and infant and cause intrauterine growth retardation. Sometimes the cause of this condition cannot be identified. Some of these children will remain small throughout life, while others may reach normal size. Because there are so many different causes of intrauterine growth retardation, no single treatment is effective in increasing the height of these individuals. Studies are underway to see if growth hormone is effective in increasing the growth rate and adult height of these children; the results are not yet known. More information about this type of short stature is available in the HGF booklet called "Intrauterine Growth Retardation" (IUGR).

Turner Syndrome

Short stature in girls may be caused by a genetic condition that affects the X chromosome. Chromosomes are small thread-like bodies in the nucleus of each cell; they contain the genetic material that determines the characteristics we inherit. Two of these chromosomes determine sexual development—the X and Y chromosomes. Boys have one X and one Y chromosome, and girls have two X chromosomes. In girls with Turner Syndrome, one of the X chromosomes is misshapen or missing in many or all body cells. Because of this, affected girls are short—they seldom reach 5 feet in height—and may have undeveloped ovaries (female sex glands that produce eggs and female hormones). Intelligence is normal. Turner Syndrome may be suspected because of the presence of certain physical features, but poor growth is sometimes the only sign. This condition is diagnosed by doing a special blood test (karyotype) to look for damaged or missing sex chromosomes. Replacement of the missing ovarian hormones enables these girls to develop normal female sexual characteristics. Treatment with biosynthetic growth hormone appears to be effective in increasing adult height in many of these young women, although long-term studies are still underway. The HGF booklet, "Turner Syndrome," supplies more information about this condition.

Precocious Puberty

One type of unusual growth pattern is caused by the early onset of adolescence. This pattern occurs more frequently in girls than boys.

The term sexual precocity is used to describe this condition, which includes early development of adult sexual characteristics. Children with sexual precocity grow rapidly and are tall for their age initially, but their bones also mature rapidly, so they stop growing at an early age and may be short as adults. A recently developed synthetic hormone (LHRH) is useful in halting this type of early sexual development and allowing additional growth. Studies are underway to determine if the addition of growth hormone to this regimen increases adult height of children with sexual precocity.

Sometimes a tumor or disease of the ovaries, adrenal glands, pituitary gland or brain will cause premature sexual development. In these cases, removal of the tumor or treatment of the disease may interrupt the rapid sexual development and result in increased adult height.

Thyroid Hormone Deficiency

Hormone deficiencies may cause growth failure in addition to other problems. A child with thyroid hormone deficiency has slow growth and is physically and mentally sluggish. Hypothyroidism, or lack of thyroid hormone, may be present at birth or develop anytime during childhood or later in life. It is very important to treat hypothyroidism promptly, especially if it occurs during the rapid growth period of infancy. Untreated hypothyroidism during this time can cause permanent damage to sensitive, rapidly growing brain cells. Thyroid hormone deficiency is easy to diagnose with a simple blood test and easy to treat with a daily pill that replaces the missing thyroid hormone. With early diagnosis and continuous treatment, these children grow and develop normally.

Growth Hormone Deficiency

Although many hormones work together to stimulate normal growth, growth hormone is one of the most important. It is produced by a bean-sized gland called the pituitary, which is located beneath a special part of the brain (hypothalamus) in the middle of the skull. The pituitary gland makes other hormones that stimulate other glands, so it is sometimes called the master gland. Pituitary abnormalities can cause a number of problems that result in poor growth: hypothyroidism, discussed earlier, may result from a pituitary malfunction, as may hypercortisolism (excess stress hormone). Growth hormone deficiency may result from abnormal formation of the pituitary

265

gland or hypothalamus, or damage to one of these areas occurring during or after birth.

Children with growth hormone deficiency grow slowly, but have normal body proportions. Without treatment, few would reach 5 feet in height as adults. A variety of tests may be necessary to diagnose this condition. A child with growth hormone deficiency also may be missing other pituitary hormones, (thyroid, adrenal or stress hormones, sex hormones). All hormones must be present in the proper

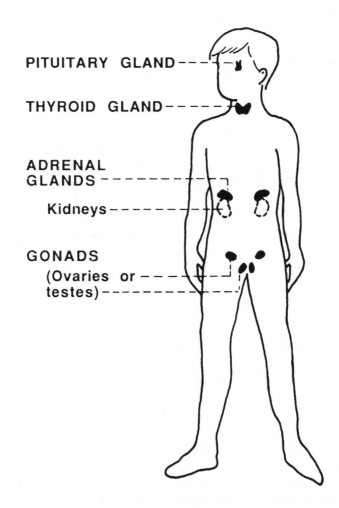

PITUITARY GLAND

THYROID GLAND

ADRENAL GLANDS

Kidneys

GONADS
(Ovaries or testes)

Figure 21.2. Location of various glands that affect human growth.

balance for normal growth to occur, so these hormones must be replaced if they are missing. Biosynthetic human growth hormone, produced by recombinant DNA technology, is available for the treatment of growth hormone deficiency. Children who are diagnosed promptly and respond well to treatment can expect to reach normal adult height. More information about this condition is presented in the HGF booklet "Growth Hormone Deficiency" [which is also reprinted in this volume].

Abnormal Tall Stature

Most tall children have tall parents and are healthy and normal, but there are some medical conditions that cause abnormal tall stature and rapid growth. A small tumor in the pituitary gland may cause too much growth hormone to be secreted, resulting in unusually fast growth and tall stature. Growth hormone excess (also called acromegaly) may be treated with medication or with surgical removal of the tumor. Some genetic conditions cause abnormal tall stature: Marfan's syndrome and Klinefelter's syndrome are two examples. These syndromes are associated with distinctive physical traits in addition to tall stature. Precocious puberty, discussed earlier, results in tall stature during childhood, although early closure of the growth plates results in short adult height.

Tall children, like short children, may stand out from their classmates and experience stress and teasing because of their size. They often look older than they are, so adults may expect too much of them. It is important for parents and teachers to be aware of the stress these children may experience as a result of looking different from their peers.

Summary

There are many causes of slow growth. Some are temporary and merely variations of normal growth patterns, and others are inherited or associated with other physical problems. These require evaluation by a doctor who can differentiate among various types of growth problems. A rule of thumb for parents who suspect a growth problem in their child is that any child who grows less than 2 inches a year after their second birthday should be seen by a physician. One of the most important things a parent can do to safeguard a child's growth and general health is to have the child examined and measured regularly by a pediatrician, family doctor, or other qualified health care provider.

Many of the conditions associated with short stature or abnormal growth can be treated. Researchers are working on developing better methods of diagnosing and treating many types of growth problems. Even though no treatment exists for some of these conditions, there are many ways a child and family may benefit from thorough evaluation of the situation. Doctors, nurses, psychologists, social workers and other professionals can work together to assist children with growth problems and their families in setting and attaining appropriate physical, emotional and educational goals. More information about the psychological and social aspects of growth problems is available in the HGF booklet called "Short & OK."

The Human Growth Foundation

The Human Growth Foundation is a national organization of parents of children with growth problems and other interested persons. Chapters of HGF are located in major cities across the nation. The members of HGF help to: educate the public about growth problems; refer children with growth problems for evaluation; provide information about growth problems to affected families; provide guidance for the physical, psychological and social development of children with growth problems; teach short children to cope with living in a bigger world; sponsor research on growth; and raise funds for these activities.

You can obtain more information about HGF activities from your local chapter or the National office by writing:

Human Growth Foundation
7777 Leesburg Pike
Falls Church, Virginia 22043
(703) 883-1773
Toll-free (800) 451-6434

Chapter 22

Growth Hormone Deficiency

Most short children do not have a serious growth problem. Many grow at a normal rate and reach an adult height that is about the same as their parents'. A child's rate of growth is an important clue to the presence or absence of a growth problem: A child who is growing at a slower than normal rate may have a serious problem, regardless of his or her height. There are many conditions and diseases that can cause poor growth; this chapter gives facts about one cause of growth failure—growth hormone deficiency.

It is estimated that 10,000 to 15,000 children in the United States have growth failure due to growth hormone deficiency. Growth hormone is a protein that is produced by the pituitary ("master") gland and is vital for normal growth. Growth hormone deficiency exists when this hormone is absent or produced in inadequate amounts. If other pituitary hormones are lacking, the condition is called hypopituitarism. When all the pituitary hormones are missing, the child has panhypopituitarism.

Control of Growth

Hormones are chemicals produced by special cells in glands and other organs of the body; most hormones are produced by cells in the endocrine glands. These hormones, which are produced in very small

Growth Hormone Deficiency ©1979, 1996 Human Growth Foundation, 777 Leesburg Pike, Falls Church, VA 22043; reprinted by permission of Human Growth Foundation, (800) 451-6434.

amounts, are released into the bloodstream and travel to the "target organ" or tissue where they exert their effect.

Several hormones are involved in regulating growth. Some act directly on target organs, while others act by triggering the production of other hormones, which activate specific organ functions necessary for growth. This finely tuned system can malfunction in several ways, causing abnormal growth.

The pituitary gland is often called the master gland because it produces several hormones that control the functions of other glands. It is located in the middle of the skull below the part of the brain called the hypothalamus. The pituitary gland has two distinct parts: An anterior (front) lobe and a posterior (rear) lobe. The pituitary gland secretes its hormones in response to chemical messages from the hypothalamus, the part of the brain to which it is connected.

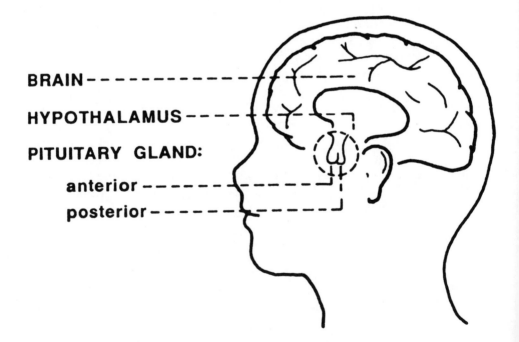

BRAIN

HYPOTHALAMUS

PITUITARY GLAND:

    anterior

    posterior

Figure 22.1. Location of the hypothalamus and pituitary gland.

Growth hormone is an anterior pituitary hormone whose main effect is to promote growth of body tissues. Other anterior pituitary hormones affect growth indirectly by working through other glands. These other hormones include:

- **Thyroid Stimulating Hormone (TSH)**— causes the thyroid gland to produce thyroid hormone, which regulates body metabolism and is essential for normal growth.

- **Adrenocorticotropic Hormone (ACTH)**—causes the adrenal glands to produce cortisol (stress hormone) and other hormones that enable the body to respond to stress. Too much cortisol will cause growth failure in a child.

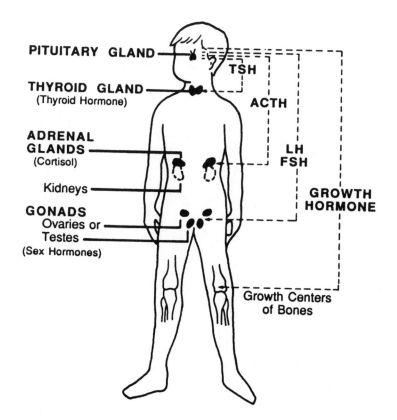

Figure 22.2. The "master gland" and the glands and organs it controls.

- **Luteinizing Hormone (LH)** and **Follicle Stimulating Hormone (FSH)**—cause the sex glands (ovaries or testes) to produce sex hormones, which are necessary for adolescent sexual development and the growth spurt that accompanies puberty.

The major hormone produced by the posterior pituitary gland is called vasopressin, or anti-diuretic hormone (ADH). It controls water output through the kidneys.

Causes of Growth Hormone Deficiency

Growth hormone deficiency may occur by itself or in combination with one or more other pituitary hormone deficiencies. It may be total (no growth hormone is produced) or partial (some growth hormone is produced, but not enough to support normal growth).

Hypopituitarism may be congenital, resulting from abnormal formation of the pituitary or hypothalamus before the child is born, or acquired, stemming from damage to the pituitary or hypothalamus during or after birth. Congenital hypopituitarism is present at birth, although it may not be apparent for many months. Acquired hypopituitarism may become evident any time during infancy or childhood, and may occur after a severe head injury or a serious illness such as meningitis or encephalitis. Many cases of acquired hypopituitarism result from a tumor called craniopharyngioma. This tumor may press on the hypothalamus or pituitary, causing one or more hormone deficiencies. Treatment consists of surgical removal of the tumor, which usually results in permanent hypopituitarism.

Sometimes no cause for hypopituitarism can be identified, or if a cause is suspected, it may be difficult to prove. Researchers are trying to learn more about the causes of growth hormone deficiency and hypopituitarism.

Diagnosis of Growth Hormone Deficiency

The child with growth hormone deficiency is often small, with an immature face and chubby body build. The rate of growth of all body parts is slow, so that the child's proportions remain normal. Intelligence usually is normal. If the child's height has been plotted on a growth chart, it will appear to be leveling off and falling away from the child's established growth curve. If growth failure has been present for a long time, the child may be much shorter than other children the same age. This is why height and weight measurements plotted on a growth chart are so important—the earlier a treatable growth problem is detected, the better the child's chance of maintaining a normal height throughout childhood and realizing his or her full growth potential.

Any child who is only as tall as children two or more years younger or who falls away from a previously normal growth curve should be evaluated by a doctor. Pediatric endocrinologists are doctors who specialize in treating children with growth and hormone problems. Depending on the situation, the doctor may measure the child over six to twelve months in order to accurately determine the child's growth rate.

The evaluation starts with gathering information on the heights of relatives and the presence of any health problems in the family. A history of early or late puberty (sexual development and growth spurt) in family members should be mentioned. The doctor will want to know about the mother's pregnancy, labor and delivery. All measurements of the child's height and weight since birth should be gathered so the doctor can plot them on a growth chart. The doctor will ask questions about the child's general health and nutritional state, past illnesses, injuries and stresses.

A thorough physical examination will be performed, and an x-ray of the hand and wrist may be obtained to see how bone development compares to height and chronologic age. A small amount of blood may be drawn to look for evidence of thyroid hormone deficiency and kidney, bone and gastrointestinal (stomach and bowel) diseases. The amount of insulin-like growth factor 1 (IGF-1) in the blood may be measured. IGF-1 is the "middle-man" in the growth process. Growth hormone stimulates the liver and other body tissues to produce IGF-1, which then acts as the link between growth hormone in the blood and the machinery inside cells that causes growth. The amount of IGF-1 in the blood provides an indirect measure of the amount of growth hormone present.

This simple evaluation often provides the doctor with enough information to identify the cause of the growth problem or to decide that no growth problem exists. If the doctor suspects that a pituitary problem may exist, further testing is necessary. A series of blood tests may be performed to measure concentrations of hormones in the blood and assess the ability of the pituitary gland to respond to various stimuli. These tests may be done in the clinic or during a brief hospitalization.

Growth hormone deficiency is moderately difficult to diagnose because the pituitary gland produces growth hormone in bursts. This means that the level of growth hormone in a single random blood sample is likely to be very low. One way of testing for growth hormone deficiency is to give the child a substance that causes the release of a growth hormone burst in normal children and measure the amount of growth hormone present in several blood samples obtained over a period of time. Since any child may not respond to any given test on a given day, more than one stimulus may be needed to evaluate the child's ability to produce growth hormone. Several growth hormone stimulators have been identified. These include vigorous exercise and several chemicals and drugs (insulin, arginine, glucagon, L-dopa, clonidine).

Another way of testing growth hormone secretion involves hospitalizing the child and measuring the amount of growth hormone present in blood samples obtained overnight during sleep or even during an entire 24 hour period. Since about two-thirds of total growth hormone production occurs during deep sleep, this test provides a better reflection of how much growth hormone the child's pituitary gland normally produces.

If several tests show that no growth hormone is present or that the amount of growth hormone being produced is not enough to support normal growth, the diagnosis of growth hormone deficiency is established. A great deal of research is being done to develop more accurate and reliable ways of diagnosing growth hormone deficiency. Even the definition of growth hormone deficiency is being revised as researchers learn more about conditions that may cause partial growth hormone deficiency.

Treatment of Growth Hormone Deficiency

Growth hormone deficiency is treated with injections of growth hormone. Most children receive six or seven injections a week because research has shown that this schedule is most effective in promoting growth. There is usually a prompt increase in growth rate after treatment starts, which may be noticeable to the child and parent in 3 to 4 months. This faster-than-normal growth rate slowly declines over time, but it continues to be greater than it would be without treatment. Many parents notice an increase in the child's appetite and a loss of body fat after treatment begins.

The treatment of a child with growth hormone deficiency usually is carried out over several years, until the child achieves normal adult height or maximum growth potential is reached. As with other conditions, children and parents may become impatient to see faster or more impressive results from therapy. They may become discouraged, even when treatment is going according to plan. It is important to

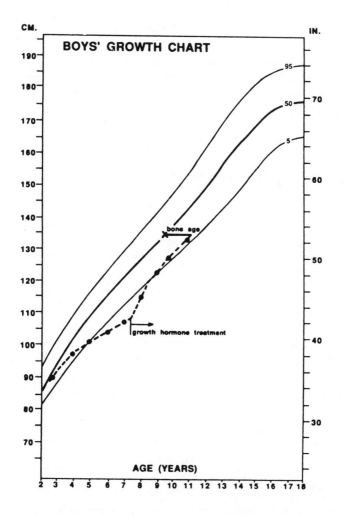

Figure 22.3. *The growth curve of a boy with growth hormone deficiency is plotted on this growth chart. His growth rate began to slow at about three years of age, but he was not evaluated by a growth specialist until his parents became concerned about his height when he entered first grade. His growth rate tripled during his first year on growth hormone therapy, and although it has slowed down since then, he is still growing at a normal rate. Because the maturity of his bones (bone age) is delayed by almost two years, his growth potential is more like a nine-year-old's than an eleven-year-old's. He has an excellent chance of reaching a normal adult height.*

275

remember that growth is a slow process that is measured over months; children who expect to grow overnight when they start treatment will be disappointed. The child's doctor will discuss realistic short and long-term expectations of therapy with the family.

If testing reveals other hormone deficiencies, medications are available to replace them; thyroid hormone, cortisol and sex hormones can be administered easily when found to be lacking. It is important that these hormones are taken as directed, because normal growth can occur only when all hormones are present in the proper amounts. Good nutrition and adequate rest are important for normal growth in all children.

Source of Human Growth Hormone

Until the early 1980s, the only source of human growth hormone was the pituitary glands of deceased people, obtained at autopsy. In April, 1985, pituitary-derived growth hormone was removed from distribution in the United States and many foreign countries following the deaths of several young adults from a very rare viral disease that may have been transmitted through the pituitary growth hormone they had received many years earlier. Fortunately, the first biosynthetic growth hormone, which is produced using recombinant DNA technology, was in the final stages of testing and was approved as safe and effective for use in growth hormone deficient children by the Food and Drug Administration in October, 1985. Because this type of growth hormone does not come from human beings, there is little possibility that human diseases can be transmitted through it.

Biosynthetic growth hormone is supplied as a powder in sterile vials. Parents and children are taught how to mix the powder into a solution and administer the injections. Treatment is continued as long as potential for growth exists and the child is responding to therapy. With early diagnosis and a good response to treatment, children with growth hormone deficiency can expect to reach normal adult height.

Psychosocial Aspects of Short Stature

Our society places great emphasis on height. Children who are short for their age sometimes have problems because playmates and teachers treat them as though they are younger rather than just smaller. Parents tend to do this too, and decrease their expectations of the child. These children then may not act their age because it's not expected of them. Teasing and name-calling may be hard to take.

276

Some of these problems may be helped by frank and open discussion with teachers and classmates.

It is very important to provide emotional support for the child with GH deficiency and to emphasize the child's many good and valuable characteristics, so that the child's stature does not limit his horizons. More about psychosocial adaptation to short stature can be learned from parents of short children and from your growth clinic doctor, nurse and psychologist.

Hope for the Future

Biosynthetic growth hormone is available in unlimited quantity for the treatment of all growth hormone deficient children. It is possible that substitutes for growth hormone may become available as research continues. These may include growth hormone releasing factor (GHRF), the hypothalamic chemical that directs the pituitary to produce growth hormone, and somatomedin, the "middle-man" that links growth hormone with linear growth.

Much research is being done to better understand the causes of growth hormone deficiency and to develop more accurate ways of diagnosing it. Many children with growth hormone deficiency can look forward to reaching normal height as a result of the research that has been done over the years and is continuing today.

The Human Growth Foundation

The Human Growth Foundation is a national organization of parents of short children and other interested people. Chapters of HGF are located in major cities across the nation. The members of these chapters help to: educate the public about growth problems; refer children with growth problems for evaluation; provide information about growth problems to affected families; provide guidance for the physical, psychological and social development of children with growth problems; help short children learn to cope with living in a bigger world; sponsor research on growth; raise funds for these activities.

You may want to obtain more information about HGF activities from your local chapter or the national office by writing:

Human Growth Foundation
7777 Leesburg Pike, Suite 202-S
Falls Church, Virginia 22043
(703) 883-1773
Toll-free: (800) 451-6434

Chapter 23

Growth Hormone Treatment: What to Expect

A doctor's recommendation to begin a child on growth hormone (GH) is based on consideration of many factors, including a complete evaluation of the child's growth pattern, general health, medical and family history, and results of laboratory tests. Parents may have many questions when they are considering a doctor's recommendation to start their child on GH. Perhaps most importantly, parents will want to understand the potential benefits and risks of GH treatment. The pediatric endocrinologist who is evaluating the child is the best person to answer these questions. This fact sheet about the possible effects of GH is intended to serve as a brief overview for parents, not as a substitute for a thorough discussion with the child's health care team. Much of the information contained here about the physical effects of GH is based on the official statement of the European Society of Pediatric Endocrinology concerning the safety and toxicity of GH, which has also been endorsed by the Lawson Wilkins Pediatric Endocrine Society in the United States.

Physical Effects of GH

GH deficient children will grow faster, often 2 to 3 times their pretreatment growth rate during the first year of therapy. This increased ("catch-up") rate wanes over time, but they should continue to grow at a normal rate while receiving therapy. GH deficient children who

An undated document produced by Human Growth Foundation; reprinted by permission of Human Growth Foundation, (800) 451-6434.

279

respond well to GH will be taller as adults than they would have been if not treated.

GH promotes the growth of muscle and bones, while the shift of lipid metabolism tends to be in the opposite direction. So, although a child's appetite often increases, body fat may decrease with GH treatment. This is because GH contributes to the breakdown of fat at the same time the child is using more calories for growth of bone, muscle and other supporting tissues.

A small percentage of children receiving GH develop a low level of weak antibodies to the medication. This means that the body recognizes the GH as a foreign protein. These antibodies are rarely of any significance, although a high level of strong antibodies can block the action of GH. If this occurs, treatment is stopped temporarily and restarted with a different brand of GH.

While GH has an anti-insulin effect, if a child is not predisposed to diabetes, blood glucose levels will remain normal. In someone with a genetic predisposition for diabetes mellitus (insulin-dependent), GH therapy may be one of multiple factors which may result in the onset of diabetes.

In some children, the need for GH therapy results from treatment they received for leukemia or a brain tumor. Based on information collected from around the world, it does not appear that GH treatment increases the risk of relapse or recurrence in these children; relapse rates are similar in children who have received GH and those who have not. GH has not been associated with an increased risk of cancer in childhood.

Several cases of benign intracranial hypertension (IC) have been reported in children starting GH treatment. IC results from increased pressure in the brain and can produce symptoms such as headaches, visual changes, nausea and vomiting. Most reported cases have occurred within the first 8 weeks of treatment and resolved after stopping GH or reducing the dose.

Slipped capital femoral epiphysis (SCFE) is a disorder of the growth plate of the hip which most often occurs during the pubertal growth spurt. Children with hormone conditions (including GH deficiency and hypothyroidism) are at increased risk for SCFE. Complaints of persistent hip or knee pain should be reported promptly to the child's doctor for evaluation.

Children with growth hormone deficiency are short, but proportionally short (e.g. length of legs is relatively consistent with the length of the trunk). During treatment, growth of bones and muscles remain proportionate.

The most serious known risk of GH treatment has been associated with the use of pituitary-derived GH; which was extracted from human pituitary glands collected at autopsy. This is the development of Creutzfeldt-Jakob Disease (CJD), a very rare, fatal neurological infection. Cases of CJD have been reported in young adults in several countries who received pituitary GH prior to 1977. The risk of infection is believed to be minimal for people who received pituitary GH in the US after 1977, when an improved purification process was introduced. Administration of pituitary-derived GH to children was discontinued in the United States in 1985 and it has not been used since then. The health of people who received pituitary GH is being followed by the National Institutes of Health. Since 1985, only recombinant DNA-derived GH has been used in the US. There is no risk of CJD for people receiving recombinant-DNA-derived GH.

Psychological Effects of GH

The overall psychological effects of GH therapy are positive; an increased growth rate, more mature appearance and the hope for an adult height within the normal range are viewed as positive by both parents and children. Even seemingly trivial milestones, such as being able to reach a light switch, give beneficial reinforcement.

Some children expect too much from GH—they think they will grow overnight or become the tallest in their class. When these expectations are not met, the child may feel disappointed, depressed, or even guilty. The response to GH is individualized and depends on many factors. It is important for the whole family to have clear and concrete information from the doctor about what is reasonable to expect in terms of increased growth rate.

Some children regret losing the special niche or role they have developed in the family or at school when they begin to grow. They may feel uncomfortable about their growing body—it's unfamiliar. They may feel like they're not special anymore when they begin to look like everyone else.

In some families, the child's growth problem may be a scapegoat. Any problems the child has had are assumed to stem from the stresses of being short. When the child begins to grow, old behavior problems may persist or new ones may develop. Although self-esteem and body image may improve as the child begins to catch up to peers in size, GH does not cure behavior problems or remove all the child's stress.

Starting to take injections is stressful for any child and family. Siblings may resent the increased attention given to the child getting shots; parents may have trouble deciding who is responsible for remembering (or forgetting!) the shots; the child getting the injections may resist them. It's not unusual for young children to regress temporarily after starting on GH (bed-wetting, thumb-sucking, irritability); older children may complain of headaches, stomachaches, or fatigue.

Summary

Many parents wrestle with the pros and cons of GH treatment. Although it is relatively safe, it is expensive and not without risks. Its use in GH deficient children is well-established; it stimulates normal growth, but it also has beneficial effects on metabolism and other bodily functions. Its effects in children who are not GH deficient are less well established. Studies have shown that it is effective in stimulating growth in girls with Turner syndrome and children with chronic renal insufficiency, but there is less information about long-term effects of treatment in these children.

GH therapy requires a long-term commitment by the child and family in order to achieve the best possible response. The medication is given by injection, with the prescribed dose divided into between three and seven shots per week. Treatment usually continues until the child has completed puberty or has stopped responding. Responsibility within the family for giving the medication may change from time to time, but it must be clearly defined.

The child's response to GH therapy should be monitored closely by a pediatric endocrinologist. This usually means visits to the doctor every three to four months with periodic laboratory and x-ray evaluations and dose changes.

GH therapy is expensive. Reimbursement may be available from health insurance, Medicaid or state children's health programs. The amount of coverage depends on individual policy guidelines and requirements. Families without insurance should explore other reimbursement sources with the home health agencies that distribute GH or with their health care team.

It is important for families to consider all aspects of GH therapy as it relates to their child's needs. Questions and concerns should be discussed with the child's health care team, and in some cases, the input of a psychologist may be helpful. Sometimes it is useful to talk with other families who have faced similar challenges; the health care team or an organization such as the Human Growth Foundation can help put families in touch with each other. Whenever GH is used, it should be one component of a treatment plan which includes attention to the child's psychological and physical well-being.

The Human Growth Foundation

The Human Growth Foundation helps individuals with growth-related disorders, their families, and health care professionals through education, research, and advocacy.

Human Growth Foundation
P.O. Box 3090
Falls Church, Virginia 22043-3090
(703) 883-1773
(800) 451-6434

—by Susan H. Parker, RN and
Patricia Rieser, FNP-C

Chapter 24

Growth Hormone Deficiency in Adults

Causes of Growth Hormone Deficiency (GHD)

Growth hormone (GH) deficient children have been treated with GH since the late 1950s, and the effects of GH deficiency in childhood are well-known. They include short stature with normal body proportions, delayed bone maturation, excess adiposity, reduced lean body mass and fasting hypoglycemia. When the children have reached final height, treatment with GH has up to now been discontinued. Although it has been recognized for many years that GH is secreted in adult life, GH deficiency in adults has remained unrecognized in endocrine clinics the world over. Only recently have the grave consequences of GHD in adults been elucidated and with the advent of recombinant human GH, the supply of the hormone has increased, making it possible to explore the effects of treating adults.

The most common causes of GH deficiency in adults are pituitary and peripituitary tumors and their treatment. In the development of hypopituitarism, the loss of hormones follow a characteristic sequence. The secretion of GH appears to be the most sensitive and is the first to disappear, followed by the secretions of gonadotropins, thyroid-stimulating hormone and finally adrenocorticotrophin. Thus, almost all patients suffering from hypopituitarism also have GHD.

From *Pituitary Patient Resource Guide*, First Annual North American Edition, ©1995 Pituitary Tumor Network Association, 16350 Ventura Blvd., Suite 231, Encino, CA 91436, (805) 499-9973; reprinted with permission.

The somatotrope cells that secrete GH make up about 50% of the hormone-producing cells of the anterior pituitary. GH is secreted in a pulsatile manner and the secretion is regulated in a complex manner by hypothalamic peptides. GH secretion decreases with age and with higher body weight. The mechanism of the decline in GH secretion with increasing age is not known. GH has both direct and indirect effect on peripheral tissues. The indirect effects are mediated mainly by insulin-like growth factor I (IGF-1). Circulating IGF-1 levels correlate to a greater or lesser degree with the GH status of the patient, with sometimes low plasma IGF-1 concentrations in patients with GHD and high concentrations in patients with acromegaly.

Effects of GHD

GH has profound effects on body composition through its anabolic, lipolytic and antinatriuretic actions. GHD in adults is associated with characteristic changes in body composition such as increased body fat and decreased lean body mass and total body water. The increase in body fat is mainly located in abdominal regions. GH replacement therapy has been shown to have profound effects on body composition. Body fat, mainly abdominal, is reduced and lean body mass is increased. Within a half year of treatment, body composition has been found to be normalized. GHD of both childhood and adult onset has been associated with low bone mass, suggesting that GH is not only important for the accumulation of bone mass up to peak bone mass, but also for the maintenance of the adult skeleton. GH has been found to increase bone mass after one to two years of treatment.

Patients with hypopituitarism on routine replacement therapy have been found to have a doubled increased mortality in cardiovascular disorders such as cerebral stroke and myocardial infarction. Untreated, GHD might explain this premature death.

GHD has been associated with a number of cardiovascular risk factors such as low HDL- and high LDL- cholesterol, increased concentrations of serum triglycerides and decreased fibrinolysis. Also, hypertension has been found to be more frequent in these patients. Treatment with GH induces favorable lipid changes such as an increase of HDL- and decrease of LDL- cholesterol concentrations. Furthermore, blood pressure has been found to decrease in response to treatment.

It was already observed many years ago that cardiac output decreased in response to hypophysectomy. Recent studies have expanded our knowledge of cardiac performance in GHD. Thus, GHD is associated with reductions in maximum oxygen uptake, maximal heart rate, cardiac wall thickness, cardiac function and physical exercise capacity. Moreover muscle strength is being reduced. Treatment has been found to normalize cardiac performance, physical exercise capacity, and muscle strength.

Quality of Life Issues

Patients with GHD often complain of fatigue, lack of concentration and memory difficulties. The fatigue reduces the working capacity, influences the professional career and impairs leisure activities. During recent years, instruments have been developed to assess "quality of life." By applying these instruments, the magnitude of problems associated with GHD in adults has been disclosed. Based on self rating questionnaires, significant impairment of "quality of life" has been found in adult patients with GHD compared to matched healthy controls. The questionnaires disclosed significant differences in energy levels and emotional reaction, as well as social isolation, implying that these patients have reduced vitality, feel less energetic and have a depressed mood and a decreased sense of well-being. Furthermore, many patients are unable to work and have disability pensions.

From a clinical point of view, the improvement of "quality of life" is the most remarkable change that is observed among the patients in response to treatment with GH. There is especially an increase in the energy level and vitality. These effects are sometimes remarkable and could be observed within the first weeks of treatment. Recently, it has been shown that HG affects the neurotransmitters in the brain suggesting that GH is of importance for brain function. Possibly these effects on the brain explain the improvement of "quality of life."

The approach to the diagnosis of adult GHD should include a high index of suspicion. Since these patients have, for the most part, hypothalamic-pituitary disease, the normal standard of care dictates that all hypothalamic-pituitary functions should be evaluated. This evaluation normally includes measurement of basal thyroid function tests, gonadotropins, gonadal steroids, prolactin, and cortisol as well as a test for hypothalamic-pituitary-adrenal reserve. The standard test which is used is the insulin tolerance test which also is the standard test for GH reserve. The measurement of serum IGF-1 may also be made but a normal IGF-1 does not exclude GHD in the adult.

GH replacement therapy is generally well tolerated, and side-effects can usually be avoided by starting with a low dose and increasing it slowly. The most common side-effects are related to fluid retention. These effects are dose-related, and respond to dose reduction.

Summary

In conclusion, evidence continues to accumulate that GH replacement therapy with GHD adults has substantial beneficial effects with improvement of body composition, skeletal mass, cardiovascular risk factors, cardiac function, exercise capacity and several aspects of "quality of life." The observed beneficial effects of GH treatment are of sufficient scale to justify considering this treatment as a routine replacement therapy in GHD adults. Recently, the regulatory authorities in Europe approved this new indication for GH therapy.

—by Bengt-Ake Bengtsson, M.D., Ph.D., Associate Professor,
Head, Division of Endocrinology
Sahlgrenska University Hospital,
Göteborg, Sweden

Chapter 25

Acromegaly

Acromegaly is a hormonal disorder that results when the pituitary gland produces excess growth hormone (GH). It most commonly affects middle-aged adults and can result in serious illness and premature death. Once recognized, acromegaly is treatable in most patients, but because of its slow and often insidious onset, it frequently is not diagnosed correctly.

The name acromegaly comes from the Greek words for "extremities" and "enlargement" and reflects one of its most common symptoms, the abnormal growth of the hands and feet. Soft tissue swelling of the hands and feet is often an early feature, with patients noticing a change in ring or shoe size. Gradually, bony changes alter the patient's facial features: the brow and lower jaw protrude, the nasal bone enlarges, and spacing of the teeth increases.

Overgrowth of bone and cartilage often leads to arthritis. When tissue thickens, it may trap nerves, causing carpal tunnel syndrome, characterized by numbness and weakness of the hands. Other symptoms of acromegaly include thick, coarse, oily skin; skin tags; enlarged lips, nose and tongue; deepening of the voice due to enlarged sinuses and vocal cords; snoring due to upper airway obstruction; excessive sweating and skin odor; fatigue and weakness; headaches; impaired vision; abnormalities of the menstrual cycle and sometimes breast

NIH Publication No. 95–3924, February 1995; and "Radiation Therapy of Acromegaly," *Pituitary Patient Resource Guide*, ©1995 Pituitary Tumor Network Association, 16350 Ventura Blvd., Suite 321, Encino, CA 91436, (805) 499-1523; reprinted with permission.

discharge in women; and impotence in men. There may be enlargement of body organs, including the liver, spleen, kidneys and heart.

The most serious health consequences of acromegaly are diabetes mellitus, hypertension, and increased risk of cardiovascular disease. Patients with acromegaly are also at increased risk for polyps of the colon that can develop into cancer.

When GH-producing tumors occur in childhood, the disease that results is called gigantism rather than acromegaly. Fusion of the growth plates of the long bones occurs after puberty so that development of excessive GH production in adults does not result in increased height. Prolonged exposure to excess GH before fusion of the growth plates causes increased growth of the long bones and increased height.

What Causes Acromegaly?

Acromegaly is caused by prolonged overproduction of GH by the pituitary gland. The pituitary is a small gland at the base of the brain that produces several important hormones to control body functions such as growth and development, reproduction, and metabolism. GH is part of a cascade of hormones that, as the name implies, regulates the physical growth of the body. This cascade begins in a part of the brain called the hypothalamus, which makes hormones that regulate the pituitary. One of these, growth hormone-releasing hormone (GHRH), stimulates the pituitary gland to produce GH. Another hypothalamic hormone, somatostatin, inhibits GH production and release. Secretion of GH by the pituitary into the bloodstream causes the production of another hormone, called insulin-like growth factor 1 (IGF-1), in the liver. IGF-1 is the factor that actually causes the growth of bones and other tissues of the body. IGF-1, in turn, signals the pituitary to reduce GH production. GHRH, somatostatin, GH, and IGF-1 levels in the body are tightly regulated by each other and by sleep, exercise, stress, food intake and blood sugar levels. If the pituitary continues to make GH independent of the normal regulatory mechanisms, the level of IGF-1 continues to rise, leading to bone growth and organ enlargement. The excess GH also causes changes in sugar and lipid metabolism and can cause diabetes.

Pituitary Tumors

In over 90 percent of acromegaly patients, the overproduction of GH is caused by a benign tumor of the pituitary gland, called an adenoma. These tumors produce excess GH and, as they expand, compress surrounding brain tissues, such as the optic nerves. This expansion causes the headaches and visual disturbances that are often symptoms of acromegaly. In addition, compression of the surrounding normal pituitary tissue can alter production of other hormones, leading to changes in menstruation and breast discharge in women and impotence in men.

There is a marked variation in rates of GH production and the aggressiveness of the tumor. Some adenomas grow slowly and symptoms of GH excess are often not noticed for many years. Other adenomas grow rapidly and invade surrounding brain areas or the sinuses, which are located near the pituitary. In general, younger patients tend to have more aggressive tumors.

Most pituitary tumors arise spontaneously and are not genetically inherited. Many pituitary tumors arise from a genetic alteration in a single pituitary cell which leads to increased cell division and tumor formation. This genetic change, or mutation, is not present at birth, but is acquired during life. The mutation occurs in a gene that regulates the transmission of chemical signals within pituitary cells; it permanently switches on the signal that tells the cell to divide and secrete GH. The events within the cell that cause disordered pituitary cell growth and GH over secretion currently are the subject of intensive research.

Non-pituitary Tumors

In a few patients, acromegaly is caused not by pituitary tumors but by tumors of the pancreas, lungs, and adrenal glands. These tumors also lead to an excess of GH, either because they produce GH themselves or, more frequently, because they produce GHRH, the hormone that stimulates the pituitary to make GH. In these patients, the excess GHRH can be measured in the blood and establishes that the cause of the acromegaly is not due to a pituitary defect. When these non-pituitary tumors are surgically removed, GH levels fall and the symptoms of acromegaly improve.

In patients with GHRH-producing, non-pituitary tumors, the pituitary still may be enlarged and may be mistaken for a tumor. Therefore, it is important that physicians carefully analyze all "pituitary tumors" removed from patients with acromegaly in order not to overlook the possibility that a tumor elsewhere in the body is causing the disorder.

How Common Is Acromegaly?

Small pituitary adenomas are common. During autopsies, they are found in up to 25 percent of the U.S. population. However, these tumors rarely cause symptoms or produce excessive GH or other pituitary hormones. Scientists estimate that about 3 out of every million people develop acromegaly each year and that 40 to 60 out of every million people suffer from the disease at any time. However, because the clinical diagnosis of acromegaly often is missed, these numbers probably underestimate the frequency of the disease.

How Is Acromegaly Diagnosed?

If a doctor suspects acromegaly, he or she can measure the GH level in the blood after a patient has fasted overnight to determine if it is elevated. However, a single measurement of an elevated blood GH level is not enough to diagnose acromegaly, because GH is secreted by the pituitary in spurts and its concentration in the blood can vary widely from minute to minute. At a given moment, a patient with acromegaly may have a normal GH level, whereas a GH level in a healthy person may be five times higher.

Because of these problems, more accurate information can be obtained when GH is measured under conditions in which GH secretion is normally suppressed. Physicians often use the oral glucose tolerance test to diagnose acromegaly, because ingestion of 75 g of the sugar glucose lowers blood GH levels less than 2 ng/ml in healthy people. In patients with GH overproduction, this reduction does not occur. The glucose tolerance test is the most reliable method of confirming a diagnosis of acromegaly.

Physicians also can measure IGF-1 levels in patients with suspected acromegaly. As mentioned earlier, elevated GH levels increase IGF-1 blood levels. Because IGF-1 levels are much more stable over the course of the day, they are often a more practical and reliable measure than GH levels. Elevated IGF-1 levels almost always indicate acromegaly. However, a pregnant woman's IGF-1 levels are two to three times higher than normal. In addition, physicians must be aware that IGF-1 levels decline in aging people and may be abnormally low in patients with poorly controlled diabetes mellitus.

After acromegaly has been diagnosed by measuring GH or IGF-1, imaging techniques, such as computed tomography (CT) scans or magnetic resonance imaging (MRI) scans of the pituitary are used to locate the tumor that causes the GH overproduction. Both techniques are excellent tools to visualize a tumor without surgery. If scans fail to detect a pituitary tumor, the physician should look for non-pituitary tumors in the chest, abdomen, or pelvis as the cause for excess GH. The presence of such tumors usually can be diagnosed by measuring GHRH in the blood and by a CT scan of possible tumor sites.

How Is Acromegaly Treated?

The goals of treatment are to reduce GH production to normal levels, to relieve the pressure that the growing pituitary tumor exerts on the surrounding brain areas, to preserve normal pituitary function, and to reverse or ameliorate the symptoms of acromegaly. Currently, treatment options include surgical removal of the tumor, drug therapy, and radiation therapy of the pituitary.

Surgery

Surgery is a rapid and effective treatment. The surgeon reaches the pituitary through an incision in the nose and, with special tools, removes the tumor tissue in a procedure called transsphenoidal surgery. This procedure promptly relieves the pressure on the surrounding brain regions and leads to a lowering of GH levels. If the surgery is successful, facial appearance and soft tissue swelling improve within a few days. Surgery is most successful in patients with blood GH levels below 40 ng/ml before the operation and with pituitary tumors no larger than 10 mm in diameter. Success depends on the skill and experience of the surgeon. The success rate also depends on what level of GH is defined as a cure. The best measure of surgical success is normalization of GH and IGF-1 levels. Ideally, GH should be less than 2 ng/ml after an oral glucose load. A review of GH levels in 1,360 patients worldwide immediately after surgery revealed that 60 percent had random GH levels below 5 ng/ml. Complications of surgery may include cerebrospinal fluid leaks, meningitis, or damage to the surrounding normal pituitary tissue, requiring lifelong pituitary hormone replacement.

Even when surgery is successful and hormone levels return to normal, patients must be carefully monitored for years for possible recurrence. More commonly, hormone levels may improve, but not return completely to normal. These patients may then require additional treatment, usually with medications.

Drug Therapy

Two medications currently are used to treat acromegaly. These drugs reduce both GH secretion and tumor size. Medical therapy is sometimes used to shrink large tumors before surgery. Bromocriptine (Parlodel®) in divided doses of about 20 mg daily reduces GH secretion from some pituitary tumors. Side effects include gastrointestinal upset, nausea, vomiting, light-headedness when standing, and nasal congestion. These side effects can be reduced or eliminated if medication is started at a very low dose at bedtime, taken with food, and gradually increased to the full therapeutic dose.

Because bromocriptine can be taken orally, it is an attractive choice as primary drug or in combination with other treatments. However, bromocriptine lowers GH and IGF-1 levels and reduces tumor size in less than half of patients with acromegaly. Some patients report improvement in their symptoms although their GH and IGF-1 levels still are elevated.

The second medication used to treat acromegaly is octreotide (Sandostatin®). Octreotide is a synthetic form of a brain hormone, somatostatin, that stops GH production. This drug must be injected under the skin every 8 hours for effective treatment. Most patients with acromegaly respond to this medication. In many patients, GH levels fall within one hour and headaches improve within minutes after the injection. Several studies have shown that octreotide is effective for long-term treatment. Octreotide also has been used successfully to treat patients with acromegaly caused by non-pituitary tumors.

Because octreotide inhibits gastrointestinal and pancreatic function, long-term use causes digestive problems such as loose stools, nausea, and gas in one third of patients. In addition, approximately 25 percent of patients develop gallstones, which are usually asymptomatic. In rare cases, octreotide treatment can cause diabetes. On the other hand, scientists have found that in some acromegaly patients who already have diabetes, octreotide can reduce the need for insulin and improve blood sugar control.

Radiation Therapy

Radiation therapy has been used both as a primary treatment and combined with surgery or drugs. It is usually reserved for patients who have tumor remaining after surgery. These patients often also receive medication to lower GH levels. Radiation therapy is given in divided doses over four to six weeks. This treatment lowers GH levels by about 50 percent over 2 to 5 years. Patients monitored for more than 5 years show significant further improvement. Radiation therapy causes a gradual loss of production of other pituitary hormones with time. Loss of vision and brain injury, which have been reported, are very rare complications of radiation treatments.

No single treatment is effective for all patients. Treatment should be individualized depending on patient characteristics, such as age and tumor size. If the tumor has not yet invaded surrounding brain tissues, removal of the pituitary adenoma by an experienced neurosurgeon is usually the first choice. After surgery, a patient must be monitored for a long time for increasing GH levels. If surgery does not normalize hormone levels or a relapse occurs, a doctor will usually begin additional drug therapy. The first choice should be bromocriptine because it is easy to administer; octreotide is the second alternative. With both medications, long-term therapy is necessary because their withdrawal can lead to rising GH levels and tumor re-expansion. Radiation therapy is generally used for patients whose tumors are not completely removed by surgery; for patients who are not good candidates for surgery because of other health problems; and for patients who do not respond adequately to surgery and medication.

Additional Information about Radiation Therapy of Acromegaly

External beam irradiation with modern equipment is available at most major medical centers. It is an important treatment of acromegaly due to pituitary adenomas secreting growth hormone that cannot be cured surgically, and has predictable effects on the growth of the adenoma and on growth hormone levels.

Control of Growth of the Pituitary Adenoma. Further growth of the tumor is prevented in more than 99% of patients, with only a fraction of a percent of patients requiring subsequent surgery for tumor mass effects, such as loss of visual function due to pressure on the optic nerve by the tumor.

Effect on Growth Hormone Levels. Growth hormone levels fall predictably with time, and by 2 years are 50% lower than the level before treatment. By 5 years after irradiation the growth hormone levels have fallen to about 25% of the baseline level before treatment. A further fall in the growth hormone level is seen at 10 and 15 years after treatment. The percentage fall in growth hormone levels is not dependent on the size of the adenoma or on the pre-radiotherapy level of growth hormone. Patients respond equally well regardless of gender, history of previous surgery, and whether high prolactin levels are

295

found. The fraction of patients achieving growth hormone levels less than 5 ng/mL approaches 90% after 15 years in our experience. Although the response to radiation is similar regardless of baseline growth hormone level, patients with initial growth hormone level greater than 100 ng/mL are significantly less likely to achieve growth hormone levels less than 5 ng/mL during long-term follow-up. Thus, surgery to remove part of an adenoma can significantly increase the long-term outcome if post-operative levels of growth hormone are below 100 ng/mL.

Effect on Pituitary Function. Hypopituitarism is the most common side effect of pituitary irradiation, and may be more likely in patients who have had surgery prior to irradiation. This complication does not appear to be more common in patients with acromegaly than in patients with other pituitary adenomas receiving similar treatment.

Side Effects. Side effects of irradiation are rare. Vision loss is extremely rare when the total dose is limited to 4680 rads given in 25 fractions over 35 days, with individual fractions not exceeding 180 rads. The reported cases have occurred almost entirely in patients who have received larger doses or higher fractional doses. The theory that patients with acromegaly are prone to radiation induced injury to the brain and optic nerves is not supported by a review of the reported cases. Other complications are also extremely rare. Given the increased mortality of acromegaly, and particularly the risk of heart disease, our approach is to normalize IGF-1 levels if possible. We recommend initial transsphenoidal adenomectomy, including partial removal of large adenomas with a low probability of surgical cure. Megavoltage irradiation is recommended to patients with persistent or recurrent growth hormone hypersecretion. Due to the delayed effects of irradiation on growth hormone secretion, we currently use bromocriptine and/or a somatostatin analogue to reduce growth hormone levels after radiotherapy. Medical therapy should be withdrawn at yearly intervals to determine whether continued medical therapy is required. Lifelong follow-up of pituitary function is indicated.

—the preceding section was prepared by Richard C. Eastman, M.D., Director, Division of Diabetes, Endocrinology and Metabolic Diseases, National Institutes of Health, NIDDK, Bethesda, Maryland

Suggested Readings

Benefits versus risks of medical therapy for acromegaly. Acromegaly Therapy Consensus Development Panel. *American Journal of Medicine* 97(5):468–473, 1994.

Eastman RC, Gorden P, Glatstein E, Roth J. Radiation Therapy of Acromegaly. *Endocrinology and Metabolism Clinics of North America* 21(3):693–711, 1992.

Ezzat S, Forster MJ, Berchtold P, Redelmeier DA, Boerlin V, Harris AG. Acromegaly. Clinical and Biochemical Features in 500 Patients. *Medicine* (Baltimore) 73(5):233–240, 1994.

Ezzat S. Living with acromegaly. *Endocrinology and Metabolism Clinics of North America* 21:753–760, 1992.

Jaffe CA; Barkan AL. Acromegaly. Recognition and treatment. *Drugs* 47(3):425–45, 1994.

Jaffe CA, Barkan AL. Treatment of acromegaly with dopamine agonists. *Endocrinology and Metabolism Clinics of North America* 21:713–735, 1992.

Krishna AY; Phillips LS. Management of acromegaly: a review. *American Journal of Medical Science* 308(6):370–375, 1994.

Melmed S. Acromegaly. *New England Journal of Medicine* 322:966–977, 1990.

Molitch ME. Clinical manifestations of acromegaly. *Endocrinology and Metabolism Clinics of North America* 21(3):597–614, 1992.

Additional Resource

Pituitary Tumor Network Association
16350 Ventura Blvd, Suite 231
Encino, CA 91436
(805) 499-9973
(805) 499-1523 Fax

Chapter 26

Pituitary Tumors

Pituitary Tumor Backgrounder

Patient Population

It is estimated that between 1% and 2% (60 million to 120 million people) of the world's population harbor clinically significant pituitary tumors. Approximately 22% of all adults have been found to harbor pituitary adenomas (tumors). While most of these tumors are thought to produce no symptoms, it is, in fact, unknown to what extent most of these tumors affect the hosts. Much still remains to be learned about pituitary functions and disease(s).

Overview

The pituitary is a peanut-shaped gland located just below the brain behind and between the eyes. The pituitary gland, long referred to as the "master gland," secretes a number of hormones that govern growth, urine output, and many other functions. Both the thyroid and adrenal glands are regulated by the pituitary gland. Pituitary tumors are usually not cancerous, but they do cause severe medical problems by pressing on the optic nerves, or by pressing on the normal pituitary, disrupting the pituitary's secretion of hormones.

Information in this chapter contains text from "Pituitary Tumor Backgrounder," *The Pituitary Patient Resource Guide*, Second Edition, ©1995, 1997 Pituitary Tumor Network Association, 16350 Ventura Blvd., Suite 231, Encino, CA 91436, reprinted with permission; and "Pituitary Tumor PDQ," National Cancer Institute, CancerNet, gopher.nih.gov/00/clin/cancernet/pdqinfo.

The symptoms of pituitary tumors vary depending on the size and location of the tumor and whether or not the tumor secretes hormones. The majority of pituitary adenomas are nonmalignant and grow slowly within the pituitary gland, inside the sella turcica, but the more aggressive and invasive of these tumors grow rapidly. They can cause blindness, increased intracranial pressure, and life-threatening endocrine abnormalities.

Some pituitary tumors stem the gland's secretion of growth hormone (GH) and cause growth arrest in children. These tumors may also limit the pituitary's secretion of the gonadotropic hormones (FSH and LH), which govern the development and function of the ovary and testis. Men may manifest testicular atrophy, decreased body hair, decreased libido, impotence and infertility. In females, the tumors often cause breast shrinkage, cessation of menstruation, decreased libido, and infertility.

Tumors that foster a lack of adrenocorticotropic hormone (ACTH) may cause low blood sugar, as well as low blood pressure, weakness and fatigue. Extreme cases can be life-threatening by causing the body to go into shock. Tumors that limit the secretion of thyroid stimulating hormone (TSH) may stunt growth and induce tiredness, constipation, dry skin, sensitivity to cold, and hoarseness. Lack of normal secretion of pituitary hormones is called hypopituitarism. If all hormones are lacking, it is called pan-hypo-pituitarism.

Other tumors induce specific symptoms by releasing an excess of pituitary hormones. Tumors that secrete the hormone prolactin can prompt the abnormal production of breast milk and the lack of menstruation in women and impotence in men. GH-secreting tumors often boost growth excessively, so that, if untreated, children may reach giant-like proportions (gigantism), a few attaining heights greater than eight feet tall and shoe sizes in the 30s. In adults, excessive GH secretion results in acromegaly. Acromegaly causes the feet, hands, nose and jaw to grow, in addition to enlarging internal organs. Gonadotropin-secreting tumors usually produce inactive hormone fragments and are associated with hypogonadism, a condition of testosterone absence or deficiency in men and estrogen deficiency in women.

ACTH-secreting tumors result in over activity of the adrenal cortex (Cushing's Syndrome), with excessive weight gain, weakness, high blood pressure, and diabetes as some of its effects. Some patients may inherit a common pituitary tumor called a craniopharyngioma. This tumor often disrupts vision by pressing on the optic nerve. Craniopharyagiomas also prompt a lack of most pituitary hormones, thereby causing a combination of many of the symptoms previously described. It often is found in children and is very difficult to treat. Rathke's cleft cyst is a close cousin of the craniopharyngioma.

Treatment

Treatment should only be undertaken by highly skilled and experienced endocrinologists and neurosurgeons. Successful outcome often rests on their specialized training.

Physicians treat pituitary tumors with surgery, radiation therapy, drugs or a combination of these treatments. Surgery is the first treatment of choice for most tumors that enlarge rapidly and threaten vision, followed by medication and finally, if other methods fail, radiation.

Pituitary Tumor PDQ

What is PDQ?

PDQ is a computer system that gives up-to-date information on cancer treatment. It is a service of the National Cancer Institute (NCI) for people with cancer and their families, and for doctors, nurses, and other health care professionals.

PDQ tells about the current treatments for most cancers. The information in PDQ is reviewed each month by cancer experts. It is updated when there is new information. The patient information in PDQ also tells about warning signs and how the cancer is found. PDQ also lists information about research on new treatments (clinical trials), doctors who treat cancer, and hospitals with cancer programs. The treatment information in this summary is based on information in the PDQ treatment summary for health professionals on this cancer.

How to Use PDQ

You can use PDQ to learn more about current treatment for your kind of cancer. Bring this material from PDQ with you when you see your doctor. You can talk with your doctor, who knows you and has the facts about your disease, about which treatment would be best for you. Before you start your treatment, you might also want to seek a second opinion from a doctor who treats cancer.

Before you start treatment, you also may want to think about taking part in a clinical trial. A clinical trial is a study that uses new treatments to care for patients. Each study is based on past studies and what has been learned in the laboratory. Each trial answers certain scientific questions in order to find new and better ways to help cancer patients. During clinical trials, more and more information is collected about new treatments, their risks, and how well they do or do not work. If clinical trials show that the new treatment is better than the treatment currently being used, the new treatment may become the "standard" treatment. Listings of clinical trials are a part of PDQ. Many cancer doctors who take part in clinical trials are listed in PDQ.

If you want to know more about cancer and how it is treated, or if you wish to learn about clinical trials for your kind of cancer, you can call the National Cancer Institute's Cancer Information Service. The number is 1-800-4-CANCER (1-800-422-6237); TTY at 1-800-332-8615. The call is free and a trained information specialist will talk with you and answer your questions.

PDQ may change when there is new information. Check with the Cancer Information Service to be sure that you have the most up-to-date information.

What Are Pituitary Tumors?

Pituitary tumors are tumors found in the pituitary gland, a small organ about the size of a pea in the center of the brain just above the back of the nose. Your pituitary gland makes hormones that affect your growth and the functions of other glands in your body.

Most pituitary tumors are benign. This means that they grow very slowly and do not spread to other parts of the body. This patient information statement covers several types of pituitary tumors. Another type of pituitary tumor, called craniopharyngioma, is covered in the patient information statements on adult or childhood brain tumors.

If you have a pituitary tumor, your pituitary gland may make too many hormones, which can cause other problems in your body. Tumors that make hormones are called functioning tumors, while those that do not make hormones are called nonfunctioning tumors.

Certain pituitary tumors can cause a disease called Cushing's disease, in which too many hormones called glucocorticoids are released into your bloodstream. This causes fat to build up in the face, back, and chest, and the arms and legs to become very thin. Other symptoms include too much sugar in the blood, weak muscles and bones, a flushed face, and high blood pressure. Other pituitary tumors can cause a condition called acromegaly. Acromegaly means that the hands, feet, and face are larger than normal; in very young people, the whole body may grow much larger than normal. Another type of pituitary tumor can cause the breasts to make milk, even though you are not pregnant; you may stop having your periods as well.

Like most tumors, pituitary tumors are best treated when they are found (diagnosed) early. You should see your doctor if you have headaches, trouble seeing, nausea or vomiting, or any of the symptoms caused by too many hormones.

If you have symptoms, your doctor may order lab tests to see what the hormone levels are in your blood. Your doctor may also order an MRI (magnetic resonance imaging) scan, which uses magnetic waves to make a picture of the inside of your brain. Other special x-rays may also be done.

Your prognosis (chance of recovery) and choice of treatment depend on the type of tumor you have, your age, and your general state of health.

Types of Pituitary Tumors

Once a pituitary tumor is found, more tests will be done to find out how far the tumor has spread and whether or not it makes hormones. Your doctor needs to know the type of tumor you have to plan treatment. The following types of pituitary tumors are found.

ACTH-Producing Tumors. These tumors make a hormone called adrenocorticotropic hormone (ACTH), which stimulates your adrenal glands to make glucocorticoids. When your body makes too much ACTH, it causes Cushing's disease.

Prolactin-Producing Tumors. These tumors make prolactin, a hormone that stimulates a woman's breasts to make milk during and after pregnancy. Prolactin-secreting tumors can cause the breasts to make milk and menstrual periods to stop when a woman is not pregnant. In men, prolactin-producing tumors can cause impotence.

Growth Hormone-Producing Tumors. These tumors make growth hormone, which can cause acromegaly or gigantism when too much is made.

Nonfunctioning Pituitary Tumors. Nonfunctioning tumors do not produce hormones.

Recurrent Pituitary Tumors. Recurrent disease means that the tumor has come back (recurred) after it has been treated. It may come back in the pituitary or in another part of the body.

How Pituitary Tumors Are Treated

There are treatments for all patients with pituitary tumors. Three kinds of treatment are used:

- surgery (taking out the tumor in an operation)
- radiation therapy (using high-dose x-rays to kill tumor cells)
- drug therapy.

Surgery is a common treatment for pituitary tumors. Your doctor may remove the tumor using one of the following operations:

- A transphenoidal hypophysectomy removes the tumor through a cut in the nasal passage.
- A craniotomy removes the tumor through a cut in the front of the skull.

Radiation therapy uses high-energy x-rays to kill cancer cells and shrink tumors. Radiation for pituitary tumors usually comes from a machine outside the body (external radiation therapy). Radiation therapy may be used alone or in addition to surgery or drug therapy.

Certain drugs can also block the pituitary from making too many hormones.

Treatment by Type

Treatments for pituitary tumors depend on the type of tumor, how far the tumor has spread into the brain, your age, and your overall health.

You may receive treatment that is considered standard based on its effectiveness in a number of patients in past studies, or you may choose to go into a clinical trial. Not all patients are cured with standard therapy and some standard treatments may have more side effects than are desired. For these reasons, clinical trials are designed to find better ways to treat cancer patients and are based on the most up-to-date information. Clinical trials are going on in some parts of the country for patients with pituitary tumors. If you want more information, call the Cancer Information Service at 1-800-4-CANCER (1-800-422-6237); TTY at 1-800-332-8615.

ACTH-Producing Pituitary Tumor

Your treatment may be one of the following:

1. Surgery to remove the tumor (transphenoidal hypophysectomy or craniotomy)

2. Radiation therapy. Clinical trials may be testing new types of radiation therapy.

3. Surgery plus radiation therapy.

4. Radiation therapy plus drug therapy to stop the tumor from making ACTH.

Prolactin-Producing Pituitary Tumor

Your treatment may be one of the following:

1. Surgery to remove the tumor (transphenoidal hypophysectomy or craniotomy).

2. Radiation therapy. Clinical trials may be testing new types of radiation therapy.

3. Drug therapy to stop the tumor from making prolactin. Clinical trials are testing new drugs for this purpose.

4. Surgery, radiation therapy, and drug therapy.

Growth Hormone-Producing Pituitary Tumor

Your treatment may be one of the following:

1. Surgery to remove the tumor (transphenoidal hypophysectomy or craniotomy).

2. Radiation therapy.

3. Drug therapy to stop the tumor from making growth hormone.

Nonfunctioning Pituitary Tumor

Your treatment may be one of the following:

1. Surgery to remove the tumor (transphenoidal hypophysectomy or craniotomy).

2. Radiation therapy alone or in addition to surgery.

Recurrent Pituitary Tumor

Treatment for recurrent pituitary tumor depends on the type of tumor, the type of treatment you already had, and other factors such as your general condition.

You may want to take part in a clinical trial of new treatments.

To Learn More

To learn more about pituitary tumor, call the National Cancer Institute's Cancer Information Service at 1-800-4-CANCER (1-800-422-6237); TTY at 1-800-332-8615. By dialing this toll-free number, you can speak with someone who can answer your questions.

The Cancer Information Service can also send you booklets. The following general booklets on questions related to cancer may be helpful:

- What You Need To Know About Cancer
- Taking Time: Support for People with Cancer and the People Who Care About Them
- What Are Clinical Trials All About?
- Chemotherapy and You: A Guide to Self-Help During Treatment
- Radiation Therapy and You: A Guide to Self-Help During Treatment
- Eating Hints for Cancer Patients
- Advanced Cancer: Living Each Day
- When Cancer Recurs: Meeting the Challenge Again

There are many other places where you can get material about cancer treatment and services to help you. You can check the social service office at your hospital for local and national agencies that help with your finances, getting to and from treatment, care at home, and dealing with your problems. The American Cancer Society, for example, has many free services. Their local offices are listed in the white pages of the telephone book.

You can also write to the National Cancer Institute at this address:

National Cancer Institute
Office of Cancer Communications
31 Center Drive, MSC 2580
Bethesda, MD 20892-2580

You can contact the Pituitary Tumor Network Association at:

Pituitary Tumor Network Association
16350 Ventura Blvd, Suite 231
Encino, CA 91436
(805) 499-2262
(805) 499-1523 fax
email: ptna@pituitary.com

Chapter 27

Pituitary Tumors in Children

Introduction

The pituitary is a peanut-shaped gland lodged in the brain behind and between the eyes. This gland secretes a number of hormones that govern growth and sexual development and functions. Although it occurs rarely, children can develop tumors in their pituitaries. These tumors are usually not cancerous, but can cause medical problems by pressing on tissues in the pituitary or adjacent to it, or by disrupting the pituitary's secretion of hormones.

Symptoms

The symptoms of pituitary tumors vary depending on the size and location of the tumor and whether the tumor secretes hormones. Headache is the most common symptom and is usually intermittent, of moderate severity, and not limited to a particular section of the head. Pituitary tumors can also cause vomiting or dizziness.

Pituitary tumors often press on the optic nerve, causing double vision, partial blindness, loss of peripheral vision, and rarely, complete loss of sight.

Pressure from pituitary tumors can also stem the gland's secretion of certain hormones. A pituitary tumor that limits the secretion

From *Pituitary Patient Resource Guide*, First Annual North American Edition, ©1995 Pituitary Tumor Network Association, 16350 Ventura Blvd., Suite 231, Encino, CA 91436, (805) 499-9973; reprinted with permission.

of growth hormone (GH) stunts the growth of children and causes low blood sugar, which can induce fainting, dizziness, anxiety and intense hunger. Tumors that foster a lack of adrenocorticotropic hormone (ACTH) also cause low blood sugar, as well as low blood pressure, which can cause dizziness when standing and fatigue. In extreme cases, the lack of ACTH can cause the body to go into shock, which can be life-threatening.

Some pituitary tumors delay or stop the sexual development of children. In post-puberty boys, the tumors cause their genitals to shrink and foster a loss of facial and pubic hair. In post-puberty girls, the tumors cause breast shrinkage, partial loss of pubic hair, and cessation of menstruation. These tumors wreak such effects by limiting the pituitary's secretion of the gonadotropin hormone, which helps govern the development and functioning of the ovary and testes.

Pituitary tumors that limit the secretion of thyroid stimulating hormone (TSH) can stunt growth, foster poor school performance, induce tiredness, constipation, dry skin, a sensitivity to cold, and cause girls to have irregular periods or not to menstruate at all. Some pituitary tumors stem the secretion of vasopressin. This hormone triggers the kidney's reabsorption of water from urine and a lack of it causes such symptoms as great thirst, excess urination, voracious appetite accompanied by emaciation, loss of strength and fainting.

Other pituitary tumors secrete an excess of pituitary hormones, which induce specific symptoms. Tumors that secrete the hormone prolactin can prompt the production of breast milk and the lack of menstruation in post-puberty girls, and impotence in post-puberty boys. An excess of prolactin can also delay or stop puberty in both sexes. A rare type of pituitary tumor causes an excess of prolactin and associated symptoms not by secreting prolactin, but by disrupting the neural pathways that inhibit prolactin secretion.

Pituitary tumors that secrete ACTH stunt growth, delay or stop puberty, and cause weight gain, acne, purple streaks in the skin, a round red face, and a bulge of fat just below the neck. These tumors can also foster weakness, depression, forgetfulness, and trigger a sudden loss of vision that can be complete or partial.

GH-secreting tumors in growing children can boost growth excessively, so that, if not treated, the children reach giant-like proportions, some attaining heights greater than eight feet tall and shoe sizes in the thirties. These tumors can also cause arthritis.

In post-puberty children whose bones have stopped growing, excess growth hormone can cause their feet and hands, lips, nose and jaws to enlarge. It can also foster excess perspiration and fatigue, a widening of the spaces between the teeth, furrows in the forehead, and weakness in the hands.

Tumors that secrete luteinizing hormone (LH) can lead to precocious puberty in children younger than age 9. In girls, the tumors foster breast development, pubic hair, and menstruation. In boys, the tumors cause their genitals to enlarge and facial and pubic hair to sprout. Tumors that secrete follicle stimulating hormone (FSH), in contrast, can retard sexual development in both sexes and stunt growth. These tumors often disrupt vision by pressing on the optic nerve.

Some pituitary tumors can disrupt the function of the thyroid gland by secreting thyroid stimulating hormone. This in turn enlarges the thyroid, causing a visibly large lump in the neck known as a goiter. These tumors also cause nervousness, a rapid pulse, weight loss, excess eating and sweating, and a sensitivity to heat.

The most common type of pituitary tumor in children is inherited and is called a craniopharyngioma. This tumor often disrupts vision by pressing on the optic nerve. Craniopharyngiomas also cause a lack of most pituitary hormones, prompting a combination of some of the symptoms previously described for tumors that induce a deficiency of single pituitary hormone.

Diagnosis

Larger pituitary tumors can be detected on an x-ray, computerized tomography scan or magnetic resonance scan. Many pituitary tumors, however, are too small to be noticeable on such images of the pituitary region of the brain. To diagnose these tumors, doctors try to detect the hormonal abnormalities they induce with various tests. Often blood or urine levels of specific hormones are measured within a few hours of giving the patient compounds known to stimulate or suppress production of the hormones.

Sometimes patients must undergo a glucose tolerance test. For this test, they fast overnight, drink a sugar solution and then the technician takes blood samples in which they measure their blood sugar levels and levels of growth hormone.

To detect pituitary tumors that foster a lack of vasopressin, patients must undergo a water deprivation test. For this test, patients are deprived of water and food for 8 hours while being monitored in a hospital. During that period of time, urine output and blood samples are collected and analyzed.

If patients are suspected of having a pituitary tumor that secretes ACTH, they might have to undergo a procedure known as bilateral inferior petrosal sinus sampling. For this test, small tubes are threaded through both jugular veins on either side of the neck until they reach the veins adjacent to the pituitary. Blood samples are taken from these two veins at the same time that a blood sample is drawn from a vein in the arm.

A greater concentration of ACTH in the pituitary veins than in the arm vein confirms that the pituitary is generating the excess ACTH and not tumors located in other organs or tissues. If one pituitary vein has a greater concentration of ACTH than the other, in addition, that indicates the tumor lies in the section of the pituitary that is closest to that vein.

Doctors treat pituitary tumors with radiation therapy, surgery, drugs, or a combination of these treatments. Surgery is the treatment of choice for tumors that enlarge rapidly and threaten vision. The treatment plan for other pituitary tumors varies according to the type and size of the tumor.

Surgical removal of large pituitary tumors must be done through a hole drilled in the skull. Infrequent complications of the surgery include stroke, brain infection, and brain damage. Often, large tumors are too close to vital regions of the brain for surgeons to safely remove them completely. A portion of the tumor is left behind, consequently, which must be treated with radiation to prevent regrowth.

Smaller tumors can be removed via an incision made through the roof of the mouth just under the lip. The latter procedure, known as transsphenoidal surgery, does not disrupt brain tissue other than the pituitary because the gland is accessed through one of the sinuses. This is considered low-risk surgery, although rare complications can develop. These complications include inflammation of the membrane that encases the brain (meningitis), brain infection, and total loss of pituitary functions, the latter of which is treated with a number of medications taken for life.

Within a day of surgery on the pituitary, some patients will develop great thirst and excess urination because the surgery has stemmed the pituitary's secretion of the hormone vasopressin. The lack of vasopressin can be effectively treated with a synthetic form of the hormone taken via a nose spray or by injection. This drug often has to be taken for just a few weeks, after which normal secretion of vasopressin is restored. Rarely, the secretion of vasopressin is permanently disrupted, in which case the drug must be taken for life.

Surgery can also transiently or permanently disrupt the secretion of other pituitary hormones. Patients with this complication are treated with drugs that replace the deficient hormones or the compounds the hormones induce the body to produce.

Radiation therapy for pituitary tumors involves directing radiation at the tumor several times a week for about 6 weeks. Side effects of the therapy can include some permanent memory loss and a permanent loss of certain pituitary hormones, which are replaced with drugs.

The treatment of choice for small tumors that secrete ACTH is removal by transsphenoidal surgery. These tumors can often be completely removed, with the surgery rarely causing a deficiency of other pituitary hormones. If surgery is not possible because the tumor is too close to critical areas of the brain, about three-quarters of the children with ACTH-secreting tumors can be effectively treated with radiation therapy.

If surgery and radiation therapy do not effectively treat ACTH-secreting tumors, the adverse effects of these tumors can often be curtailed by surgically removing the adrenal glands. ACTH's stimulation of these glands, which are lodged above the kidneys, cause most of the symptoms associated with pituitary tumors that secrete ACTH.

Patients whose adrenals are removed, however, must permanently take the drugs cortisone and aldosterone to replace some of the hormones the adrenals secrete, including those vital for maintaining blood pressure and salt retention. In less than one quarter of the patients treated with this surgery, the pituitary tumor grows to a large enough size within ten years that vision is threatened and the tumor must be removed by transsphenoidal surgery or shrunk via radiation therapy.

ACTH-secreting pituitary tumors can also be treated with a number of drugs taken orally such as nicotane, aminoglutethimide, metyrapone, trilostane, and ketoconasole. These drugs often cause serious or debilitating side effects including skin rashes, gastrointestinal disorders, dizziness and inflammation of the liver. For this reason, drug therapy for ACTH-secreting pituitary tumors is usually only given for a few months to relieve symptoms until patients can be treated with surgery or radiation.

Doctors usually treat tumors that secrete prolactin with the drug bromocriptine, which is taken orally each day. This drug causes the tumor to shrink. Patients often have to take it for several years to be permanently cured of their tumors. Bromocriptine's main side effects are stomach irritation and drowsiness, which is countered by taking the drug at bedtime.

Bromocriptine also sometimes effectively treats pituitary tumors that secrete growth hormone, as well as those that induce excess prolactin by disrupting the neural pathways that inhibit prolactin secretion.

Tumors that secrete GH, TSH, LH or FSH and craniopharyngio- mas are usually treated with radiation therapy if surgery cannot re- move all of the tumor. Some patients with growth hormone-secreting tumors are treated with a drug that inhibits the release of the hor- mone until radiation therapy is completed. Many doctors prefer to treat all patients with radiation therapy following surgical removal of craniopharyngiomas to reduce the risk of recurrence.

Patients with pituitary tumors that foster a lack of certain hor- mones are usually treated with drugs that replace these hormones or the compounds the hormones induce the body to produce. Most of these drugs are taken orally each day for the rest of the patient's life, although some must be given by injection or via a nasal spray.

— by Margie Patlak,
National Institute of Child Health
and Human Development
National Institutes of Health
Bethesda, Maryland

Chapter 28

TSH (Thyroid Stimulating Hormone)-Secreting Pituitary Tumors

If you, or a member of your family, have been diagnosed with a TSH pituitary tumor, this chapter will summarize the main points necessary to understand this disease and its treatment.

Definition

A TSH (Thyroid-Stimulating Hormone) pituitary tumor arises from one of the TSH-secreting cells localized in the anterior pituitary. This tumor secretes an excess of TSH (sometimes even more active than the normal TSH) and often also alpha-subunit (one of the two components of TSH). The cells secreting the other pituitary hormones usually have a normal function; however, in some cases, the tumor can secrete one or more other hormones (active or not).

Frequency

TSH pituitary tumors are rare; they represent about 2% of all pituitary tumors.

Cause

Right now, the cause is unknown; no familial predisposition has been found. Scientists work hard to identify the factors called

From *Pituitary Patient Resource Guide*, First Annual North American Edition, ©1995 Pituitary Tumor Network Association, 16350 Ventura Blvd., Suite 231, Encino, CA 91436, (805) 499-9973; reprinted with permission.

oncogenes that transform a normal cell into a tumorous cell. In the future, when these factors are identified, we hope that specific treatment will be able to target the oncogenes, and reverse the tumoral transformation.

Pathology

The tumors are overwhelmingly benign adenomas (very few will have a malignant transformation, with the possibility of distant metastases, like in any cancer.)

Natural Evolution

Even if the pathology of the tumor is benign, we know that the local evolution can be very aggressive, with extension toward the optic chiasm (crossing of both optic nerves), with the potential risk of sight impairment or even blindness, or toward other important brain structures. There is not much room around the pituitary gland, so it is understandable that if the tumor keeps on growing, there can be serious consequences.

Size

The exact size is better evaluated by the surgeon: if the tumor is less than 1 cm, it is a micro-adenoma; if it is more than 1 cm, it is a macro-adenoma. The smaller tumors are less likely to be invasive or complicated and are more often cured by surgery alone. Unfortunately, diagnosis is often made at the stage of macro-adenoma.

Symptoms

The symptoms occur insidiously, and it sometimes takes years before you realize that there is something wrong.

- *Symptoms related to the secretion of excess TSH:* TSH is the hormone that drives the thyroid gland; an excess of TSH will result in excessive production of thyroid hormones, called hyperthyroidism. The main symptoms are: palpitations, fast heart beats, tiredness, increased frequency of bowel movements, weight loss, nervousness, heat intolerance, excess sweating, irregular periods in women.

- *Symptoms related to the tumor itself (shared by all other pituitary tumors)*: headaches, visual defects (serious complication of a big tumor with upward extension.)

- *Other:* if another hormone is secreted at the same time, you can experience other symptoms of hormonal imbalance: for example, in the case of secretion of GH (growth hormone), symptoms of acromegaly.

Diagnosis

Your Endocrinologist will coordinate your work-up in order to confirm the diagnosis, eliminate other causes of hyperthyroidism and inappropriate secretion of TSH and have a good idea of the extension and sometimes complications of your tumor.

The extent of the work-up depends on the center where you will be evaluated and treated. Research centers will run more sophisticated tests that are not mandatory for the diagnosis but will help to better understand TSH-pituitary tumors and eventually find a more specific treatment. The minimal work-up should include:

Hormonal Work-up

- Level of TSH and alpha subunit in the basal situation and usually after stimulation by TRH (TRH-TSH Releasing Hormone is the hormone that drives the secretion of TSH by the pituitary).

- Level of thyroid hormones

- Level of the other pituitary hormones to check if their secretion is increased (if the tumor secretes more than one hormone) or impaired (a big tumor can compress and compromise the function of the adjacent normal pituitary). It is important to know it before surgery.

Other Pre-Surgical Tests

- Visualization of the tumor by MRI or CT-scan of the pituitary. This will provide information on the size and extension of the tumor.

- Visual fields, to check if there is any sight impairment.

Treatment

TSH-pituitary tumors are rare and can be locally aggressive in their evolution. After thorough evaluation, you need to be treated and followed by a specialized team that is experienced in dealing with TSH-pituitary tumors (remember, all pituitary tumors are not alike): Besides your endocrinologist, the team should include outstanding neurosurgeon and radiation therapy specialists. The three main tools for treatment are:

Surgery

Surgery is the treatment of choice. The procedure is called transsphenoidal surgery. The surgeon will try to remove selectively the adenoma, sparing the normal pituitary. In the case of well-encapsulated tumors, cure is possible with surgery alone, mainly in the case of micro-adenoma. However, only a prolonged follow-up will confirm the cure. In the case of an invasive tumor, the surgeon can remove as much as is safely possible, thus improving the efficacy of subsequent external radiation and/or octreotide treatments. The procedure is minimally traumatic with a low risk of complications in expert hands: a leak of cerebral fluid with its risk of infection (meningitis), damage of the normal pituitary or a transient water imbalance (diabetes insipidus or the opposite, retention of water) are possible.

External Radiation

If the surgeon knows that there are tumorous cells left (invasive tumor) or in the case of recurrence after surgery, external radiation is necessary. The radiation destroys residual tumor; however, the effect is slow and some patients will need medication (octreotide), while waiting the full effect of radiation. Unfortunately, normal pituitary cells also are sensitive to radiation, meaning that normal pituitary function can be compromised in the following years. Another good reason to have continuing endocrine follow-up is so that replacement hormones can be introduced when necessary. If you have not yet completed your family, it is important for you to know that radiation will progressively decrease your fertility, and the possible therapeutic options should be discussed. Lastly, in the long run, some patients may develop memory problems as a consequence of this irradiation.

Medical Treatment

The majority of TSH pituitary tumors are sensitive to an analog of somatostatin (octreotide). This drug has recently been approved by the FDA for acromegaly, but not yet for TSH-pituitary tumors; as such, it may only be administered by certain research centers. It is the drug of choice if surgery and/or external radiation are not curative. This drug is palliative and cannot cure the disease, but it can decrease the secretion of TSH and stop the growth of the tumor. At high doses, a shrinking of the tumor may occasionally occur. Octreotide is given by subcutaneous injections, two to three times a day. Possible side effects include stomach problems with diarrhea (which usually improve after a few injections) and gallbladder stones.

Hormonal replacement is sometimes necessary, if pituitary function is impaired. Anti-thyroid medications (PTU or Tapazole) or destruction of the thyroid by radioactive iodine usually have no place in the treatment of TSH-pituitary tumors because TSH levels go up when thyroid hormones decrease and tumor growth may be stimulated.

Follow-up

A long follow-up is necessary, even when surgery seems to have been curative. Here again, because of the aggressiveness and rare nature of the tumor, it should only be managed by an experienced team. Your endocrinologist will look for signs of recurrence, and also screen for possible complications of your treatment (i.e., pituitary insufficiency after external radiation, gall bladder stones on octreotide.)

Reviews should be more frequent at the beginning and then on a yearly basis when you are stable. Again, it should include blood work (hormonal evaluation), MRI or CT scan of the pituitary and visual fields testing, plus an ultrasound of the gallbladder to screen for stones, if you are on octreotide.

Suggested References

B.D. Weintraub, P.A. Petrick, N. Gesundheit and E.H. Oldfield. TSH-secreting pituitary adenoma. In *Frontiers in Thyroidology*, 1986, vol. 1, 71-77, Ed. G. Medeiros-Neto and E. Gaitan (Plenum publishing corporation)

N. Gesundheit, P. Petrick, M. Nissim et al. TSH-secreting pituitary adenomas: clinical and biochemical heterogeneity: case reports and follow-up of nine patients. *Annals of Internal Medicine* 1989; 111:827-835

Ph. Chanson, B.D. Weintraub and A. Harris. Octreotide therapy for TSH-secreting pituitary adenomas: a follow-up of 52 patients. *Annals of Internal Medicine* 1993

— by Francoise Brucker-Davis, M.D., Visiting Associate,
NIDDK Molecular and Cellular Endocrinology Branch,
National Institutes of Health, Bethesda, Maryland

Chapter 29

Detecting Gonadotropin-Secreting Pituitary Tumors

A new method for detecting gonadotropin-secreting pituitary tumors has shown that they are far more common in women than was previously believed, according to a group of Pennsylvania researchers. Once thought to be rare and to primarily affect men over 50, these noncancerous tumors known as gonadotropin adenomas now are being recognized with increasing frequency in both men and women. Gonadotroph adenomas are so named because they secrete hormones targeted to the gonads: the ovaries and testes.

Unlike other types of pituitary tumors, gonadotropin adenomas rarely betray their presence by dramatically altering blood levels of pituitary hormones, according to Dr. Peter J. Snyder, professor of medicine at the University of Pennsylvania School of Medicine in Philadelphia. "As a result these adenomas usually go unrecognized until they become large, so large that they compress the optic nerve and impair vision," he says. By that point the tumor may be about the size of a walnut or larger, and surgical removal is the preferred treatment.

Dr. Snyder and his colleagues found a way to induce telltale elevations of two gonadotropic hormones, follicle-stimulating hormone (FSH) or luteinizing hormone (LH), without surgically removing the tumor in most patients who have gonadotropin adenomas. The investigators discovered that patients who have gonadotroph adenomas often have a paradoxical response to thyrotropin-releasing hormone

"Research Highlights," *Research Resources Reporter*, January/February 1993.

(TRH), a hormone secreted by the hypothalamus. TRH normally stimulates release of a thyroid-targeted pituitary hormone. Tumorous gonadotropin cells, however, secrete gonadotropins or their subunits in response to TRH, the scientists say. Exactly how these cells acquire TRH receptors is still unknown.

Tumors can arise from any of five types of hormone-secreting cells of the anterior pituitary gland. In most cases pituitary tumors oversecrete characteristic hormones and produce striking clinical

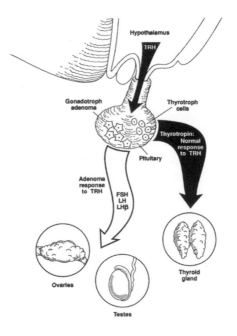

Figure 29.1. Tumorous gonadotropin cells often have an abnormal response to thyrotropin-releasing hormone (TRH). By testing for this anomalous response, Dr. Snyder and his colleagues can identify gonadotropin adenomas without removing pituitary tissue. TRH normally stimulates thyrotroph cells in the pituitary to secrete thyrotropin, a hormone that targets the thyroid gland. Gonadotroph adenomas, however, secrete low levels of follicle-stimulating hormone (FSH), luteinizing hormone (LH), and the LHβ subunit in response to TRH. Administering TRH to patients who have gonadotropin adenomas can boost the abnormal anomalous response, producing telltale elevations of LHβ in the blood.

320

symptoms, such as enlarged fingers and toes in the case of a growth-hormone-secreting tumor, or the premature cessation of menses in women who have prolactin-secreting tumors.

In contrast, gonadotropin adenomas rarely generate hormone-related syndromes. Because these tumors secrete gonadotropins in such low concentrations, they are often mistakenly identified as nonsecreting tumors. But when excised and studied in cell culture, many apparently nonsecreting pituitary tumors in fact secrete the products of gonadotropin cells, Dr. Snyder says. By administering TRH to men who have pituitary tumors and then tracking blood levels of the gonadotropic hormones, Dr. Snyder and other investigators identified more than half of the patients who had gonadotropin adenomas, as later confirmed by studying surgically removed tumor cells. Healthy individuals and most patients who have other types of pituitary tumors have no aberrant response to TRH, Dr. Snyder says.

"Once we began to understand the characteristics of gonadotropin adenomas in men, we decided to apply these characteristics to recognizing gonadotropin adenomas in women," he says. Few such cases had been reported, but it was unclear whether this rarity was due to a lower incidence or to the greater difficulty of detecting these tumors in women.

"This was clearly a more difficult problem," says Dr. Snyder, "especially because when a woman is postmenopausal, which is the age at which most of these adenomas are recognized, elevated levels of FSH or LH could be a normal consequence of menopause and not an indicator of a gonadotropin adenoma." During menopause the ovaries produce less estrogen. As a result the gonadotropin cells in the pituitary gland step up production of FSH and LH in a futile attempt to stimulate estrogen secretion.

"Initially there appeared to be no way to identify gonadotropin adenomas in women based on blood hormone levels alone," says Dr. Snyder. "But then I realized that one possibility would be to use the TRH test."

The scientists administered TRH intravenously to 16 women who were diagnosed as having nonsecreting pituitary tumors based on blood hormone concentrations, 16 healthy age-matched women, and 10 women who had pituitary tumors that secreted prolactin, growth hormone, or corticotropin. Among the patients who had nonsecreting tumors, 14 were postmenopausal and most initially sought medical treatment because of vision loss. Many of these patients had been referred to the study by a team of neuro-ophthalmologists at the Wills Eye Hospital in Philadelphia. The investigators sampled the patients' blood before and after administering TRH and then measured serum levels of FSH, LH, and their subunits.

A subunit of luteinizing hormone known as LHß was found to be a useful marker for gonadotropin adenomas, the scientists note. Among the 16 patients who were judged to have nonsecreting tumors, 11 showed a significant increase in LHß after receiving TRH. In contrast, none of the other women who had hormone-secreting tumors and none of the healthy control subjects had a significant LHß response to TRH. After the nonsecreting adenomas were surgically removed and established in cell culture, secretions of FSH, LH, and LHß *in vitro* roughly corresponded to the patients' hormonal responses to TRH *in vivo*.

Based on this and other studies, Dr. Snyder and his colleagues conclude that about three-quarters of the apparently nonsecreting pituitary adenomas in women are actually of gonadotropin cell origin, and most of these can be recognized *in vivo* by administering TRH. Gonadotroph adenomas, unheard of two decades ago, may in fact comprise about 40 percent of all benign pituitary tumors in both men and women, Dr. Snyder says.

Administration of TRH will not likely lead to earlier detection of gonadotropin adenomas, however, since these tumors are such inefficient hormone producers, Dr. Snyder says. "The tumor will have to be of a certain size to noticeably change the blood concentration of the various compounds we measure," he points out. Visual disturbances or other indicators of a large tumor will still be the first symptoms that call attention to the problem, "but once someone is found to have an adenoma, this test can tell us what kind of adenoma it is, even when previously employed blood tests would not. Once we recognize the cell type of origin we can start to direct treatment against that type of cell," Dr. Snyder says.

Today the preferred treatment for most gonadotropin adenomas is surgical removal, which often restores vision. But surgery is a risky and expensive procedure, Dr. Snyder says. "Surgery is not often successful in removing all of the adenoma, and the tumor may grow back if not further treated. " Administration of TRH can be used periodically to track the success of surgery and also to evaluate the effectiveness of nonsurgical treatments.

"Radiation therapy is sometimes successful in reducing the size of gonadotroph adenomas, but it may take months or years to work, so it's often used as adjunctive treatment following surgery," he says. Dr. Snyder and his coworkers are now testing the effectiveness of a drug known as Nal-Glu-GnRH as a treatment for gonadotroph adenomas. This drug hinders the action of the hypothalamic hormone known as gonadotropin-releasing hormone (GnRH), which stimulates hormone secretion by normal gonadotropin cells in the pituitary gland.

"We have already shown that when Nal-Glu-GnRH is given to men who have gonadotropin adenomas and higher-than-normal FSH concentrations, these concentrations return to normal within 1 week. We are now attempting to determine if repetitive administration will reduce the size of the adenoma itself."

—by Victoria L. Contie

Additional Reading

1. Daneshdoost, L, Gennarelli, TA, Bashey, HM, et al., Recognition of gonadotropin adenomas in women. *New England Journal of Medicine* 324:589-594, 1991.

2. White, MC, Daniels, M, Newland, P, et al., LH and FSH secretion and responses to GnRH and TRH in patients with clinically functionless pituitary adenomas. *Clinical Endocrinology* 32:681-688, 1990.

3. Daneshdoost, L, Pavlou, SN, Molitch, ME, et al., Inhibition of follicle-stimulating hormone secretion from gonadotropin adenomas by repetitive administration of a gonadotropin-releasing hormone antagonist. *Journal of Clinical Endocrinology and Metabolism* 71:92-97, 1990.

4. Snyder, PJ, Gonadotroph cell pituitary adenomas. *Endocrinology and Metabolism Clinics* 16:755-764,1987.

The research described in this article was supported by the General Clinical Research Centers Program of the National Center for Research Resources and by the National Institute of Diabetes and Digestive and Kidney Diseases.

Chapter 30

Pituitary Tumors and the Reproductive System

Functioning and non-functioning pituitary tumors affect the reproductive system. The pituitary tumor may compromise the function of the remaining pituitary gland resulting in decrease in other hormones normally secreted by the pituitary. After pituitary surgery or irradiation, normal pituitary cells may be damaged which will lead to the deficiency of other pituitary hormones. The symptoms of hormone deficiency may become apparent only after many months or years.

In the human, the testes and the ovary are mainly controlled by two pituitary hormones: luteinizing hormone (LH) and follicle-stimulating hormone (FSH). In men, LH controls the secretion of the male hormone testosterone from the testes. FSH regulates the production of sperm by the testes. In women, FSH helps the follicle (which contains the egg) to develop and to produce female hormones including estradiol. LH in the female controls the rupture of the follicle releasing the mature egg (ovulation). It also promotes the function of the corpus luteum to produce another female hormone, progesterone. Progesterone from the corpus luteum supports early pregnancy.

Possible Reproductive Problems in Men with Pituitary Tumors

If the pituitary hormone LH is low, testosterone production by the testes is decreased. Low testosterone levels are associated with decreased

From *The Pituitary Patient Resource Guide*, Second Edition, © 1995, 1997 Pituitary Tumor Network Association, 1630 Ventura Blvd., Suite 231, Encino, CA 91436; reprinted with permission.

sexual function, in particular, loss of sexual desire. Other long-term effects of low testosterone include decrease in beard growth, loss of body hair, decrease in muscle mass and strength, osteoporosis, and decrease in red cell mass. Deficiency in testosterone can be remedied by replacement in the form of intramuscular injections of the hormone dissolved in oil once every 2 to 3 weeks. Transdermal delivery systems are also available which can be applied to the scrotum or other parts of the body. Newer preparations of the male hormone under development include: sublingual natural testosterone tablets, longer acting intramuscular injections, and creams/gels. Before testosterone replacement, a thorough physical examination including a rectal examination to exclude prostate disease must be done. Blood tests are recommended to exclude liver dysfunction, lipid abnormalities, and prostate disease. Regular follow-up to assure adequate replacement is required after stabilization of the dose at 6 monthly or yearly intervals. Testosterone replacement will not make a man fertile. Deficiency of the secretion of FSH may be an additional cause of low sperm production. If fertility is desired, an endocrinologist should be consulted and hormone replacement should be altered to human chorionic gonadotropin as a substitute for LH and human menopausal gonadotropin for FSH as necessary. Recombinant human FSH and LH may be available soon.

Possible Reproductive Problems in Women with Pituitary Tumors

Prolactin can be secreted by a pituitary tumor either alone or sometimes together with growth hormone. This increase in prolactin may cause menstrual irregularities and milk production by the breast (galactorrhea). Bromocriptine, or the recently approved carbergoline, is highly effective in decreasing prolactin levels to the normal range and can restore normal reproductive function in both women and men.

Untreated acromegaly or Cushing's Disease can also be associated with the occurrence of excessive and coarse body hair in women (hirsutism). Hirsutism in Cushing's Disease is due to excessive production of male hormones by the adrenal glands. Hirsutism in acromegaly can be due to excessive production of male hormones (androgens) from the ovary or the adrenals.

In acromegaly the associated increase in production of insulin-like growth factor 1 (IGF-I) in these organs may be one of the causes of excess androgens. The hirsutism associated with Cushing's Disease or acromegaly will usually decrease in severity with lowering of cortisol or growth hormone levels that occur after treatment of the pituitary tumor.

Most frequently, in association with secreting or non-secreting tumors, the levels of the other pituitary hormones such as luteinizing hormone and follicle stimulating hormone are decreased. This will lead to abnormal development of the ovarian follicles, decreased ovarian hormone secretion (estrogens and progestins) and disturbed ovulation. If the female hormone secretion is low, symptoms such as vaginal dryness, skin changes, smaller and softer breasts, and other long-term risk factors such as loss of bone mass (osteoporosis) and increased risks of coronary heart disease may develop. Estrogen replacement therapy should be used with progestins to counteract the effect of estrogens alone on the endometrium. Combinations of estrogens and progestins can be used in cyclical manner or continually. The schemes of hormone replacement therapy are the same as those used for post-menopausal women. If the woman desires fertility, then she should consult an endocrinologist or reproductive endocrinologist. The endocrinologist should be consulted since the pituitary tumor may enlarge during pregnancy and treatment of the tumor should be completed before pregnancy occurs. If there is no ovulation, induction of ovulation can be initiated with follicle stimulating hormone (human menopausal gonadotropins or human follicle stimulating hormone) to induce the development of the follicles containing the egg and luteinizing hormone (human chorionic gonadotropin) to induce ovulation. If pregnancy occurs, progestins are used to support the endometrium until the embryo is implanted into the endometrium. These hormones should be administered in a sequential manner and must be monitored by ultrasound examination of the ovary, and blood hormone levels, usually under the supervision of a reproductive endocrinologist. The success of ovulation induction is usually high in patients with pituitary tumors.

— by Christina Wang MD., Director,
Clinical Study Center,
Harbor-UCLA Medical Center.

Chapter 31

Prolactinomas

What Is a Prolactinoma?

A prolactinoma is a tumor in the pituitary gland which secretes a hormone called prolactin. Pituitary tumors are clinically evident in about 14 people in 100,000. However in postmortem studies about 1 in 20 subjects have a small prolactinoma. This tumor is in over 99% of cases benign. It is the most common type of pituitary tumor.

Prolactin is the milk hormone and levels of this hormone in the blood rise during pregnancy to stimulate and prepare the breast for lactation. After delivery of the baby the prolactin levels will fall unless breast feeding takes place. However if the baby is allowed to suckle then the mother's prolactin will rise in response to the suckling to maintain milk production.

What Is the Cause of Prolactinomas?

While research continues to unravel the mechanisms of disordered cell growth in the pituitary, the cause of pituitary tumors remains unknown. Most pituitary tumors are sporadic in nature and are not genetically transmitted from parents to offspring.

From *Pituitary Patient Resource Guide*, First Annual North American Edition, ©1995 Pituitary Tumor Network Association, 16350 Ventura Blvd., Suite 231, Encino, CA 91436, (805) 499-9973; reprinted with permission.

Where Is the Pituitary Gland?

The pituitary gland sits virtually in the middle of the head. The pituitary gland sits in a bony box (sella turcica (saddle)). The eye nerves sit right above the pituitary gland. If a pituitary tumor expands the size of the pituitary it may give rise to local symptoms such as headache or visual disturbance. The visual disturbance is due to pressure on the eye nerves. Tumors may over secrete a hormone. Prolactinomas over secrete prolactin giving rise to elevated levels of prolactin in the blood (hyperprolactinemia). Disturbances of other pituitary functions may also arise.

What Is the Importance of Hyperprolactinemina?

Women who develop hyperprolactinemia usually notice that they have a change in the pattern of their menstrual cycles. They may lose their periods altogether (amenorrhea), their periods may become irregular or their periods may become very heavy (menorrhagia). They may notice that the breasts secrete milk inappropriately (galactorrhea). In addition they often notice a reduction in their sex drive (libido) which may be associated with pain on intercourse due to vaginal dryness.

Men with hyperprolactinemia may develop hypogonadism and galactorrhea. However the onset is very insidious and since men do not have any objective measure to observe (like periods in women) they often deny that they have a problem. In this situation their partner is usually a more objective assessor of their sexual performance. Thus most men only present very late in the course of their disease with symptoms of the large tumor; they usually complain of headaches and/ or visual disturbances. After they are treated, then they recognize that their sexual function was abnormal.

What Is the Differential Diagnosis?

Elevated levels of prolactin can occur from multiple different causes. The most frequent cause is the taking of medications which act by blocking the effects of dopamine at the pituitary or depleting dopamine stores in the brain. These include major tranquilizers such as trifluoperazine (Stelazine) and haloperidol (Haldol), and metoclopramide (Reglan). Less frequently, drugs such as alpha methyldopa, and reserpine may elevate prolactin levels. Another cause of hyperprolactinemia is any disease within the pituitary fossa which may interfere with the delivery of dopamine from hypothalamus to the prolactin secreting cells. Thus, non functioning tumors and actively secreting tumors (causing acromegaly and Cushing's Syndrome) may also cause mild hyperprolactinemia. The way these are distinguished is usually by the degree of elevation of prolactin and the size of the tumor as visualized on MRI scan or CT scan.

Breast manipulation and stimulation as well as chest wall injury may cause hyperprolactinemia by reflex stimulation. However prolactin elevation from this cause is usually modest.

How Is Prolactinoma Treated?

The first line of treatment for a prolactinoma is medical rather that surgical. Approximately 80% of patients may expect their prolactin levels to be restored to normal with return of normal gonadal function. The size of pituitary tumor will also be reduced by medical treatment.

Medical treatment consists of the prescription of a dopamine agonist drug. The first effective dopamine agonist drug for this condition was bromocriptine. It is the first line of treatment. It is critical that treatment is initiated slowly, since this will prevent the development of side effects. Thus, many authorities recommend that treatment is initiated with a quarter of a 2.5 mg tablet taken on going to bed in the evening together with a glass of milk and a cookie. In this way the absorption of the drug from the gut is slowed and no side effects usually develop. The dose is increased every three days to one quarter of a tablet with breakfast and on retiring, and then increased to half a tablet at night and a quarter with breakfast. The dose is then increased to half a tablet twice a day; then one tablet at night and half with breakfast and finally one tablet twice a day. Serum prolactin is checked when the patient is on one tablet twice a day. If it is not normal a third tablet is added at lunch time by first taking half a tablet; and then if this is well tolerated, the dose is increased to a full tablet.

Other regimens of bromocriptine administration are used by physicians, but the one listed above is the one least likely to cause side effects. Bromocriptine is the only dopamine agonist which is approved for the treatment of hyperprolactinemia and for the treatment of infertility associated with it. Pergolide, another dopamine agonist, is available in the United States. It is not approved for this indication. The dose usually needed to treat hyperprolactinemia is either 50 micrograms once a day, or 100 micrograms once a day.

The most common side effects are nausea and vomiting and dizziness particularly on standing up. These usually do not occur if the therapy is initiated as described above. If they do occur the patient should back off to the previous dose which was not associated with side effects. It is important to recognize that tolerance to side effects occurs even though the prolactin lowering effects are preserved. This means that over time the side effects will disappear even though the patient continues to take the medication.

Is Surgery Ever Warranted for Prolactinoma?

If medical therapy cannot be tolerated or if it is unsuccessful then surgery should be considered. If medical therapy has been continued for a year and the prolactin levels are still elevated, and gonadal function has not been restored, then medical therapy can be considered to have failed. It may be considered to be partially successful if prolactin levels are lowered by >80% even though levels are still elevated. In this situation medical therapy should be continued possibly with the addition of surgery or radiation therapy. Similarly, if the size of the pituitary tumor on MRI has not reduced in size within a year, or has increased in size, this also can be considered as failure of medical therapy.

The results of surgery are very dependent on the skill and experience of the neurosurgeon. If the serum prolactin is less than 250 ng/ml in the best centers there is an 80% chance of normalization of the serum prolactin. The higher the prolactin the lower the chance of normalization of the serum prolactin by surgery. Depending on the size of the tumor and completeness of surgical resection, studies show that 20-50% of subjects will experience a recurrence of hyperprolactinemia. When this occurs, it is usually within 5 years from the time of surgery. However following removal of a large portion of the tumor it may be possible to normalize the serum prolactin by medical therapy, while this may have not been possible prior to surgery.

How Does a Patient Choose an Appropriate Neurosurgeon?

It is important for the patient to discuss with the surgeon the number of operations to remove pituitary tumors that he/she has performed and what the expected results are in his hands and in the major centers. The best results come from surgeons who have completed many hundreds or thousands of such operations.

What Evaluation of Pituitary Function Is Necessary?

The anterior pituitary gland produces a variety of hormones which affect many different endocrine functions. These include ACTH, or corticotropin, which stimulates the adrenal glands to produce cortisol; thyrotropin, which stimulates the thyroid gland to produce thyroid hormone; the gonadotropins LH and FSH, which stimulate the ovaries to regulate ovulation and the testes in men to regulate spermatogenesis and testosterone production. In addition, prolactin and growth hormone are produced by the pituitary gland to regulate lactation and growth, respectively. These pituitary functions are usually normal in patients who have a prolactinoma. These can be evaluated by a simple blood test which measures not only the hormone which is produced from the pituitary, but that which is produced by the target gland in response; for example, TSH is measured as well as serum thyroxin or free thyroid hormone levels.

How Can the Pituitary Tumor Be Visualized?

The pituitary and pituitary tumors can be visualized by one of two techniques, either Computer Assisted Tomography (CAT Scan) or by Magnetic Resonance Imaging. Magnetic Resonance Imaging, or MRI, is the preferential method for identifying pituitary tumors. This test should be performed in any patient who is suspected of having a pituitary tumor. If a pituitary tumor is found, and is then either followed or treated medically or surgically, it is probably advisable to repeat the scan at one year. Many physicians repeat the scan annually, while others repeat the scan based on clinical symptoms and signs. Another practice is to double the interval between scans, so that after the first year, it may be another two years before the scan is repeated, and then four years, etc. in the asymptomatic patient.

What Is the Relationship of Prolactinomas to Pregnancy and Oral Contraceptives?

If the woman has a microprolactinoma, then there is no reason that she cannot conceive and have a normal pregnancy after successful medical therapy. The risk of swelling of the pituitary, giving rise to symptoms from hypopituitarism or compression of vital structures is less than one percent. In patients with macroadenomas, the risk is greater, and some people consider it as high as twenty-five percent. The important issue is that the patient should be carefully evaluated prior to becoming pregnant, and should have an MRI scan and plotting of objective visual fields. During pregnancy, if there is no swelling of the pituitary, pregnancy should be uneventful, but the patient should consult their endocrinologist if they should develop symptoms, particularly headache, nausea, vomiting, excessive thirst or urination or extreme lethargy. Most endocrinologists see patients at two-monthly intervals through the pregnancy. If a patient has completed a successful pregnancy, the chance for completing further successful pregnancies is extremely high. As soon as a patient is pregnant, it is usually advised that she stop taking bromocriptine or dopamine agonist drug, and this is only re-started if the patient develops symptoms from expansion of the tumor during pregnancy.

Oral contraceptives were at one time considered to be involved in the development of hyperprolactinemia. However, this has since been proven to be untrue, and therefore patients who have hyperprolactinemia who have been treated with bromocriptine or other dopamine agonists may also take an oral contraceptive for contraceptive purposes. Similarly, post-menopausal estrogen replacement is quite safe to take in patients with prolactinoma, providing that the prolactinoma is treated with medical therapy or surgery.

What is the Risk of Osteoporosis in Hyperprolactinemia?

Hyperprolactinemia does not cause osteoporosis unless hypogonadism is also present. All patients who are hypogonadal have an increased risk of development of osteoporosis. The usual recommendation is that the patient should be treated for the hyperprolactinemia so that gonadal function is restored to normal. In addition, they should take the appropriate amount of calcium (1 gm calcium gluconate or carbonate), exercise, and other general preventive measures used in prevention of osteoporosis.

*—by Michael O. Thorner, M.D., D.Sc., FRCP,
Professor of Medicine, University of Virginia,
Health Sciences Center, Charlottesville, Virginia*

Chapter 32

Medications for Pituitary Diseases

Patients with pituitary tumors often require medication therapy to suppress hormonal hyper secretion, to replace the missing hormone(s), or to accomplish both tasks. It is absolutely imperative for the patient to participate actively in the choice of therapy and to comply with the treatment protocol.

An active discussion of the reasons for a particular treatment, the goals to be accomplished, and the potential pitfalls is a necessary prerequisite for successful cooperation between a knowledgeable endocrinologist and an intelligent patient.

Replacement Therapy

The pituitary tumor itself or its treatment (surgery and/or radiation) can irreparably damage the proper function of the healthy pituitary cells. While surgical damage occurs right away (and thus is easy to detect), radiation causes delayed damage whose results may not be obvious for years. This requires a life-long follow-up to detect the earliest signs of the incipient pituitary failure.

Clinical pictures, as well as hormonal tests, play equally important roles and sophisticated stimulation tests are sometimes needed. As a rule of thumb, there is a particular order in the disappearance of pituitary hormones. Growth hormone is the most sensitive one and vanishes first, followed by gonadotropins (LH and FSH), then ACTH and later TSH. In practice, however, the patient may develop a loss of only one hormone, or the order of disappearance may be broken with bizarre combinations and permutations.

Growth Hormone Deficiency

GH deficiency should definitely be treated in children to assure proper statural growth. This should be done only by a qualified pediatric endocrinologist. Currently, four preparations are available in the United States: Protropin® by Genentech, Genotropin® by Pharmacia & Upjohn, Humatrope® by Lilly, and Norditropin® by Novo-Nordisk. All are exceedingly expensive (approximately $20,000 per year) and require daily injections. Fortunately, other companies are poised to capture a slice of the market, and the price will inevitably fall. GH replacement for adult hypopituitary patients is officially approved by the FDA and should be covered by the insurance companies. Recent studies have suggested that adult hypopituitary patients may benefit from GH replacement in terms of normalization of bone density, muscle strength, general energy, etc. Whether GH replacement in adults can prevent cardiovascular complications and/or extend life span, is unknown. The conclusive studies are not yet available and there are some potential complications of GH therapy. This treatment has to be administered under close medical supervision by a qualified endocrinologist. The benefits of GH replacement in the elderly non-hypopituitary patients are uncertain and the side effects may be more severe in this group. This indication is not approved by the FDA. Apparently, GH can be bought for this purpose on the "black market" or through chains of the "for profit" establishments in Mexico, that advertise GH as a "Fountain of Youth" type innocuous drug. Talk to your endocrinologist before using it!

Gonadotropin Deficiency

In men, restoration of potency, and prevention of bone and muscle loss are accomplished by the intramuscular injections of Depot-Testosterone. The drug is given every 2-3 weeks, 200-300 mg. per injection. The existing oral preparations are totally ineffective and may cause liver damage. Testosterone skin patches and new oral androgens are under continuous development: ALZA Corporation has released its new Testoderm®, a scrotal patch, and Smith-Kline Beecham has released Androderm®, patches that can be worn on the arms, legs, back or abdomen. Transdermal testosterone replacement offers no physiological advantage *vs.* intramuscular injections, is much more expensive and often causes skin irritation.

In women, estrogen in different forms (Estraderm® patches, Estrace®, and Premarin® or Ogen® tablets) are equally effective and the choice is dictated by the financial considerations and convenience (patches in some patients cause skin irritation, for example). If a woman has a uterus, periodic administration of progestagen (Provera® tablets) is needed. Fertility can be restored in both sexes by hCG/hMG therapy and should be done only by reproductive endocrinogists or gynecologists. In women, this should be closely monitored by ultrasound and estrogen measurements to avoid potentially severe (and occasionally fatal) complications. Treatment with clomiphene or GnRH pumps is usually ineffective in patients with pituitary damage.

ACTH Deficiency

This is by far the most important deficit to treat. Unrecognized or untreated, this condition may result in death during severe stressful illnesses (heart attack, pneumonia, etc.). Cortisone acetate (~37.5 mg/day), hydrocortisone (~25 mg/day) or prednisone (~7.5 mg/day) are usually given for life. During stressful illnesses (flu, for example) the dose should be doubled by the patient for the duration of acute disease. If an illness is accompanied by vomiting and/or diarrhea, the absorption of the oral drug may be impaired and this would require an injection. Contact your doctor immediately! Identification bracelets are mandatory: this is your best insurance policy in case you are brought to the hospital while unconscious.

TSH Deficiency

This results in hypofunction of the thyroid gland. Replacement therapy with levothyroxine is easy, reliable, cheap and 100% effective. Several good brand name preparations are available and all are equally effective: Synthroid®, Levoxyl®, and Levothroid® are practically interchangeable. Avoid generics; some are very unreliable. Also, steer away from older preparations such as desiccated thyroid, Proloid®, Ecthroid®, or Thyrolar®.

Prolactin Deficiency

This of no practical importance in men. In women this will result in the inability to lactate (produce milk) but this is of little concern, since artificial baby foods are widely available.

Vasopressin Deficiency

Vasopressin deficiency causes diabetes insipidus. If mild, this may be left untreated as long as water is freely available. DDAVP is a synthetic hormone that is given by nasal sprays or tablets. The dose should be adjusted by your endocrinologist.

Overall, proper replacement therapy is highly effective and, while being a chore at the beginning, soon becomes routine and doesn't appreciably affect the quality of life.

Another group of medications (unfortunately very small) is directed toward suppression of persistent hormone hypersecretion. Bromocriptine (Parlodel®) is highly effective for suppression of prolactin hypersecretion and shrinks a large proportion of prolactin-secreting tumors. The latter may obviate pituitary surgery or radiation. The doses may range from 2.5 mg to more than 20 or 40 mg per day. Stopping the drug will almost inevitably result in re-expansion of the tumor and restoration of prolactin hypersecretion. Some patients cannot tolerate the drug because of nausea, abdominal pain or lightheadedness. In some women, these side effects may be ameliorated by the vaginal route of administration. Pergolide (Permax®) is not approved for treatment of hyperprolactinemia but is very effective. It may be an alternative for some patients who are intolerant to bromocriptine. Other medications are being developed and Parlodel-LAR®, an indictable form of bromocriptine (one injection per month) is undergoing trials.

Cabergoline (Dostinex® has recently been approved for treatment of hyperprolactinemia (Pharmacia & Upjohn). It needs to be taken orally once or twice a week and may have less side effects than bromocriptine. The choice between different preparations is dictated by their efficacy and side effect profile in an individual patient as well as by the price.

Most importantly, remember that not every case of hyperprolactinemia results from a pituitary prolactinoma. All too often it is due to some other pituitary disease, medications, thyroid disease, renal failure or even chest wall damage. Every case of hyperprolactinemia should be investigated by a qualified endocrinologist before the final decision about treatment is made.

Bromocriptine is less effective for acromegaly. Even though the doses are usually higher, GH normalizes only in about 10% of patients and tumor shrinkage is rare. Nevertheless, for a responsive patient, this may be an excellent choice.

Octreotide® (Sandostatin) is highly effective in acromegaly. It normalizes GH secretion in ~60-80% of patients, and shrinks tumors measurably in a significant proportion of them. It is approved by the FDA, and the insurance companies will reimburse the cost at least partially. This is not an ideal medication: it requires 3-4 daily injections, it causes diarrhea and abdominal cramps, it may cause gallstones (a gall bladder surgery may be needed) and occasionally it may worsen the pre-existent diabetes. Only physicians thoroughly familiar with this drug should direct the treatment. A long-acting indictable preparation (once a month) is in the works. Octreotide is successfully used in some patients with TSH-producing pituitary tumors.

Lanreotide (Ipsen) is another somatostatin analogue that is available in Europe. It is as good as octreotide and a choice between the two will be decided solely by the price.

Unfortunately, there is no specific medication therapy for patients with LH/FSH secreting tumors or for ACTH-secreting tumors (Cushing's disease). In the latter, however, adrenal overproduction of cortisol may be chronically normalized by an anti-yeast medication, Ketoconazole.

Any patient diagnosed with pituitary disease or who is suspected to have one should be seen by an endocrinologist with expertise in this field. This will give the best chance for appropriate and speedy diagnosis, immediate therapy and successful long-term follow-up.

— by Ariel L. Barkan, M.D.,
Pituitary and Neuroendocrine Center,
University of Michigan, Ann Arbor, Michigan

Part Five

Thyroid and ParathyroidDisorders

Chapter 33

Thyroid Information

Hypothyroidism

More than half the people suffering from an underactive thyroid don't know it and have never been treated.

In this condition, usually caused by chronic inflammation (thyroiditis), also called Hashimoto's disease, your thyroid gland puts out too little thyroid hormone. As a result, your whole metabolism is "low"— you may feel run down, slow, depressed, sluggish, constipated, cold, and tired. Your hair may be brittle; your skin dry and itchy, your muscles cramp.

Diagnosis. A diagnosis can easily made with a simple blood test measuring the amount of thyroid stimulating hormone (TSH) from the pituitary gland. A high TSH shows that the pituitary is trying to tell your thyroid to raise your hormone level—and that it needs raising. If your TSH is high, other tests measuring thyroid hormone levels can sort out the severity of the condition.

Treatment. Treatment is also straightforward. The missing thyroid hormone is replaced in pill form, usually as pure thyroxine. Once the body has the hormone it needs, you should feel well. Rechecking the TSH level periodically will tell whether your thyroid dose is right.

Information in this chapter was prepared by the Thyroid Foundation of America, Inc, Ruth Sleeper Hall, RSL 350, 40 Parkman Street, Boston, MA 02114-2698, (800) 832-8321; reprinted with permission.

In rare cases, the pituitary gland is the problem, not the thyroid. Here, treatment must be directed toward the pituitary in addition to supplying the needed thyroid hormone.

Iodine Deficiency. This can be a cause of hypothyroidism and other serious physical and mental problems if the diet is deficient and iodine is not available through iodized salt and other sources. Not a problem in the USA, but serious worldwide.

Elderly People. Elderly people are at risk of having this problem occur unrecognized later in life. 17% of women and 9% of men have hypothyroidism by age 60.

Newborns. At birth, babies are now tested in the USA so thyroid difficulties are caught early. An under performing or missing thyroid gland can be supplemented with the needed thyroxine. One in 4,000 babies born in the U.S. today needs treatment.

Other Family Members. Family members may share the inheritance that leads to hypothyroidism. This means they are more likely to have thyroid problems, and also related conditions like diabetes, pernicious anemia, depression, arthritis, a variety of skin disorders— even carpal tunnel syndrome.

Hyperthyroidism

An overactive thyroid involves perhaps 5 to 7 million people in the U.S. Either the whole thyroid, or a "hot nodule" inside the gland, produces too much hormone, and too much hormone causes body-wide stimulation of every cell and function. You may experience rapid heartbeat, tremors, weakness, heat intolerance, weight loss, mood swings, and problems with digestion.

Causes. Causes range from autoimmune stimulation which causes the whole gland to make too much hormone, to a condition where lumps or nodules in the thyroid become overactive.

Graves' Disease. Also known as Diffuse Toxic Goiter, is the most common form of hyperthyroidism. Not only does the excess hormone cause all kinds of difficulties, but the same autoimmune process may cause tissue behind the eyes to swell, pushing the eyes forward, a condition called "exophthalmos."

Diagnosis. Your diagnosis will include a test for thyroid hormone in the blood (T4) which will be high; as well as for thyroid stimulating hormone (TSH) from the pituitary which will be low since it is turned off by the high level of thyroid hormone.

A picture of what is going on inside the gland may also be needed, to determine whether "hot nodules" are present. Pictures are made with a radioactive scan, or by ultrasound.

Treatment. The focus may be on:

- making the body less responsive to the stimulus given by the thyroid hormone, or
- cutting down the gland's ability to make too much hormone, or
- removing the gland altogether.

Beta adrenergic blocking agents are drugs which block the action of thyroid hormone. Other drugs known as antithyroid agents, such as methimazole or propylthiouracil, work to shut off iodine from the gland, which then makes less hormone.

Radioactive iodine may be given in a sufficient dose to damage many of the gland's hormone-making cells. The thyroid shrinks in size and production of hormone drops off, while the radioactive iodine is quickly excreted. Your hormone level then often falls below normal, but can be supplemented easily.

Less often, surgery may remove a hyperactive nodule or part of an overactive gland.

Goiter

This is a bulge in your neck caused by an enlarged thyroid gland. It does NOT mean that there is cancer in the gland.

The gland may enlarge when it is becoming overactive—that is, when you are hyperthyroid. Or, it may signal that the gland is failing and the pituitary is telling it work harder. The goiter may be a sign of inflammation, sometimes caused by infection, sometimes not. A form called simple—or nontoxic—or multinodular goiter, may just mean the gland has become bigger or lumpy but is not making you sick.

Thyroid Lumps or Nodules

Many people have these in their gland without problems. A few lumps are involved in overproduction of hormone and need to be

345

treated. Even fewer are cancerous—these must be properly diagnosed and treated.

Postpartum Thyroiditis

Five percent of women may be either hypo- or hyperthyroid after pregnancy. If they have other autoimmune conditions, like diabetes, this figure may rise to a quarter of new mothers. The problems often right themselves with time, but it is still important to treat them, so that the new mother is healthy.

Thyroid Cancer

This is rare. It accounts for 0.6% of cancers in men, 1.6% of cancers in women. Because the thyroid is the only part of the body that uses iodine, a dose of short-lived radioactive iodine is often given to kill thyroid cancer cells. Most thyroid cancers can be treated—and cured—with surgery and/or radioiodine.

See Your Doctor. If any of these symptoms describe your condition, see your doctor. Most thyroid tests are quick and easy. Most treatment is very effective.

Where Your Doctor Looks for Answers

Basic information on the functioning of the thyroid is straightforward. A TSH blood test tells whether the thyroid hormone levels are normal. If not, measurement of the hormones T3 and T4 can define the severity of the problem.

If you have a lump (nodule), or a goiter, it can often be felt in your neck by your doctor. Various ways of picturing it are available, including a radioactive scan or ultrasound. Neither of these is painful or harmful.

If you have a thyroid nodule, yet none of the foregoing tests can rule out cancer, your doctor will likely recommend a thyroid biopsy to obtain a small amount of tissue to examine for cancer cells.

What Kind of Doctor Can Help Me?

Your family doctor will probably be the first person to determine that you have a problem with your thyroid. He or she may send you for a complete evaluation to a thyroid specialist. Such a doctor is likely to be an endocrinologist, and a member of the American Thyroid Association, the Endocrine Society and/or the American Association of Clinical Endocrinologists.

Radiologists and specialists in nuclear medicine may administer such tests as ultrasound or radioactive scan.

The endocrinologist will usually perform a thyroid biopsy. If you need part or all of the thyroid removed, your physician will recommend a surgeon experienced in thyroid operations.

Additional Information

The Thyroid Foundation of America, Inc., provides support and information to you and the millions of Americans who have thyroid disease. The services include:

- Educational brochures about important thyroid disorders.

- Thyroid books which explain how your thyroid works in understandable terms.

- Newsletters with articles by thyroid experts to bring you continuing education (remember, thyroid problems are life-long and treatment may change).

- Referrals to thyroid specialists in your area for consultation or a second opinion.

If you are facing thyroid surgery or concerned about a related topic, the foundation can offer help. You may contact them at:

The Thyroid Foundation of America, Inc.
Ruth Sleeper Hall, RSL 350
40 Parkman Street
Boston, MS 02114-2698
617-726-4136 (Fax)
800-832-8321

Chapter 34

What Is Thyroid Disease?

What Is the Thyroid?

The thyroid is a small, butterfly-shaped gland just below the Adam's apple. This gland plays a very important role in controlling the body's metabolism, that is, how the body functions. It does this by producing thyroid hormones (T4 and T3), chemicals that travel through the blood to every part of the body. Thyroid hormones tell the body how fast to work and use energy.

The thyroid gland works like an air conditioner. If there are enough thyroid hormones in the blood, the gland stops making the hormones (just as an air conditioner cycles off when there is enough cool air in a house). When the body needs more thyroid hormones, the gland starts producing again.

The pituitary gland works like a thermostat, telling the thyroid when to start and stop. The pituitary sends thyroid stimulating hormone (TSH) to the thyroid to tell the gland what to do.

About 20 million Americans have some form of thyroid disease. The thyroid gland might produce too much hormone (hyperthyroidism), making the body use energy faster than it should, or too little hormone (hypothyroidism), making the body use energy slower than it should. The gland may also become inflamed (thyroiditis) or enlarged (goiter), or develop a single lump (nodule).

What Is Hyperthyroidism?

Hyperthyroidism makes the body speed up. It occurs when there is too much thyroid hormone in the blood ("hyper" means "too much"). Nearly 10 times more frequent in women, it affects about 2% of all women in the United States.

The most common form of hyperthyroidism, Graves' disease, is caused by problems with the immune system and tends to run in families. It affects at least 2.5 million Americans, including Olympic athlete Gail Devers who won a gold medal in track after being diagnosed with and treated for Graves' disease.

Symptoms include:

- fast heart rate
- nervousness
- increased perspiration
- muscle weakness
- trembling hands
- weight loss
- hair loss
- change in skin thickness
- increased frequency of bowel movements
- decreased menstrual flow and less frequent menstrual flow
- goiter
- eyes that seem to be popping out of their sockets

The symptoms of hyperthyroidism rarely occur all at once. However, if you have more than one of these symptoms, and they continue for some time, you should see your doctor.

What Is Hypothyroidism?

Hypothyroidism causes the body to slow down. It occurs when there is too little thyroid hormone in the blood ("hypo" means "not enough"). Hypothyroidism affects more than 5 million people, many of whom don't know they have the disease. Women are more likely than men to have hypothyroidism.

Also, one out of every 4,000 infants is born with the condition. If the problem is not corrected, the child will become mentally and physically retarded. Therefore, all newborns in the United States are tested for the disease.

Symptoms include:

- feeling slow or tired
- feeling cold
- depression
- drowsy during the day, even after sleeping all night
- slow heart rate
- poor memory
- difficulty concentrating
- muscle cramps
- weight gain
- husky voice
- thinning hair
- dry and coarse skin
- heavy menstrual flow
- milky discharge from the breasts
- infertility
- goiter

Many of the symptoms of hypothyroidism can occur normally with aging, so if you have one or two of them, there is probably no reason to worry. However, if you are concerned about any of these symptoms, you should see your doctor.

What Is Thyroiditis?

Thyroiditis is an inflammation of the thyroid gland and the most common cause of hypothyroidism. When patients with thyroiditis have any symptoms, they are usually the symptoms of hypothyroidism. It is also common to have an enlarged thyroid that may shrink over time.

The type of thyroiditis seen most often is Hashimoto's thyroiditis, a painless disease of the immune system that runs in families. Hashimoto's thyroiditis affects about 5% of the adult population, increasing particularly in women as they age.

Another form of thyroiditis affects women of childbearing age. Postpartum thyroiditis occurs in 5%-9% of women soon after giving birth and is usually a temporary condition.

Viral and bacterial infections can also cause thyroiditis.

What Is a Goiter?

A goiter is an abnormal swelling in the neck caused by an enlarged thyroid gland. It can become quite large. The problem occurs in at least 5% of the population.

Worldwide, the most common cause of a goiter is lack of iodine, a chemical which the thyroid uses to produce its hormones. About 100 million people don't get enough iodine in their diets, but the problem has been solved in North America and Western Europe by adding iodine to salt. Even with the right amount of iodine, the thyroid gland can swell, creating a goiter. This can occur in any type of thyroid disease, including hyperthyroidism, hypothyroidism, thyroiditis, and thyroid cancer. Many goiters develop with normal thyroid hormone levels and do not require treatment.

Are All Thyroid Lumps Cancerous?

Thyroid lumps (also called nodules) are growths in or on the thyroid gland. They occur in 4%-7% of the population. More than 90% of these lumps are benign (not cancerous) and usually do not need to be removed. Thyroid cancer is found in only about 8,000 people each year and causes about 1,000 deaths per year.

Thyroid cancer is more common in patients who have had radiation to the head or neck. A thyroid nodule might cause your voice to become hoarse, or it could make breathing or swallowing difficult. However, it usually produces no symptoms and is discovered incidentally by you or your physician.

How Is Thyroid Disease Discovered?

As with any disease, it is important that you watch for the early warning signs. However, only your doctor can tell for sure whether or not you have thyroid disease. He or she can measure the amount of thyroid hormones in your blood, as well as look at the structure and function of your thyroid gland. If a nodule is found, your doctor can test whether or not it is cancerous.

How Is Thyroid Disease Treated?

If you have thyroid disease, your doctor can discuss which treatment is right for you. There are several types of treatment:

- Radioactive iodine is used to shrink a thyroid gland that has become enlarged or is producing too much hormone. It may be used on patients with hyperthyroidism, a goiter, or some cases of cancer.

- Surgery is normally used to remove a cancer and may also be used to remove a large goiter.

- Thyroid hormone pills are a common treatment for hypothyroidism, for patients with a goiter, and for patients who have had thyroid surgery. The pills provide the body with the right amount of thyroid hormone.

What Is The Thyroid Society for Education and Research?

The Thyroid Society for Education & Research is a national, not-for-profit organization whose mission is to pursue the prevention, treatment, and cure of thyroid disease. To accomplish this mission, The Thyroid Society participates in, and raises funds for, patient and community education programs, professional education, and scientific research. The work of The Thyroid Society is supported by various grants and by individual contributions.

For further information contact:

The Thyroid Society for Education and Research
7515 South Main Street, Suite 545
Houston, TX 77030
1-800-THYROID (1-800-849-7643)
(713) 799-9909

Chapter 35

Thyroid Tests and Treatments

What Is the Thyroid?

The thyroid is a small, butterfly-shaped gland just below the Adam's apple. This gland plays a very important role in controlling the body's metabolism, that is, how the body functions. It does this by producing thyroid hormones (T4 and T3), chemicals that travel through the blood to every part of the body. Thyroid hormones tell the body how fast to work and use energy.

What Are the Signs and Symptoms of Thyroid Disease?

When your doctor examines you for thyroid disease, he or she should first ask about your symptoms and then check the physical signs. Your doctor will ask questions about your memory, emotions, and (in women) menstrual flow and check your heart rate, muscles, skin, and thyroid gland.

Our board of medical advisers [The Thyroid Society for Education and Research] has reviewed this information. However, this brochure does not take the place of personal health care by your doctor. If you think you may have some form of thyroid disease, please see your doctor for an examination.

Which Blood Tests Will My Doctor Use?

After a physical examination, your doctor may examine certain hormone levels in your blood. The most common tests check the levels of thyroid hormones (T4 and T3) and thyroid stimulating hormone (TSH). Another commonly performed test, the T3 Resin Uptake, is used to calculate the Free Thyroxine Index (FTI). In addition, your doctor may perform a test with an injection of thyrotropin releasing hormone (TRH). If your doctor suspects Hashimoto's thyroiditis or Graves' disease, he or she will probably test you for antithyroid antibodies or thyroid stimulating antibodies.

What Does the Radioactive Iodine Uptake Show?

Iodine is an important building-block for thyroid hormones. Your doctor may give you a small amount of radioactive iodine and then measure the amount absorbed by the thyroid gland. If the thyroid absorbs a lot of this iodine, you may be hyperthyroid. Low iodine uptake may signal hypothyroidism or thyroiditis.

Why Is the Structure of My Thyroid Important?

Examining the structure of your thyroid gland and the surrounding area tells your doctor about enlargement of the thyroid (goiter) or a lump (nodular) which may be cancerous.

Which Tests Look at the Structure of My Thyroid?

- A thyroid image (or scan) shows the size, shape, and function of the gland. It uses a radioactive chemical, usually iodine or technetium, which the thyroid absorbs from the blood. A special camera then creates a picture, showing how much chemical was absorbed by each part of the gland. The test shows the size of the thyroid and tells whether lumps are hot (usually benign) or cold (either benign or malignant). The scan is frequently done at the same time as the radioactive iodine uptake.

- In needle aspiration biopsy, a small needle is inserted into the nodule in an effort to suck out (aspirate) cells. If the nodule is a fluid-filled cyst, the needle often removes some or all of the fluid. If the nodule is solid, several small samples are removed for examination under the microscope. Over 90% of the time, this testing tells the doctor whether the nodule is cancerous or not.

- Ultrasound uses high-pitch sound waves to find out whether a nodule is solid or filled with fluid. About 10% of nodules are fluid-filled cysts, and they are usually not cancerous. Ultrasound may also detect other nodules that are not easily felt by the doctor. The presence of multiple nodules reduces the likelihood of cancer.

How Is Thyroid Disease Treated?

The two basic goals for treating thyroid disease are to return thyroid hormone levels to normal and to remove potentially cancerous lumps. Treatments include radioactive iodine, antithyroid drugs, beta-blocking drugs, thyroid hormone pills, and surgery.

Radioactive Iodine

How Does Radioactive Iodine Work?

The thyroid gland absorbs iodine from the blood. When radioactive iodine enters your thyroid, it slowly shrinks the gland over a period of weeks or months.

The treatment is safe, simple, convenient, and inexpensive. It is usually given only once, rarely causes any pain or swelling, and does not increase the risk of cancer. However, it must be avoided during pregnancy or nursing, and patients should not become pregnant for six months after treatment.

When Is Radioactive Iodine Used?

Radioactive iodine is the most common treatment for hyperthyroidism. It does not require hospitalization. About 95% of patients need only one treatment. They usually start getting better in three to six weeks, and most are cured within six months.

This treatment may also be used after surgery for thyroid cancer. Radioactive iodine dissolves any cancer tissue that could not be removed by surgery. The dose of radioactive iodine is larger in this case, and patients usually stay in the hospital for a day or two.

Antithyroid Drugs

What Do Antithyroid Drugs Do?

Antithyroid drugs block pathways leading to thyroid hormone production. They may be used to prepare hyperthyroid patients for treatment with either radioactive iodine or surgery. They may also be used as the sole treatment for hyperthyroidism. The two antithyroid drugs available in the United States are propylthiouracil (PTU) and methimazole (Tapozole®).

Antithyroid drugs have a relatively low success rate when they are used alone to treat hyperthyroidism. They are particularly useful in a few special situations: to treat children, to control hyperthyroidism during pregnancy, and to prepare certain patients for radioactive iodine therapy or surgery.

Are There Any Side Effects?

Antithyroid drugs cause side effects in about 10% of patients. Reactions can include:

- skin rash
- swollen, stiff, painful joints
- sore throat and fever
- low white blood count, which can lead to serious infections
- jaundice (yellow coloring of the skin) and, rarely, liver failure.

Most side effects clear up once the drugs are stopped. If you think you are having a reaction to antithyroid drugs, call your doctor immediately.

Beta-blocking Drugs

When Are Beta-blocking Drugs Used?

Beta-blocking drugs, also called beta blockers, treat the symptoms of hyperthyroidism. They do not significantly affect the gland or the levels of thyroid hormones in the blood. Instead, they "block" the effects of thyroid hormones.

Beta blockers are most useful for patients whose hyperthyroidism makes them uncomfortable. High hormone levels can cause a faster heart rate and trembling. Beta-blocking drugs help control these symptoms.

Thyroid Hormone Pills

When Are Thyroid Hormone Pills Used?

Thyroid hormone pills provide the body with the right amount of thyroid hormone when the gland is not able to produce enough by itself. The pills are frequently needed after surgery or radioactive iodine therapy.

Thyroid hormone tablets are the standard treatment for hypothyroidism. While symptoms usually get better within a few months, most patients must take the pills for the rest of their lives. This is especially true for hypothyroidism caused by Hashimoto's thyroiditis or radioactive iodine treatment.

If the entire thyroid gland has been surgically removed, thyroid hormone tablets replace the body's own source of the hormone. If only a part of the gland has been removed, the pills may keep the remaining gland from working too hard. This decreases the chance that the thyroid gland will grow back.

How Much Hormone Do I Need?

The preferred hormone for treatment is levothyroxine (T4). You should use only the brand-name that your doctor prescribes, since generic brands may not be as reliable. Name-brand levothyroxine pills include Synthroid®, Levoxyl®, and Levothroid®.

Patients sometimes take more pills than they should, trying to speed up the treatment or lose weight. However, this can lead to hyperthyroidism and long-term complications, such as osteoporosis. You should take the pills as your doctor prescribes.

At different times in your life, you may need to take different amounts of thyroid hormone. Therefore, you should see your doctor at least once a year to make sure everything is all right.

Are Thyroid Hormone Pills Needed after Treatment for Hyperthyroidism?

Many patients treated for hyperthyroidism become hypothyroid. They will need to take thyroid hormone pills for the rest of their lives. In addition, they will need to see their doctor at least once a year.

Surgery

When Is Surgery Performed?

Surgery (thyroidectomy) is the primary treatment for suspected thyroid cancer and can be used to treat hyperthyroidism. Surgery is used to remove large goiters that make breathing or swallowing difficult. Occasionally, a goiter may be removed for cosmetic reasons.

Can You Tell Me More about Cancer Surgery?

If thyroid cancer is suspected, your doctor will recommend surgery. The surgeon usually removes only one lobe of the thyroid, unless cancer is confirmed at surgery. A section of the gland is tested during surgery (frozen section) to tell the surgeon whether it is cancerous (malignant) or not cancerous (benign). If it is malignant, all or most of the thyroid is removed. If the cancer has spread outside of the thyroid, lymph nodes in the neck may also have to be removed. In addition, radioactive iodine therapy may be needed six weeks after surgery to destroy any remaining cancer tissue.

How Is the Operation Done?

The operation is usually performed under general anesthesia and takes about two hours. After surgery, patients may stay in the hospital for up to four days. They may also need to take some time off from work (a week or two for a desk job and three to four weeks for physical labor).

Are There Any Risks?

Thyroid surgery is a safe treatment. However, as with any surgery, there are risks. About 1% of patients develop problems with normal speech caused by damage to nerves leading to the voice box, which lies very close to the thyroid. Occasionally, there may be damage to the parathyroid glands, which control the level of calcium in the blood. If this happens, the patient will need to take calcium and other medicines to prevent future problems. Minor risks of surgery include infection, bleeding, and a scar. The chance of death is very small.

What is The Thyroid Society for Education & Research?

The Thyroid Society for Education & Research is a national, not-for-profit organization whose mission is to pursue the prevention, treatment, and cure of thyroid disease. To accomplish this mission, The Thyroid Society participates in, and raises funds for, patient and community education programs, professional education, and scientific research. The work of The Thyroid Society is supported by various grants and by individual contributions.

For further information, call or write: The Thyroid Society for Education and Research, 7515 South Main Street, Suite 545, Houston, TX 77030; 1-800-THYROID (1-800-849-7643) or (713) 799-9909.

Chapter 36

How a Physician Makes a Clinical Evaluation of Goiter Size

Clinical Scenarios—How Large Are These Thyroid Glands?

For each of the following patients, assessment of thyroid size is an important part of the clinical examination. In case 1, a 32-year-old woman presents with symptoms and findings consistent with hyperthyroidism, but she has no exophthalmos and has always been anxious. In case 2, a 55-year-old man has a diagnosis of Graves' disease, and the choice is made for radioactive iodine ablation therapy. In case 3, a 64 year-old man has a goiter that causes discomfort on swallowing, and thyroxine is to be administered in an attempt to shrink the thyroid gland.

Why Assess the Thyroid Gland for Size?

A goiter is simply an enlargement of the thyroid gland and may result from hormonal or immunological stimulation of gland growth or the presence of inflammatory, proliferative, infiltrative, or metabolic disorders. A common error among those first learning about the thyroid is to associate thyroid size with function; a goiter, however, can be present in hyperthyroidism, hypothyroidism, or in a euthyroid state. Determining whether a thyroid is enlarged can aid in diagnosis,

Kerry Siminoski, M.D., "The Rational Clinical Examination: Does This Patient Have a Goiter?" *JAMA*, March 8, 1995, Vol. 273, No. 10; reprinted with permission.

differential diagnosis, and decisions about laboratory testing; in determining specific therapy and therapeutic dosing; and subsequently in monitoring of the clinical course. For example, when a patient presents with symptoms that could be caused by hyperthyroidism, the detection of a goiter increases the likelihood that thyrotoxicosis is present. If the patient described in the first case had an enlarged thyroid, hyperthyroidism would be a likely diagnosis. On the other hand, if her gland were of normal size, anxiety might be the explanation for her symptoms. Determination of thyroid size also is useful once a specific disease is diagnosed. In patients with Graves' disease, for example, thyroid size may be a factor in determining choice of treatment, since patients with smaller glands are more likely to go into immunologic remission during antithyroid drug therapy. If radioiodine is the chosen treatment, as in the second case, the size of the gland is often used in calculating the dose to be administered. Finally, responses to various therapies can be monitored clinically by assessing thyroid size, such as the attempt to shrink a large goiter with thyroid hormone administration in the third case.

The Anatomic Basis of Thyroid Examination

Landmarks and Relation to Other Structures

The thyroid gland is located in the anterior neck and usually consists of two lobes connected at their lower midregions by a transverse isthmus. The most prominent structure in the anterior neck is the thyroid cartilage. Inferior to the thyroid cartilage lies the cricoid cartilage, and inferior to this lies the isthmus of the thyroid gland, as low as the level of the fourth tracheal ring. Each thyroid lobe lies against the sides of the trachea, extending up from the isthmus to the region of the cricoid and thyroid cartilages and downward toward the clavicles. The posterior portion of each lobe lies beneath the belly of the ipsilateral sternocleidomastoid muscle. Since the fascial envelope of the thyroid gland is continuous with the pretracheal fascia of the cricoid cartilage and hyoid bone, the thyroid ascends and descends along with the laryngeal structures during swallowing.

How Large Is the Normal Thyroid?

The thyroid size in a population is largely determined by the supply of iodine in the diet, with a tendency to larger glands in iodine-deficient areas. Consequently, studies of clinically normal thyroid glands have demonstrated sizes that span an extreme range in euthyroid individuals, differing by geographic location and varying through time within a given region as iodine supplementation has been instituted. Until the middle of this century most authors considered a typical thyroid gland to be about 20 to 25 g, and a commonly accepted upper normal size was 35 g. More recent studies in iodine-supplemented populations have reported mean weights of 10 g or less and an upper normal size of 20 g. While a value of 35 g may still apply in iodine-deficient areas, an upper normal weight of 20 g is probably appropriate for most parts of the Western world and will be used for this analysis. Using this definition, the prevalence of goiter is typically 2% to 5% in iodine replete regions.

How to Examine the Thyroid Gland to Determine Size

The normal thyroid, due to its relatively small size, partial concealment by the sternocleidomastoids, and soft texture, is rarely visible and may be marginally palpable. Enlargement is initially noted as an increase in the size of the lateral lobes to palpation. Further growth results in a gland visible in the anterior neck on careful inspection from the side and from the front with the neck extended. With increasing size, the gland becomes even more prominent on inspection from the side and visible from the front with the head in a normal position. Ultimately, a very large goiter is easily palpable, has prominence from the side of greater than 1 cm, and is visible from the front at a distance.

As a result of observations on these patterns of enlargement, various systems have been described to size a thyroid gland based on (1) the estimated weight; (2) the volume relative to the size of normal glands; (3) the presence or absence of palpable or visible enlargement; (4) the degree of visible prominence when the neck is viewed laterally; (5) neck circumference determined by tape measure; (6) the surface area of the gland projected onto the skin; and (7) the maximum width of the lower poles using a ruler or calipers. Many of these rating scales were developed for epidemiologic studies of goiter in endemic areas and were intended to classify significant goiters rapidly (with examination time in some studies averaging only 18 seconds per subject). As a result, many are of little use for the smaller thyroid glands seen in regions without significant levels of endemic goiter. Most studies from which data for accuracy and precision of goiter determination can be derived do not report specifics of thyroid examination technique. Consequently, there is no objective evidence to support the use of one examination method over another. Many of the variations are minor, though, and shared features will be described.

The patient should be comfortably positioned, either standing or seated, with the neck in a neutral position or slightly extended. The region of the neck below the thyroid or cricoid cartilage should be observed from the front, with good cross-lighting to accentuate shadows and highlight masses. If an abnormality is suspected, the neck should be moved as appropriate to alter the prominence of the area under suspicion. A particularly useful maneuver is fully extending the neck for inspection. This position stretches superficial tissues over the thyroid gland, which is pressed against the relatively unyielding trachea, and visibility of the gland is enhanced. Another aspect of thyroid inspection that is often neglected is to observe the neck from the side, looking for a prominence protruding from the normally smooth and straight contour between the cricoid cartilage and the suprasternal notch. The amount of prominence should be measured using a ruler. This requires a certain degree of guesswork in deducing where the normal neck contour would lie, but the measurement can provide information useful for ruling in the presence of a goiter, as will be discussed herein. There is no particular spot to place the ruler—it merely serves as a visual guide to estimating the degree of protrusion.

Following inspection the gland is palpated, and this is where the greatest differences in methods arise. Authors vary as to whether they prefer palpation using fingers or thumbs, an approach from the front or from behind—the patient, and whether each lobe is palpated by the ipsilateral hand or the opposite hand. In the absence of data to support a specific method, though, examiners should use the approach with which they are most comfortable. Regardless of the technique used, it is often useful to first attempt to locate the thyroid isthmus by palpating between the cricoid cartilage and suprasternal notch. An isthmus may not be felt, but if it is, this can help locate the gland. When palpating the lobes, it is beneficial to relax the sternocleidomastoids. To better feel the left lobe, for example, the neck can be slightly flexed and rotated to the left, both to relax the left sternocleidomastoid and to make space for the palpating fingers or thumb between the sternocleidomastoid and trachea. There are certain additional maneuvers that may be useful, such as measuring neck circumference or the dimensions of a lobe using calipers, but no information is available to assess accuracy or precision of these techniques. Other elements of the thyroid examination that are carried out concomitantly with size assessment include determining gland texture, gland mobility, tenderness, and the presence of nodularity. Auscultation also may be performed for the presence of bruits. These features have their own implications but are not central to determining the presence of a goiter, so are beyond the scope of this discussion. If no thyroid is detected in the neck, it may be maldescended or intrathoracic. Methods of examining for these variants will not be discussed here, since, again, no information is available to analyze the reported techniques.

Dogma holds that the thyroid examination is improved by having the patient swallow during both inspection and palpation. Indeed, it has been stated that swallowing increases sensitivity of inspection alone to that of inspection combined with palpation. No study, however, has actually analyzed whether a swallowing maneuver is of benefit, although most examiners believe it is. The movement resulting from swallowing accomplishes several things. First, it changes the shadowing of any mass, enhancing visual detection of a bulge in the neck contour that may be too subtle to be detected otherwise. Second, movement of the thyroid raises a low-placed gland up from below the sternal notch or lower sternocleidomastoid, making it accessible when it may not have been previously. Third, as in any palpation technique, movement of the object against the palpating hand increases definition. Finally, since only the larynx, upper trachea, and thyroid gland move with swallowing, this maneuver can aid in anatomical localization. Swallowing has thus become an integral part of the thyroid examination, based on common sense and experience but no formal study. One final point is that the degree of excursion of the thyroid on swallowing is proportional to the size of the bolus swallowed, so the patient should be given a sip of water.

When examining the thyroid to determine the presence of a goiter, the goal is estimating gland size. Most endocrinologists express findings in absolute mass or as relative to an upper normal-sized gland, such as "normal" or "two to three times normal size." Many nonendocrinologists have some difficulty quantifying thyroid mass, but this ability is crucial in accurately classifying a gland, as will be seen later in the analysis of accuracy.

False-Positive and False-Negative Goiters

Finding a goiter when one is not present may simply be an error in detection. There are, however, several common causes of a false-positive goiter or pseudo goiter. One is simply an easily palpable gland in a thin individual. Since the entire thyroid is so accessible, the tendency is to interpret this accessibility as being due to an enlarged gland rather than the true reason, a decrease in interfering tissues that normally block access to the gland. A second cause is a variant of the normal placement of the thyroid gland in the neck. In some individuals, the gland is higher than usual, and this prominence is again attributed to enlargement. A third anatomical variant has been termed "Modigliani syndrome." This is where the thyroid actually lies in normal position below the cricoid cartilage, but such individuals possess long, curving necks that enhance the prominence and palpability of the gland. A fourth condition producing pseudo goiter is a fat pad in the anterior and lateral neck. While this may be more common in obese individuals, it can also be found in those of normal weight, particularly young women. With experience, examiners can learn to differentiate this from true thyroid tissue by the differing textures and shapes and the lack of movement of a fat pad with swallowing. Another cause involves the thyroid being pushed forward by lesions behind it, making it more easily palpable. Finally, any enlargement in the vicinity of the thyroid gland may be mistaken for an enlarged thyroid gland, particularly if it is adherent to the thyroid or larynx and so moves with swallowing.

There are three principle causes of false-negative goiter detection in addition to true misclassification. The first and probably most common cause, of course, is an inadequate physical examination. In some circumstances an imperfect examination is unavoidable, as when a patient is intubated. In most cases, however, with a little effort, a good examination can be performed on virtually all patients. Second, some individuals, particularly the obese, the elderly, or those with chronic pulmonary disease, have very short and thick necks, obscuring the thyroid. Some patients also have an atypical thyroid placement, such as a retrosternal location, or lobes that are lateral and obscured by the sternocleidomastoids, making palpation difficult.

Precision of Estimating Thyroid Size

Interobserver Variability

Data on interobserver precision in estimating thyroid size are available both for rating scales that attempted to place glands in one of three or four categories based on palpability and visibility and for simple estimation of the presence or absence of a goiter. Agreements were good to very good in both cases.

As might be expected, the majority of disagreements between observers involved smaller glands and those near the cutoff for goiter determination, and most disagreed by only one stage in classifications. Agreement may be better between examiners with greater experience than between those with differing levels of training.

Intraobserver Variability

In two studies examiners placed thyroid size in categories of enlargement, and repeated the examination on a separate occasion. Intraobserver agreement was slightly better for the inspection component of the examination than for palpation.

Accurancy of Estimating Thyroid Size

Three criterion standards have been used in assessing the accuracy of thyroid size determination: weight measured after surgical or postmortem removal, ultrasound assessment, and nuclear scintigraphy. Ultrasound assessments of thyroid weight correlate well with true gland weight as determined following excision (r=0.88 to 1.00), although there is lack of agreement as to the best formula to use for estimating size. Nuclear scan determination is a little less reliable but acceptable (r=0.77 to 0.98). Again, different formulas have been used to translate the scintigraphic profile to thyroid volume.

Combining data from nine studies of detection of goiter by physical examination, the sensitivity from combined data was 0.70 (95% CI, 0.68 to 0.73) with a specificity of 0.82 (95% CI, 0.79 to 0.85). If a goiter was clinically detected, the positive likelihood ratio of one being present was 3.8 (95% to CI, 3.3 to 4.5) Conversely, if a goiter was not felt to be clinically present, the negative likelihood ratio was 0.37 (95% CI, 0.33 to 0.40). These likelihoods are comparable with, or better than, those for many other physical signs and were not affected by the presence of single or multiple nodules. Experienced examiners were somewhat more accurate in their assessments than more junior colleagues.

Some authors have defined specific stages of thyroid enlargement, based on the usual sequence of changes that occur as the thyroid gland increases in size. Since some of these staging classifications incorporate observations not normally used in simply estimating thyroid mass, they can significantly enhance the predictive abilities of the clinician. In the combined data from four studies, when a clinician felt that a thyroid gland was of normal size, the positive likelihood ratio of goiter being present was 0.15 (95% CI, 0.10 to 0.91). If classified as one to two times normal size, the positive likelihood ratio was 1.9 (95% CI, 1.1 to 3.0), and for greater than two times normal, the positive likelihood ratio was 25.0 (95% CI, 3.6 to 175).

Certain staging methods for thyroid enlargement can help clarify the true status of some of the patients with glands felt to be in the range of one to two times normal size after routine inspection and palpation. The amount of prominence of the thyroid on lateral inspection, for example, resulted in a high likelihood of goiter if it was greater than 2 mm. Of further utility was finding that a gland was not visible with the neck extended, a result that effectively ruled out a goiter.

Bias in Estimating Thyroid Size

When the results from four different studies estimating thyroid gland weights were combined, a regression line was produced describing the tendency to bias in gland size determination. This clearly shows that smaller glands are routinely overestimated in size, while larger glands are underestimated. The size at which this crossover occurs corresponds to about 2½ times upper normal size. The practical application of this finding is that glands in the one to two times normal size category fall in the range in which size is typically overestimated.

The Bottom Line

To determine whether a goiter is present, follow these steps:

1. Examine the thyroid gland by inspection and palpation.

2. Categorize thyroid size as normal or goiter. Subcategorize goiter as small goiter (one to two times normal) or large goiter (greater than two times normal).

3. If you placed the thyroid in the small goiter category, consider whether you overestimated the size; determine whether there is any prominence in the profile of the neck in the region of the thyroid when viewed laterally (classify the prominence as £2 mm or ³2 mm) and determine if the gland is not visible from the front with the neck extended.

4. Place your patient in one of the following categories: "goiter ruled out": normal thyroid size or thyroid considered to be not visible with neck extended; "goiter ruled in": large goiter present or lateral prominence greater than 2 mm or "inconclusive": all other findings.

—by Kerry Siminoski, M.D.

Chapter 37

Thyroid Disease and Pregnancy

Why Are Women More Likely to Get Thyroid Disease?

In general, women are much more likely than men to become hyperthyroid or hypothyroid and to get Hashimoto's thyroiditis. The reason for this is uncertain.

Women are also more vulnerable to autoimmune diseases. Two of the most common thyroid diseases, Hashimoto's thyroiditis and Graves' disease, are caused by problems with the body's immune system. Normally, the immune system defends the body against germs and viruses. In autoimmune diseases, the system attacks the body's own tissues. Diseases of the immune system tend to run in families.

What Is Special About Thyroid Disease and Pregnancy?

Hyperthyroidism or hypothyroidism can affect a woman's ability to become pregnant. They may also cause a miscarriage if they are not quickly recognized and properly treated.

Women who become pregnant may not notice signs of thyroid disease because similar symptoms can occur in a normal pregnancy. For example, patients may feel warm, tired, nervous, or shaky. In addition, enlargement of the thyroid (goiter) commonly occurs during pregnancy.

A pregnant woman is treated differently than is a nonpregnant woman or a man. For example, radioactive materials commonly used in diagnosing and treating many thyroid diseases are never used in pregnant women. The timing of a biopsy or surgery for a thyroid nodule and the choice of drugs for hyperthyroidism may be different in a pregnant woman. These issues require careful consultation with your doctor.

What Is Postpartum Thyroiditis?

Postpartum thyroiditis is a temporary form of thyroiditis. It occurs in 5%-9% of women soon after giving birth (postpartum). The effects are usually mild. However, the disease may recur with future pregnancies.

The symptoms usually last for six to nine months. First, the damaged thyroid gland may release its stored thyroid hormones into the blood, causing hyperthyroidism. During this time, you can develop a goiter, have a fast heart rate, and feel warm or anxious. Then, a few months later, you will either return to normal or become hypothyroid. Hyperthyroidism occurs because the thyroid has been damaged and its hormone reserves used up. If this happens, you may feel tired, weak, or cold. The hypothyroidism usually lasts a few months until the thyroid gland completely recovers. Occasionally the hypothyroidism may be permanent.

How Do Doctors Test for Thyroid Disease?

As with any disease, it is important that you watch for the early warning signs of thyroid disease. However, only your doctor can tell for sure whether or not you have the disease. Your doctor may examine:

- your history and physical appearance
- the amount of thyroid hormones, thyroid stimulating hormone (TSH), and antithyroid antibodies in your blood.

How Is Thyroid Disease Treated?

Pregnancy places some limits on the treatments which you can receive, because your doctor must also look out for the safety of your child. A common treatment for hyperthyroidism is radioactive iodine, but it must be avoided by women who are pregnant or nursing a baby. Surgery to remove a goiter or cancer may also be delayed until after the pregnancy. However, needle aspiration biopsy of a thyroid nodule may be safely done during pregnancy.

Treatments which may be used for thyroid disease during pregnancy include:

- antithyroid drugs, which block the production of thyroid hormone
- thyroid hormone pills, which provide the body with the right amount of thyroid hormone when the gland is not able to produce enough by itself.

Postpartum thyroiditis may or may not be treated during the hyperthyroid stage, depending upon its severity. If the patient later becomes hypothyroid, her doctor may prescribe thyroid hormone pills.

What About My Child?

If you or a blood relative have Hashimoto's thyroiditis or Graves' disease, there is a chance that your children will inherit the problem. These diseases are also linked to other autoimmune conditions, such as premature gray hair, diabetes mellitus, arthritis, and patchy loss of skin pigment (vitiligo). You should tell your child's doctor, so that the appropriate examinations can be performed.

Also, one out of every 4,000 infants is born without a working thyroid gland. If the problem is not corrected, the child will become mentally and physically retarded. Therefore, all newborns in the United States are tested for the disease. Once the problem is discovered and corrected, the child can grow up normally.

What Is the Thyroid?

The thyroid is a small, butterfly-shaped gland just below the Adam's apple. This gland plays a very important role in controlling the body's metabolism, that is, how the body functions. It does this by producing thyroid hormones (T4 and T3), chemicals that travel through the blood to every part of the body. Thyroid hormones tell the body how fast to work and use energy.

What Is The Thyroid Society for Education and Research?

The Thyroid Society for Education & Research is a national, not-for-profit organization whose mission is to pursue the prevention, treatment, and cure of thyroid disease. To accomplish this mission, The Thyroid Society participates in, and raises funds for, patient and community education programs, professional education, and scientific research. The work of The Thyroid Society is supported by various grants and by individual contributions. For more information, contact:

The Thyroid Society for Education and Research
7515 South Main Street, Suite 545
Houston, Texas 77030
1-800-THYROID (1-800-849-7643)
(713) 799-9909

Chapter 38

Hyperthyroidism

What Is Hyperthyroidism?

Hyperthyroidism makes the body speed up. It occurs when there is too much thyroid hormone in the blood ("hyper" means "too much"). The disease affects nearly 2.5 million Americans. Five to 10 times more common in women, it affects about 2% of all women in the United States.

What Causes Hyperthyroidism?

There are several different causes of hyperthyroidism:

- The entire thyroid gland may be overactive, producing too much hormone. Doctors call this problem diffuse toxic goiter, or Graves' disease.

- One or more lumps (also called nodules) in the gland may be overactive. A single lump is called a toxic autonomous nodule, and several lumps are called a toxic multinodular goiter.

- The gland may be inflamed, a condition called thyroiditis. It can release the thyroid hormone that was stored in the gland, causing hyperthyroidism that lasts for a few weeks or months.

- Some patients may take more thyroid hormone pills than needed or prescribed.

- Some drugs, such as Quadrinal®, amiodarone (Cordarone®), and Lugol's solution, contain large amounts of iodine, a chemical the thyroid uses to produce its hormones, and may cause the thyroid to produce too much hormone.

What Is Graves' Disease?

Graves' disease is the most common form of hyperthyroidism. It affects many Americans, including Olympic athlete Gail Devers, who won a gold medal in track after being diagnosed with and treated for Graves' disease.

Graves' disease is caused by problems with the immune system. Normally, the immune system defends the body against germs and viruses. In autoimmune diseases such as Graves', the immune system attacks the body's own tissues. In Graves' disease, the body produces antibodies which make the thyroid gland produce too much thyroid hormone.

Diseases of the immune system tend to run in families and are about five times more common in women. Graves' is linked to other autoimmune conditions, such as Hashimoto's thyroiditis, premature gray hair, diabetes mellitus, arthritis, and patchy loss of skin pigment (vitiligo).

What Is Exophthalmos?

Hyperthyroidism from any cause can make the upper eyelids pull back, but Graves' disease often causes one or both eyes to bulge out of their sockets. This condition, known as exophthalmos, can cause loss of eye muscle control, double vision, and (rarely) loss of vision. Most cases require no treatment, but some patients may need to see an eye doctor (ophthalmologist) for specialized treatment. This may include steroids, radiation, or surgery.

How Do Doctors Test for Hyperthyroidism?

As with any disease, it is important that you watch for the early warning signs of hyperthyroidism. However, only your doctor can tell for sure whether or not you have the disease. Your doctor may examine:

- your history and physical appearance

- the amount of thyroid hormones, thyroid stimulating hormone (TSH), and thyroid stimulating antibodies in your blood

- the structure and function of your thyroid gland, using thyroid imaging, which takes a picture of the gland after you have been given a small amount of radioactive iodine.

How Is Hyperthyroidism Treated?

The basic goal of treatment is to return thyroid hormone levels to normal. Patients who are hyperthyroid from taking too much thyroid hormone need only to have their dosage properly adjusted. Patients whose hyperthyroidism is caused by thyroiditis usually do not require any of the treatments described below, since their condition gets better on its own.

Treatment for hyperthyroidism from Graves' disease, toxic autonomous nodule, or toxic multinodular goiter may include one or more of the following:

- Radioactive iodine to shrink an enlarged thyroid or toxic nodule or nodules that are making too much thyroid hormone. This treatment is safe and is widely used in adults with hyperthyroidism.

- Surgery.

- Antithyroid drugs, such as propylthiouracil (PTU) and methimazole (Tapozole®), for patients with Graves' disease and, less commonly, in other hyperthyroid patients.

- Beta-blocking drugs to treat the symptoms of hyperthyroidism while waiting for one of the above treatments to work.

Your doctor will be able to discuss the benefits and risks of each treatment.

Many patients treated for hyperthyroidism become hypothyroid. They will need to take thyroid hormone pills for the rest of their lives. In addition, they will need to see their doctor at least once a year.

What Is the Thyroid?

The thyroid is a small, butterfly-shaped gland just below the Adam's apple. This gland plays an important role in controlling the body's metabolism, that is, how the body functions. It does this by producing thyroid hormones (T4 and T3), chemicals that travel through the blood to every part of the body, telling it how fast to work and use energy.

What Are the Signs and Symptoms of Hyperthyroidism?

Signs and symptoms may include:

- fast heart rate (100-120 beats per minute or higher)
- slightly elevated blood pressure
- nervousness or irritability
- increased perspiration
- muscle weakness (especially in the shoulders, hips, and thighs)
- trembling hands
- weight loss, in spite of a good appetite
- hair loss
- fingernails partially separated from fingertips (onycholysis)
- swollen fingertips (achropachy or clubbing)
- retracted (pulled back) upper eyelids
- change in skin thickness
- increased frequency of bowel movements
- goiter (an abnormal swelling in the neck caused by an enlarged thyroid gland)
- in women, decreased menstrual flow and less frequent menstrual flow
- in men, slight swelling of the breasts
- in Graves' disease: thick or swollen skin over the shin bones (pretibial myxedema); eyes that seem to be popping out of their socket (exophthalmos).

Most of these conditions will return to normal after the hyperthyroidism is treated. Certain others may be treated separately.

What Is The Thyroid Society for Education & Research?

The Thyroid Society for Education & Research is a national, not-for-profit organization whose mission is to pursue the prevention, treatment, and cure of thyroid disease. To accomplish this mission, The Thyroid Society participates in, and raises funds for, patient and community education programs, professional education, and scientific research. The work of The Thyroid Society is supported by various grants and by individual contributions.

For more information, call or write: The Thyroid Society for Education and Research, 7515 South Main Street, Suite 545, Houston, TX 77030; 1-800-THYROID (1-800-849-7643) or (713) 799-9909.

Chapter 39

Commonly Asked Questions about Graves' Disease

The leading cause of hyperthyroidism, Graves' Disease represents a basic defect in the immune system, causing production of immuno-globulins (antibodies) which stimulate and attack the thyroid gland, causing growth of the gland and overproduction of thyroid hormone. Similar antibodies may also attack the tissues in the eye muscles and in the pretibial skin.

Facts

- Graves' Disease occurs in less than one fourth of one percent of the population.
- Graves' Disease is more prevalent among females than males.
- Graves' Disease usually occurs in middle age, but also occurs in children and adolescents.
- Graves' Disease is not curable, but is a completely treatable disease.

Symptoms

- Fatigue
- Weight loss
- Restlessness
- Tachycardia
- Changes in libido
- Muscle weakness

An undated publication of the National Graves' Disease Foundation, 320 Arlington Road, Jacksonville, FL 32211 (904) 724-0770; reprinted with permission.

- Heat intolerance
- Tremors
- Enlarged thyroid gland
- Heart palpitations
- Increased sweating
- Blurred or double vision
- Nervousness and irritability
- Eye complaints, e.g. redness and swelling

- Hair changes
- Restless sleep
- Erratic behavior
- Increased appetite
- Distracted attention span
- Decrease in menstrual cycle
- Increased frequency of stools

Who Develops Graves' Disease?

Although Graves' Disease most frequently occurs in women in the middle decades (8:1 more than men), it also occurs in children and in the elderly. There are several elements contributing to the development of Graves' Disease. There is a genetic predisposition to autoimmune disorders. Infections and stress play a part. Graves' Disease may have its onset after a severe external stressor. In other instances, it may follow a viral infection or pregnancy. Many times the exact cause of the onset of Graves' is simply not known. It is not contagious, although it has been known to occur coincidentally between husbands and wives. Of research importance, the Graves' gene in DNA has not yet been identified.

How Is Graves' Disease Treated?

There are three standard ways of treating Graves' Disease. The choice of treatment varies to some degree from country to country, and among particular physicians as well. The decision should be made with the full knowledge and informed consent of the patient, who is the primary member of the treatment team. The selection of treatment will include factors such as age, degree of illness, and personal preferences. Generally speaking, from least invasive to most invasive, the treatments include:

1. Anti-thyroid drugs which inhibit production or conversion of the active thyroid hormone;

2. Radioactive iodine (I-131), which destroys part or all of the thyroid gland and renders it incapable of overproducing thyroid hormone; or

3. Sub-total thyroidectomy in which a surgeon removes most of the thyroid gland and renders it incapable of overproducing thyroid hormone.

The first treatment is about 20-30% effective, and the latter two treatments result in about a 90-95% remission rate of the disease. In a few cases, the treatments must be repeated. In all cases, lifetime follow-up laboratory studies must be done, and in almost all cases, lifetime replacement thyroid hormone must be taken.

Are There Any Alternatives to These Treatments of Graves' Disease?

There are a number of things that you can do to assist your body in healing. However, the state of science as we know it indicates there is no "natural" way to "cure" Graves' Disease. For instance, although there are no specific foods that will change your thyroid function, the more healthy, nutritionally dense foods you consume, the better your body will be able to fight against infection and further insult. Equally, many of the treatments like acupuncture, exercise, meditation, and various mind-body therapies may provide comfort measures and relief, but are not a substitute for standard medical treatment. Be sure to consult and collaborate with your physician when embarking on additional therapies. There are many studies of other autoimmune disorders that indicate that the more input and control a patient has in their care, the more rapid their recovery will be. It is of interest to all who are hopeful of more, effective, additional treatment modalities in the future that the National Institute of Health is trying to adequately research and evaluate the hard data of alternative therapies.

What Are the Complications?

Graves' Disease usually responds to treatment, and after the initial period of hyperthyroidism, is relatively easy to treat and manage. There are some exceptions to this, and for some, treatment and subsequent stabilization are much more challenging, both to the patient and the treating team of physicians. The more serious complications of prolonged, untreated, or improperly treated Graves' Disease include weakened heart muscle leading to heart failure, osteoporosis, and/or severe emotional disorders.

Where Can I Get More Information?

The National Graves' Disease (NGDF) is a lay organization that provides patient education and support. Membership entitles you to the newsletter, bulletins, discounts at the annual national conference and contribute to the continuation and availability of the Foundation to others with Graves' Disease. All our materials are prepared by experts in their field and carefully monitored for accuracy. The information is not a substitute for medical care.

For more information, contact:

National Graves' Disease Foundation
320 Arlington Road
Jacksonville, FL 32211
(904) 724-0770

Chapter 40

Living with Graves' Disease

Many people ask: "What can I do about my Graves' Disease?" When one feels helpless and powerless, a sense of hopelessness sets in. Although your Graves' Disease will not go away, there are many things you can do to have a greater sense of mastery in your life. What you eat, what you do, what you think, and what you know—all these things can effect your health.

Medical Care

First and foremost, adequate health care is a must! Select your physician with care. Ask questions. Although your physician may not be able to spend hours with you, your questions deserve answers. If there are no answers (which in many instances there are none) you deserve that information, too. Your medication is essential. It is a replacement for the thyroid hormone that your body once manufactured. When your thyroid was overactive, there was too much of the hormone circulating. That is the cause of your symptoms of insomnia, anxiety, jitteriness, heat intolerance, fatigue, heart racing and weight loss. When your thyroid was surgically removed or deactivated by radioactive iodine treatments, your body's supply of thyroid hormone was instantly or progressively ended. Your doctor will perform the blood tests to determine the level of thyroxine you need. If your blood level is too high, you will begin to experience similar symptoms as when

©1991, 1997 National Graves' Disease Foundation, 320 Arlington Road, Jacksonville, FL 32211, (904) 724-0770; reprinted with permission.

you were hyperthyroid. If the blood level of the hormone is too low, you will experience hypothyroid symptoms: slow heart rate, hair and nail changes, dry skin, sensitivity to cold, joint pains, hoarseness, weight gain, loss of appetite, difficulty concentrating, depression, constipation, muscle weakness or muscle cramps, puffy eyes. If you begin to feel any of these symptoms, contact your doctor. A simple blood test will clarify if your medication needs adjusting. You are not "bothering" the doctor. If your blood levels are satisfactory, there may be other medications that will take care of the symptoms.

The remainder of your care is up to you, however.

Nutrition

There are a number of nutritional concepts that you need to become familiar with and keep in mind when you plan your meals. Weight control is usually important to people with Graves' Disease. Your thyroid controls metabolism, and you may now have a tendency to gain weight. Eating to reduce caloric intake while maintaining high nutrition requires more effort than you may be accustomed to. Focus on fresh fruits and vegetables—those will give you the most vitamins and minerals for your efforts, and offer the balance you need. The preservatives ("sodium") in canned and frozen foods may contribute to swelling, and since swelling is frequently a problem for Graves' Disease, you may now need to be more aware of your salt intake. Since, for reasons unknown, people with Graves' Disease sometimes develop problems with an elevated cholesterol, you may have to become aware of your fat intake. Fish and chicken will be better for you than excessive amounts of pork and beef. Limit rich sauces and cheeses. Learn about nutrition. There are many resources. Both the American Heart Association and the American Diabetes Association have excellent, nutritional food plans, as does Weight Watchers, your local hospital dietitians, and registered dietitian consultants. Fad diets are not healthy—avoid them.

Exercise

You will feel better if you develop a regular exercise program. No one expects you to be an Olympic athlete, but exercise that strengthens your heart and improves circulation and muscle tone which are needed to keep your cardiovascular system functioning well, and keep you physically fit.

Studies show that exercise reduces appetite and increases your energy level. Concentrate on activities you already know how to do, as well as learning new ones. Have a variety of physical activities to avoid boredom, as well as the limitations of weather. Walking continues to be the most overall beneficial physical activity, and it is available to everyone! If you can't walk, bike or swim—rock! Vigorous rocking in a stable rocking chair uses all the muscles in the body!

Relaxation

Learning to relax refers to reducing the muscular tension in order to increase effective circulation, as well as mental calmness. It is not only an "attitude," but a learnable skill. Relaxation is more than just "getting away"—it is a positive and satisfying experience that gives peace of mind. It is well documented that Graves' Disease is also a stress-related illness. The "stress" is often simply a result of the fast-paced, action-packed lifestyle we lead.

Relaxation may take many forms: learning new things, exercising, gardening, walking in the woods, creative activities, soft lighting, soft music, a bubble bath, a good book.

If you are interested in some of the mental exercises to create peace of mind and relaxed bodies, there are many to chose from. You might prefer the systematic tensing and letting go of specific muscle groups—known as progressive muscle relaxation or you might like imagining beautiful scenes. There is considerable research being done on the efficacy of mental imagery (visualization) and its effect on the immune system. Yoga, Tai Chi, and meditation are all ways to practice relaxation and visualization.

Relaxation exercises must be practiced daily. When you discover your favorite activities, plan to devote at least one half hour each day. You have to make a personal commitment to yourself. The National Institute of Mental Health says: "Remember, finding effective techniques for relaxation is not merely a pastime for the idle rich. It is essential for everyone's physical and mental well-being."

Support System

A support system may be defined as those caring, available people in your life who will listen, who will tell it like it is, and who allow you to reciprocate that caring, sharing dialogue. It is important that people in your support system be available, that is, live near you. Long-distance friends are good to have, but do not substitute for a support system near at hand. Listening is important. Many times you do not need advice, you just need to say what you are thinking and feeling out loud, and have those thoughts and feelings acknowledged. You need to discuss things, not necessarily have problems solved. One of the purposes of the National Graves' Disease Foundation is to establish support groups in as many places as possible. That way, people with Graves' Disease can talk with others who understand. There is significant evidence that support groups are one of the most powerful institutions for specific groups. Support groups provide the essential ingredient that is needed for everyone who has to live with a disorder—hope, and a sense of humor!

—by N.H. Patterson, Ph.D.,
Executive Director,
National Graves' Disease Foundation,
President, Counseling Services, Inc.

Chapter 41

Graves' Eye Disease

The eye changes associated with Graves' disease can be called either Graves' ophthalmopathy, Graves' orbitopathy, or Graves' eye disease. Approximately 50% of the patients with Graves' disease develop some eye disease, but the eye changes may be so subtle that patients are unaware of them. For most patients with Graves' disease, eye involvement is minimal. Severe orbitopathy occurs in less than 5% of patients with Graves' disease.

Graves' eye disease is not caused by thyroid dysfunction. Graves' disease is an autoimmune disease that affects the eyes and the thyroid gland independently of each other. Thus, the hyperthyroidism may improve with therapy, while the eye disease stays the same or gets worse. Even though the thyroid disease and the eye disease run independent courses, it is important to treat the hyperthyroidism associated with Graves' disease.

An ophthalmologist is usually involved in the treatment of Graves' eye disease. Most thyroidologists and endocrinologists should be able to recommend an ophthalmologist experienced in the treatment of Graves' eye disease. In addition, The Thyroid Society maintains a list of such ophthalmologists throughout the country.

Symptoms of Graves' eye disease may include a feeling of irritation or sand in the eyes, double vision (diplopia), and excessive tearing. Inflammation and swelling behind the eye may cause actual

Thyroid Signpost, Vol I, No. 6, May 1996, ©1996 The Thyroid Society for Education and Research, 7515 S. Main Street, Suite 545, Houston, TX 77030, (800) THYROID; reprinted with permission.

protrusion of the eyeball from the orbit. When this protrusion occurs, it is called exophthalmos or proptosis.

When the eye changes are severe, there may be marked swelling of the eye, inability to move an eye, corneal ulceration, and in extreme cases, loss of vision. Fortunately, these severe changes occur infrequently, but when they do occur, consultation with an ophthalmologist is essential. Graves' eye disease usually affects both eyes, although each eye may be affected to a different degree. In some cases, only one eye is affected.

The course of Graves' eye disease is unpredictable. The initial, or active, phase of Graves' eye disease may last for eighteen to twenty-four months. During this time period, the eye signs and symptoms may change considerably. For this reason, physicians are reluctant to use certain treatments, such as surgery, during this phase, fearing that ongoing inflammation will cause the eyes to change again after surgery. Thus, most physicians advise patients to defer treatments such as surgery until the eye disease goes into an inactive phase. Of course, if a patient's symptoms are severe or if loss of vision is threatened, then all available treatments will be used at any time, even during the active phase.

Most patients will receive only symptomatic treatment during the active phase of Graves' eye disease (see following list). Most importantly, it should be stressed that smoking aggravates Graves' eye disease.

Physicans may advise the following to relieve symptoms associated with Graves' eye disease:

- discontinue smoking
- avoid smoke-filled rooms
- use lubricating eye drops
- cover eyes while sleeping
- wear wrap-around dark glasses outdoors during the day
- elevate the head of the bed to reduce overnight eye swelling
- wear prism glasses, or cover one eye with a patch, to relieve double vision
- turn ceiling fans off before going to bed
- avoid exposure to strong sunlight
- avoid or limit wearing contact lenses
- take diuretics temporarily to relieve swelling around the eyes

When symptoms of inflammation are severe, either steroids in large doses or radiation therapy may be advised. Surgery (orbital decompression) is sometimes recommended when the inflammation is so severe that loss of vision is threatened. The choice of therapy among steroids, radiation, and surgery (used individually or in combination) and the timing of therapy require a great deal of thought on the part of the team caring for the patient with Graves' eye disease.

Once the inflammation in the eyes has stabilized, or entered the inactive phase, patients may then have surgery to relieve signs and symptoms, such as lid retraction, swelling around the eyes, or double vision. Ophthalmologists specializing in plastic surgery of the eye perform the surgery to relieve lid retraction and swelling around the eyes. Sometimes other ophthalmologists who specialize in diseases of the muscles of the eye perform the operation(s) to relieve double vision.

Medical and Surgical Treatment Options For Graves' Eye Disease

- steroids
- radiation therapy
- surgical adjustment of eyelid placement
- plastic surgery for swelling around the eye(s)
- eye muscle surgery for realignment of the eye(s)
- orbital decompression

Thyroid Signposts

Thyroid Signposts are patient information sheets focusing on a specific thyroid-related topic and are a public education service of:

The Thyroid Society for Education and Research
7515 South Main Street, Suite 545
Houston, TX 77030
(800) THYROID

Chapter 42

Treatment Options for Hyperthyroidism and Graves' Disease

Hyperthyroidism makes the body work too fast because there is too much thyroid hormone in the blood. Graves' disease is the most common cause of hyperthyroidism. Graves' disease occurs because of a problem in the body's immune system—antibodies are produced that overstimulate the thyroid gland. The main objective in treating hyperthyroid patients is to stop the production of too much thyroid hormone. There are four basic treatment options:

- radioactive iodine (I^{131})
- antithyroid drugs: Propylthiouracil (PTU); Tapazole®
- surgery (thyroidectomy)
- refusal of treatment.

Radioactive Iodine (I^{131}). This is the treatment of choice for the majority of the endocrinologists in this country. It is an effective, simple, safe way to treat patients with Graves' disease or other forms of hyperthyroidism. Patients often have fears and misconceptions about using radioactive iodine.

- Studies have been done since the 1940s on patients receiving this treatment, their children, and their grandchildren. There has been no increased incidence of cancer, leukemia, etc.

Thyroid Signpost, Vol I, No. 4, Revised May 1996, ©1996 The Thyroid Society for Education and Research, 7515 South Main Street, Suite 545, Houston, TX 77030, (800) THYROID; reprinted with permission.

- There are no increased instances of birth defects in children born to mothers who have had this treatment and waited the recommended time before becoming pregnant. (Pregnancy should be avoided for six months after the treatment.) As a matter of fact, fertility is often restored to women whose infertility is due to hyperthyroidism. Treating the disease also lessens the chance of miscarriage.

- Pregnant women should not be given radioactive iodine for any reason. If a patient has any doubt as to whether she is pregnant, treatment (and testing) with radioactive iodine should be delayed.

- Hospitalization is not required in order to treat hyperthyroidism with radioactive iodine.

- Radioactive iodine treatment ablates the thyroid gland (turns it into something like a dried-up raisin). Patients wishing to avoid destruction of the gland should know that the thyroid gland frequently "burns out" within 15 years even without treatment.

- Radioactive iodine does not cause a person to gain weight. However, because Graves' disease increases the metabolism, patients should keep in mind that they cannot continue to eat the way they did while hyperthyroid. Because of changes in the metabolism after hyperthyroidism is treated, many patients will gain weight. This weight can be lost through diet and exercise once the thyroid levels are normalized.

What Can Be Expected with Radioactive Iodine Treatment?

- It is usually given in liquid form or as a capsule. The dose can range from 4 to 29 millicuries.

- It is tasteless.

- There are almost never any side effects. In some rare cases, there can be an inflammation of the thyroid gland causing a sore throat and discomfort.

- Radioactive iodine not taken up by the thyroid gland is excreted in urine and saliva. There is no evidence that the small amount of I^{131} excreted in the urine and saliva is harmful. Nonetheless, prudent nuclear medicine experts have recommended a wide variety of precautions. While these recommendations are sometimes confusing and inconsistent, it may be appropriate to take a few simple measures to avoid unnecessary exposure of infants and children to I¹³¹. Treated patients should rinse out their glasses or cups and eating utensils immediately after drinking and eating. The toilet should be flushed immediately after use, and the rim of the bowl should be wiped dry, if necessary.

- It is advisable to drink two to three extra glasses of water a day during the four-to seven-day period following radioactive treatment so that radioactive material will not collect in the bladder for a long period of time.

- Because radioactive iodine passes into breast milk, breast feeding mothers are asked to wean their babies before treatment.

- It typically takes six weeks before thyroid hormone production is noticeably reduced. The average length of time for the thyroid hormone levels to become normal is about three to four months. If thyroid levels are not considerably reduced six months after treatment, the doctor might suggest repeating the treatment. Ninety percent of the time only one treatment is required, however, it might take as many as three attempts. The patient could be advised to take beta blockers and other medications the doctor believes are necessary until normal thyroid hormone production is restored.

- Many patients treated with radioactive iodine become hypothyroid. This may happen within weeks, months, or years of treatment. Therefore, patients should be aware of the signs and symptoms of hypothyroidism and their physicians should monitor their thyroid hormone levels regularly. When the patient becomes hypothyroid, thyroid hormone replacement begins and continues for life—one pill a day.

Antithyroid Drugs. The more popular antithyroid drugs used in this country are Propylthiouracil (PTU) and Tapazole®. Some physicians will recommend antithyroid medication as a first line of treatment to see if the patient is one of the lucky 30% of patients who go into a remission after taking antithyroid medication for one to two years. (Patients are said to be in remission if their hyperthyroidism does not recur after discontinuing the antithyroid drugs.) If antithyroid drugs do not work for the patient, then the physicians will recommend radioactive iodine.

Antithyroid drugs are also used to treat very young children, older patients with heart conditions, and pregnant women. For severe or complicated cases of hyperthyroidism, especially in older patients, PTU or Tapazole® can be given for four to six weeks to bring the hyperthyroidism under better control prior to administering radioactive iodine treatment. In cases when women are diagnosed with Graves' disease while they are pregnant, PTU is prescribed. The smallest dose possible is given because the medication does cross over to the fetus. The mother should be checked every three to four weeks during the pregnancy so that the lowest possible dose can be given. Too much PTU can cause fetal goiter, hypothyroidism, and mental retardation.

What Can Be Expected with Antithyroid Drug Treatment?

- Several pills are taken from one to four times a day, every day for six to 18 months.

- Some patients complain that the pills have an unpleasant smell and taste.

- There is usually some symptom relief within one to two weeks, depending upon how much thyroid hormone the thyroid gland has stored. In some cases, it can be several months to delete this oversupply.

- Antithyroid drugs have a relatively low success rate. While PTU or Tapazole® may correct the problem temporarily or for a few years, the chances of a permanent remission are less than 30% once the drugs are stopped.

- The likelihood of achieving a permanent remission is increased if the patient takes the medication for one to two years.

- There are side effects in 10% of the people treated with Tapazole® or PTU. These are:
  - skin rash over most of the body
  - swollen, stiff, painful joints
  - sore throat and fever (the white blood cell count is reduced in patients on the medication). If this happens, the antithyroid drugs should be stopped immediately and the physician contacted.
  - jaundice
  - liver damage, which is fatal in rare cases

- Because antithyroid drugs pass into breast milk, only PTU in a dosage less than 200 mg a day is advised if the baby is not weaned.

- Within 15 years, the thyroid gland may burn out, resulting in hypothyroidism and the patient will need thyroid hormone replacement.

Thyroid Surgery or Thyroidectomy. This is seldom recommended for the treatment of hyperthyroidism today because of the effectiveness and safety of radioactive iodine therapy. Surgery is the most expensive option for the treatment of hyperthyroidism; however, it may be used for:

- a pregnant women in her second trimester who cannot tolerate antithyroid drugs;

- a patient who also has a thyroid nodule suspicious for cancer;
- a patient who has a coexisting problem for which surgery in the neck is necessary.

What Can Be Expected with Thyroid Surgery?

- Patients will be in the hospital for one to three days.

- Surgery is usually done under general anesthesia and lasts about two hours.

- A small cut approximately three to four inches long is made along the natural crease of the neck, and the surgeon removes enough of the thyroid gland to prevent recurrence of the disease.

- After going to the recovery room for a few hours, patients are returned to their rooms. Patients can usually get out of bed, eat, and have visitors the evening of the surgery.

- It can take up to a year for the scar to heal and the redness to disappear.

- Because most of the thyroid gland is removed, some patients will have to begin lifelong thyroid hormone replacement.

What Are the Possible Complications of Thyroid Surgery?

- The four parathyroid glands located around the thyroid gland can be accidentally damaged causing low calcium levels that can lead to muscle spasms, convulsions, and the formation of cataracts, if untreated.

- Minor voice changes are not uncommon, but only 1% of those operated on have major voice problems. The nerves from the larynx (voice box) are very near the thyroid gland and sometimes pass through the gland. It is sometimes unavoidable that they are damaged during surgery.

- As with any surgery, there is the risk of surgical death, bleeding, and infection.

Refusing Treatment. Patients always have this as an option, but should be aware of the consequences.

- Untreated hyperthyroidism can cause heart problems.

- Weight loss and/or diarrhea can become so severe that patients become incapacitated.

- An excess of thyroid hormones over an extended period of time can lead to osteoporosis.

- Behavior changes such as irritability, nervousness, and paranoia increase, making it appear that the patient is suffering from a severe mental disorder. There have even been cases where patients have been placed in mental institutions.

- Patients' ability to maintain jobs and relationships can be severely compromised.

- The thyroid gland frequently burns out within 15 years resulting in hypothyroidism, even if no treatment is given.

Chapter 43

Hypothyroidism

What Is Hypothyroidism?

Hypothyroidism causes the body to slow down. It occurs when there is too little thyroid hormone in the blood ("hypo" means "not enough"). Hypothyroidism affects more than 5 million Americans, many of whom don't know they have the disease. Women are more likely than men to have hypothyroidism.

What Causes Hypothyroidism?

There are several different causes of hypothyroidism:

- An inflammation of the thyroid gland called thyroiditis can lower the amount of hormones produced. The number one cause of hypothyroidism is Hashimoto's thyroiditis, a painless disease of the immune system that runs in families. Another form of thyroiditis, postpartum thyroiditis, occurs in 5%-9% of women soon after giving birth and is usually a temporary condition.

- Thyroid surgery or radioactive iodine treatment may cause hypothyroidism.

- One out of every 4,000 infants is born without a working thyroid gland. If the problem is not corrected, the child will become mentally and physically retarded.

- About 100 million people around the world don't get enough iodine in their diets. Iodine is a chemical which the thyroid uses to produce its hormones. The problem has been solved in North America and Western Europe by adding iodine to salt.

Some other possible causes of hypothyroidism are radiation therapy to the head and neck, birth defects, certain drugs, problems with the pituitary gland, and a gradual wearing out of the thyroid gland.

What Is Hashimoto's Thyroiditis?

Hashimoto's thyroiditis is the most common form of thyroiditis and the leading cause of hypothyroidism. It affects about 5% of the adult population, increasing particularly in women as they age.

Hashimoto's thyroiditis is caused by problems in the body's immune system. Normally, the immune system defends the body against germs and viruses, but in diseases such as Hashimoto's, the system attacks the body's own tissues by mistake. Hashimoto's thyroiditis causes the immune system to produce certain antithyroid antibodies, which damage the gland and keep it from producing enough hormones.

Diseases of the immune system tend to run in families and are more common in women than in men. Hashimoto's is linked to other autoimmune conditions, such as Graves' disease, premature gray hair, diabetes mellitus, and arthritis.

How Do Doctors Test for Hypothyroidism?

As with any disease, it is important that you watch for the early warning signs of hypothyroidism. However, only your doctor can tell for sure whether or not you have the disease. Your doctor may examine:

- your history and physical appearance
- the amount of thyroid hormones, thyroid stimulating hormone (TSH), and antithyroid antibodies in your blood.

How Is Hypothyroidism Treated?

The standard treatment for hypothyroidism is thyroid hormone pills. The pills provide the body with the right amount of thyroid hormone when the gland is not able to produce enough by itself. While the symptoms of hypothyroidism are usually corrected within a few months, most patients need to take the pills for the rest of their lives.

The preferred thyroid hormone for treatment is levothyroxine (T4). You should use only the brand-name that your doctor prescribes, since generic brands may not be as reliable. Name-brand levothyroxine pills include Levothroid®, Synthroid®, and Levoxine®. (®Levothroid is a registered trademark of Forest Pharmaceuticals; ®Synthroid is a registered trademark of Boots Pharmaceuticals; and ®Levoxine is a registered trademark of Daniels Pharmaceuticals.)

Patients sometimes take more pills than they should, trying to speed up the treatment or lose weight. However, this can lead to hyperthyroidism, a disease in which there is too much thyroid hormone in the blood, and to long-term complications, such as osteoporosis. You should take the pills as your doctor prescribes.

At different times in your life, you may need to take different amounts of thyroid hormones. Therefore, see your doctor once a year to make sure everything is all right.

What Is the Thyroid?

The thyroid is a small, butterfly-shaped gland just below the Adam's apple. This gland plays a very important role in controlling the body's metabolism, that is, how the body functions. It does this by producing thyroid hormones (T4 and T3), chemicals that travel through the blood to every part of the body. Thyroid hormones tell the body how fast to work and use energy.

What Are the Signs and Symptoms of Hypothyroidism?

Possible effects of hypothyroidism are:

- slow heart rate (less than 70 beats per minute)
- elevated blood pressure
- feeling slow or tired
- feeling cold
- drowsy during the day, even after sleeping all night
- poor memory
- difficulty concentrating
- muscle cramps; numb arms and legs
- weight gain
- puffy face, especially under the eyes

- husky voice
- thinning hair
- dry, coarse, flaky, yellowish skin
- in children, short height
- constipation
- heavy menstrual flow
- milky discharge from the breasts
- infertility
- goiter (an abnormal swelling in the neck caused by an enlarged thyroid gland).

What Is the Thyroid Society for Education and Research?

The Thyroid Society for Education & Research is a national, not-for-profit organization whose mission is to pursue the prevention, treatment, and cure of thyroid disease. To accomplish this mission, The Thyroid Society participates in, and raises funds for, patient and community education programs, professional education, and scientific research. The work of The Thyroid Society is supported by various grants and by individual contributions.

For more information, call:

The Thyroid Society
7515 South Main Street, Suite 545
Houston, TX 77030
1-800-THYROID (1-800-849-7643)
(713) 799-9909

Chapter 44

Recognizing Early Hypothyroidism

Underactive Thyroid

Your thyroid weighs less than an ounce. But this tiny butterfly-shaped gland located just below your Adam's apple has an enormous effect on your health. All aspects of your metabolism, from the rate at which your heart beats to the speed at which you burn calories, are regulated by thyroid hormones.

As long as your thyroid makes the right amount of hormones, your metabolism runs normally. In hyperthyroidism, your thyroid releases an excessive amount of hormones, speeding metabolic activity as much as 60 to 80 percent. More frequently, however thyroid troubles involve hypothyroidism, in which your thyroid fails to make and release enough hormones.

About 6 to 7 million Americans, mainly women older than age 40, are affected by an underactive thyroid. Because initial symptoms are often subtle, only about half of all cases are diagnosed early.

However, the sensitivity of thyroid function tests has gradually improved over the last 20 years, Diagnosing mild disease before symptoms worsen is now easier. Once an underactive thyroid is diagnosed, treatment is simple and generally trouble-free.

"Underactive Thyroid: This Common Condition Can Be Easy to Miss," *Mayo Clinic Health Letter*, Vol. 14, No. 3, March 1996, ©1996 Mayo Foundation for Medical Education and Research, 200 First St. SW, Rochester, MN 55905; reprinted with permission.

Running at Low Speed

Your thyroid gland makes and releases two major iodine-containing hormones, thyroxine (T4) and triiodothyronine (T3). As they circulate in your blood, these hormones regulate your metabolism. They maintain the rate at which your tissues use fats and carbohydrates, help control your body temperature, influence your heart rate and help regulate production of protein.

To maintain your body's normal metabolism, your thyroid must release the right amount of hormones at all times. In your brain, the hypothalamus and pituitary gland monitor hormone levels and control the rate of hormone release.

Thyroid-stimulating hormone (TSH), released by the pituitary, regulates the rate at which your thyroid makes hormones. When the blood level of thyroid hormones increases, the pituitary lowers TSH production, reducing thyroid hormone release. If the level of thyroid hormones in your blood drops, the pituitary releases more TSH, stimulating your thyroid to secrete more hormones.

If your thyroid becomes underactive, the delicate balance of chemical reactions regulated by the hormones goes awry, slowing your metabolism and causing a host of symptoms.

A Slow and Subtle Start

Early symptoms of an underactive thyroid, such as sluggishness and fatigue, are often vague. It can be easy to discount them as simply "getting older."

As your metabolism continues to slow, you may develop signs such as chronically cold hands or feet, constipation, pale and dry skin, a puffy face, and a hoarse voice.

People often attribute weight gain to an underactive thyroid. But the weight gain is usually limited to 10 to 20 pounds, most of which is fluid retention.

An underactive thyroid also causes elevated blood levels of cholesterol. Levels continue to increase as the disease progresses.

If hypothyroidism isn't treated, symptoms gradually become more noticeable and severe. Constant overstimulation of your thyroid to release more hormones can lead to an enlarged thyroid (goiter). Forgetfulness and slowing of your thought processes can also develop.

Advanced or extreme hypothyroidism, called myxedema (mik-suh-DE-muh), is rare and usually results from long-term, undiagnosed disease. Myxedema can cause life-threatening coma.

Your Immune System Is Often to Blame

Most common causes of an underactive thyroid include the following.

Autoimmune disorder. In this condition, your immune system produces antibodies that attack your thyroid tissue. This sets up an inflammatory process that eventually can destroy the gland.

Treatment with radioactive iodine. Use of radioactive iodine to control an overactive gland can result in an underactive thyroid. The radioactive material becomes concentrated in the gland and slowly reduces its function.

Radiation therapy. Exposing your thyroid to radiation during treatment for cancers of the head and neck may also lead to hormone deficiency.

Thyroid surgery. Removing all or a large portion of your thyroid to treat thyroid cancer can slow or halt hormone production.

Less often, hypothyroidism may result from the following.

Congenital disease. Approximately 1 in 5,000 newborns has a defective thyroid gland or no gland at all. All babies now receive thyroid tests at birth.

Pituitary disorder. About percent of cases of hypothyroidism occur when an insufficient amount of TSH is released by a defective pituitary gland.

Iodine deficiency. Before the 1920s, an underactive thyroid sometimes resulted from consuming too little iodine. But the addition of iodine to some common foods has eliminated iodine deficiency in the United States.

Restoring Normal Speed

Because underactive thyroid disease is more prevalent in older women, some experts recommend women age 60 and older be screened for the disorder during routine annual physical examinations. However, Medicare doesn't cover the cost of screening.

In general, your doctor may test for an underactive thyroid if you're feeling progressively tired, if you have signs such as dry skin or a hoarse voice, or if you've had previous thyroid problems.

Diagnosis of the disease is based on your symptoms and the results of blood tests that measure thyroxine and TSH levels. Low levels of thyroxine and high levels of TSH signal an underactive thyroid.

Treatment for an underactive thyroid is straightforward daily use of levothyroxine (Levothroid, Levoxine, Synthroid) made from synthetic thyroid hormones. The oral medication restores adequate hormone levels, speeding chemical processes and shifting your body back into normal gear.

After just a few days of treatment, physical symptoms such as fatigue start to subside. The medication also gradually lowers cholesterol levels elevated by the disease. Treatment with levothyroxine is usually lifelong.

To determine the right dosage of levothyroxine, your doctor generally checks your TSH level every two to three months. Then an annual blood test is usually adequate to ensure maintenance of the right dosage. Excessive amounts of the hormone can accelerate bone loss, which may worsen osteoporosis or add to your risk of this disease.

If you have coronary artery disease or severe hypothyroidism, your doctor may start treatment with a small amount of medication and gradually increase the dosage. Progressive hormone replacement allows your heart to adjust to the increase in metabolism.

Levothyroxine causes virtually no side effects and is relatively inexpensive. You're generally advised to avoid generic forms of the drug because some can vary in strength. If you change brands, let your doctor know to ensure you're still receiving the right dosage. Also, don't skip a day or stop taking the drug because you're feeling better. Sluggishness will gradually return.

Solution in a Shaker

In the early 1900s, hypothyroidism and development of goiter were common in Switzerland and in the Midwest and Great Lakes regions of the United States, where water and soil lack iodine. Without enough dietary iodine, your thyroid can't make iodine-containing hormones.

After scientists recognized iodine deficiency as the cause of hypothyroidism, iodized salt was introduced in Switzerland in 1922. In 1924, the Michigan Department of Health was first to permit sale of iodized salt in the United States.

Since then, surgery to remove large goiters, once common, is now rarely necessary. However, iodine deficiency still remains a problem in some countries.

In the United States, even if you don't use iodized table salt, you're ensured an adequate amount of iodine because of the addition of iodized salt to many processed foods and enriched breads. Water, dairy products and seafood also contain iodine naturally.

Chapter 45

What Is Thyroiditis?

Thyroiditis is an inflammation of the thyroid gland. It affects about 12 million people in the United States. Thyroiditis can cause either hyperthyroidism or hypothyroidism, or one followed by the other. It can also cause a goiter, an abnormal swelling in the neck due to an enlarged thyroid.

What Are the Main Types of Thyroiditis?

Chronic thyroiditis, called Hashimoto's thyroiditis, is by far the most common form. It begins so slowly that most people don't know anything is wrong. Over time, the disease destroys thyroid tissue until permanent hypothyroidism results. Some patients with Hashimoto's have normal thyroid functions (euthyroidism) with a goiter.

Subacute thyroiditis is the second most common form, with far fewer cases than in chronic thyroiditis. Often caused by a viral infection, the disease lasts for several months. At first, gland destruction causes the release of stored thyroid hormones, inducing temporary

---

hyperthyroidism. A month or two later, the patient may become hypothyroid, because the thyroid has been damaged and its hormone reserves used up. Most patients return to normal within six to nine months, but the hypothyroidism could be permanent.

There are two types of subacute thyroiditis. *Painful* subacute thyroiditis causes a tender, swollen thyroid gland with pain throughout the neck. The pain usually responds to treatment with aspirin or other anti-inflammatory drugs. *Painless* subacute thyroiditis causes a painless swelling of the thyroid gland. When this disease occurs after pregnancy, it is called postpartum thyroiditis.

Acute thyroiditis, a rare disease, is caused by an acute infection. Patients with the disease become very sick and have a high fever. The neck is red, hot, and very tender. Acute thyroiditis is a medical emergency and must be treated with antibiotics and surgery.

What Is Hashimoto's Thyroiditis?

Hashimoto's thyroiditis, also called chronic thyroiditis, is named for the Japanese doctor who discovered it. It affects about 5% of the adult population, increasing particularly in women as they age. Hashimoto's, the most common form of thyroiditis, is the leading cause of hypothyroidism.

Hashimoto's thyroiditis results from problems with the body's immune system. Normally, the immune system defends against germs and viruses, but in diseases such as Hashimoto's, the immune system attacks the body's own tissues. Hashimoto's thyroiditis makes the immune system produce antithyroid antibodies, which damage the gland and keep it from producing enough hormones.

Diseases of the immune system tend to run in families and are about five times more common in women than in men. Hashimoto's is linked to other autoimmune conditions, such as Graves' disease, premature gray hair, diabetes mellitus, arthritis and patchy loss of pigment of the skin (vitiligo).

What Is Postpartum Thyroiditis?

Postpartum thyroiditis is a temporary form of painless subacute thyroiditis. It occurs in 5%-9% of women soon after giving birth (postpartum). The effects are usually mild. However, the disease may recur with future pregnancies.

How Do Doctors Test for Thyroiditis?

As with any disease, it is important that you watch for the early warning signs of thyroiditis. However, only your doctor can tell for sure whether or not you have the disease. Your doctor may examine:

- your history and physical appearance
- the amount of thyroid hormones, thyroid stimulating hormone (TSH), and antithyroid antibodies in your blood
- your sedimentation rate, a blood test useful in diagnosing thyroiditis
- the radioactive iodine taken up by your thyroid

How Is Thyroiditis Treated?

If thyroiditis makes you temporarily hyperthyroid, your doctor may ask you to take a beta-blocking drug. This medicine helps control the symptoms, such as rapid heart rate and tremors.

Thyroid hormone pills are the standard treatment for permanent hypothyroidism caused by Hashimoto's thyroiditis. The pills provide the body with the right amount of thyroid hormone when the gland is not able to produce enough by itself. Most patients need to take the pills for the rest of their lives.

Levothyroxine (T4) is the thyroid hormone of choice for treating hypothyroidism. You should use only the brand-name that your doctor prescribes, since generic brands may not be as reliable. Examples of name-brand levothyroxine pills are Levoxyl®, Levothroid®, and Synthroid®. (®Levoxyl is a registered trademark of Daniels Pharmaceuticals; ®Levothroid is a registered trademark of Forest Pharmaceuticals; ®Synthroid is a registered trademark of Knoll Pharmaceuticals.)

You should take your thyroid hormone pills only as your doctor prescribes. Patients sometimes take more pills than they should, trying to speed up the treatment or lose weight. However, this can lead to hyperthyroidism or long-term complications, such as osteoporosis.

At different times in your life, you may need to take different amounts of thyroid hormones. Therefore, you should see your doctor once a year to make sure everything is all right.

What Is the Thyroid?

The thyroid is a small, butterfly-shaped gland just below the Adam's apple. This gland plays a very important role in controlling the body's metabolism, that is, how the body functions. It does this by producing thyroid hormones (T4 and T3), chemicals that travel through the blood to every part of the body. Thyroid hormones tell the body how fast to work and use energy.

What Are the Signs and Symptoms of Thyroiditis?

Thyroiditis can cause either hyperthyroidism or hypothyroidism, or one followed by the other.

Common signs and symptoms of hyperthyroidism include:

- fast heart rate (100-120 beats per minute, or higher)
- nervousness or irritability
- increased perspiration
- muscle weakness (especially in the shoulders, hips, and thighs)
- trembling hands
- weight loss, in spite of a good appetite.

Common signs and symptoms of hypothyroidism include:

- slow heart rate (less than 70 beats per minute)
- feel slow or tired
- drowsy during the day, even after sleeping all night
- poor memory
- difficulty concentrating
- muscle cramps, numb arms and legs
- weight gain
- constipation
- heavy menstrual flow.

What Is The Thyroid Society for Education and Research?

The Thyroid Society for Education & Research is a national, not-for-profit organization whose mission is to pursue the prevention, treatment, and cure of thyroid disease. To accomplish this mission, The Thyroid Society participates in, and raises funds for, patient and community education programs, professional education, and scientific research. The work of The Thyroid Society is supported by various grants and by individual contributions. For more information, contact: The Thyroid Society, 7515 South Main Street, Suite 545, Houston, Texas 77030; 1-800-THYROID (1-800-849-7643) or (713) 799-9909.

Chapter 46

Hashimoto's Disease

In 1912 Dr. H. Hashimoto, a Japanese pathologist, described four patients with enlargement of their thyroid glands. He examined the thyroids of these patients with a microscope and found that their thyroid tissue was invaded by white blood cells known as lymphocytes. In addition, he described degeneration and scarring within the gland, features which suggested tissue destruction by some underlying process.

Thyroiditis is the general term used to describe disorders in which the thyroid gland becomes inflamed. In some forms of thyroiditis (acute and subacute thyroiditis) the inflammation appears to be caused by or associated with a bacterial or viral infection. In contrast, in chronic lymphocytic thyroiditis, also known as Hashimoto's Disease, the inflammation appears to be due to the action of antibodies produced by the lymphocytes which Dr. Hashimoto observed in his patients so long ago. Because the inflammation is so mild, patients who are developing the condition tend to have few symptoms until so much of the thyroid has been destroyed that hypothyroidism develops.

A Common Disorder

Although Hashimoto's Disease was initially felt to be fairly rare, physicians have come to realize that it is actually extremely common.

From *The Bridge*, The Thyroid Foundation of America, Inc., Ruth Sleeper Hall, RSL 350, 40 Parkman St., Boston MA 02114-2698, (800) 832-8321; reprinted with permission.

Studies of large numbers of people suggest that 10% of women over the age of fifty become hypothyroid due to this condition. In fact it may be even more widespread, for other studies have shown that 16% of women over fifty have antibodies against thyroid tissue in their blood. It seems likely that these antibodies reflect the presence of chronic thyroiditis. Follow-up studies of these patients have shown that they are at increased risk for hypothyroidism in later years.

If you begin to develop the low grade thyroid inflammation of chronic lymphocytic thyroiditis you will likely feel perfectly well and have no symptoms or physical evidence of a thyroid problem for many years. Your thyroid hormone levels will be normal and the subtle changes within your thyroid gland do not produce any noticeable enlargement or goiter. Therefore, you probably won't have difficulty swallowing. You are not likely to have any symptoms until the inflammation within your thyroid gland damages enough thyroid tissue so that your thyroid is no longer able to make normal amounts of thyroid hormones. At that point your physician may suspect a thyroid problem during your annual physical examination because a slight enlargement of your thyroid gland may be evident. Alternatively, your thyroid may become lumpy or "nodular" and the condition may be detected in a thyroid biopsy done to evaluate one of your thyroid nodules. Some patients with Hashimoto's disease, however do not have any thyroid enlargement or lumps.

As the disease progresses, you may also begin to have symptoms of thyroid hormone deficiency or hypothyroidism. Many patients feel tired, cold, or mentally down. You may also experience constipation, dry skin, dry and brittle hair, and muscle cramps.

At that point a blood test will probably show a low level of the thyroid hormone Thyroxine (T4) and an increase in your Thyroid Stimulating Hormone (TSH) confirming hypothyroidism.

Treatment

If Hashimoto's Disease is causing only slight thyroid enlargement or nodularity, your physician may not treat you with thyroid hormone. Instead, he or she may simply monitor your condition with periodic examinations and measurements of your thyroid blood tests.

On the other hand, if your thyroid inflammation has progressed to the point of causing hypothyroidism, your physician will probably prescribe treatment with thyroid hormone tablets in gradually increasing doses until your thyroid levels are normal, at which time your symptoms should disappear.

Most physicians monitor treatment by periodically measuring the levels of thyroid hormone and TSH in your blood. If your thyroid hormone level is normal, your TSH level will also be normal. If you're not taking enough thyroid hormone, your pituitary will increase its production of TSH and your TSH blood level will be above normal. On the other hand, if you are taking too much thyroid hormone the level of TSH in your blood will be below normal. Your physician will use the results of blood tests to be sure that your medication dosage is appropriate.

Related Conditions

Hashimoto's Disease tends to occur in families. In these families some relatives may also have hypothyroidism, while others may have the type of hyperthyroidism known as Graves' Disease. Still other individuals may have different antibody-mediated "autoimmune" diseases including, insulin-dependent diabetes, pernicious anemia, patchy hair loss known as alopecia areata, white spots on the skin known as vitiligo, and prematurely gray hair.

If some of these conditions occur in your family, your physician may elect to perform thyroid blood tests in older family members, especially in women over fifty, in an effort to detect mild hypothyroidism due to Hashimoto's Disease before it causes serious illness. Such screening techniques are being used increasingly since the symptoms of mild early hypothyroidism can often be mistakenly attributed to aging. Needless to say, it is gratifying for a patient to find that some of their fatigue and lethargy are due to hypothyroidism, which can be treated, rather than to the aging process.

It is fortunate that we have developed these sensitive techniques for diagnosing and treating Hashimoto's Disease and the hypothyroidism which it can produce. If it has caused you to become hypothyroid, you should have no cause for concern, as long as you see your physician regularly for thyroid examinations, blood tests, and treatment.

— by Lawrence C. Wood, M.D., Massachusetts General Hospital, Boston, Massachusetts

Chapter 47

Cancer of the Thyroid

The diagnosis of cancer is terrifying for most patients because it has become associated in our minds with pain and death. But, in fact, the outlook for patients with thyroid cancer is usually excellent because 1) most thyroid cancer is easily curable with surgery, 2) it causes little pain or disability, and 3) novel and effective means of diagnosis and therapy are available for several kinds of thyroid cancer.

Thyroid cancer usually presents itself as a lump or nodule in the thyroid gland. However, it should be emphasized that most thyroid nodules (90% or more) are benign. Unfortunately, it may be difficult to distinguish a benign from a malignant nodule on the basis of history and physical examination, even with the help of laboratory tests including blood hormone levels and scans (images) of the thyroid gland. Biopsy of thyroid nodules usually provides the most valuable information in helping a physician to decide whether a surgical operation is necessary.

Occasionally, a thyroid cancer can present as a swollen lymph node in the neck, as hoarseness due to pressure from the tumor on the nerve to the voice box (recurrent laryngeal nerve), or as difficulty in swallowing or breathing due to a tumor obstructing the esophagus or windpipe.

In this review, we will discuss the most common types of thyroid malignancy.

From *Thyroid Topics* ©1995 The Thyroid Foundation of America, Inc. Ruth Sleeper Hall, RSL350, 40 Parkman Street, Boston, MA 02114-2698; reprinted with permission.

411

What Is Well-Differentiated Thyroid Cancer?

A cancer is a malignant tumor which grows in the body. A well-differentiated cancer is one which superficially looks like the normal parent tissue, in this case the thyroid gland. There are two types of well-differentiated thyroid cancer: papillary and follicular.

Well-differentiated thyroid cancers account for about 90% of all thyroid malignancies and usually they are associated with an excellent outlook. Although we do not know exactly what causes these well-differentiated cancers to grow, we do know that they are more likely to develop in patients who have received x-ray treatments in childhood for enlarged tonsils, enlarged thymus glands, acne, and occasionally for other malignancies such as Hodgkin's disease. Routine diagnostic x-rays (like chest x-rays, dental x-rays, or thyroid scans) do not cause such thyroid cancer.

What Is Papillary Thyroid Cancer?

A papilla is a nipple-like projection. Papillary cancers have multiple projections giving them a fern or frond-like appearance under the microscope. Tiny areas of papillary cancer can be found in up to 10% of "normal" thyroid glands, when thyroid tissue is carefully examined with a microscope. The more carefully a pathologist looks for these tiny cancers, the more commonly they are found. These microscopic cancers seem to have no clinical importance and are more a curiosity than a disease. In other words, there does not seem to be a tendency for these small cancer-like growths to enlarge and become more serious malignant tumors.

On the other hand, when papillary cancer grows enough to form a lump in the thyroid gland, we consider it clinically important, for it is likely to continue to enlarge and may spread elsewhere in the body. Papillary tumors make up about 70% to 80% of all thyroid cancers, and can occur at any age. There are only about 12,000 new cases of papillary cancer in the United States each year, but because these patients have such a long life expectancy, we estimate that one in a thousand people have or have had this form of cancer.

Papillary cancer tends to grow slowly and to spread by means of the lymphatic system to lymph glands in the neck. In fact, in about one third of the patients who undergo surgery for papillary cancer, the tumor has already spread to surrounding lymph glands (Lymph node metastasis). Fortunately, the generally excellent outlook is usually not altered by lymph gland metastases. The papillary cancer may also spread from one side of the thyroid to the other through the lymphatic system, again without affecting the patient's prognosis.

What ultimately determines the outlook for patients with papillary thyroid cancer is largely the extent of the original disease. As noted above, the presence or absence of lymph gland involvement usually does not affect the prognosis. The 85% of patients with papillary carcinoma who have a primary tumor that is intrathyroidal (confined to the thyroid gland itself) have an excellent outlook: the 25-year mortality rate from cancer in this situation is about 1% This means that only 1 out of every 100 such patients have died of thyroid cancer by 25 years later. By that time the vast majority of them have been permanently cured. The prognosis is not quite as good in patients over the age of 50, or in patients with tumors larger than 4 centimeters (1½ inches) in diameter.

Since the outlook in patients with intrathyroidal primary tumors is so favorable, it is important that therapy not be hazardous. Radical surgery is almost never indicated for this mild type of papillary cancer. Although up to 10% of patients with intrathyroidal papillary cancer will have a recurrence of tumor, recurrences are generally due to the growth of tumor cells within lymph glands in the neck and are not life-threatening. They are usually removed surgically.

The prognosis is not as good in patients where the cancer has grown through the thyroid into surrounding tissues. Specially, this means spread through the fibrous capsule that surrounds the thyroid gland into the tissues of the neck, and not the lymph node involvement discussed above. In a very small percentage of patients (about 5%), the cancer eventually spreads through the blood stream to distant sites, particularly the lungs and bones. These distant tumor sites (metastases) can often be treated successfully with radioactive iodine (see below). Although young patients who have papillary thyroid cancer generally have an excellent outlook, patients under the age of 20 have a somewhat higher risk of spread to lungs.

What Is Follicular Thyroid Cancer?

The normal thyroid gland is made up of sphere-shaped the structures called follicles. When a thyroid cancer contains these normal structures, the cancer is called a follicular cancer. Follicular cancer makes up about 10-15% of all thyroid cancers in the United States, and tends to occur in somewhat older patients than papillary carcinoma.

Follicular cancer of the thyroid is considered to be more aggressive than papillary cancer. In about one-third of patients with follicular

413

thyroid cancer, the tumor is minimally invasive and tends not to spread. The prognosis is excellent in this situation. In the other two-thirds of patients, the follicular cancer is more invasive. It may grow into blood vessels and from there spread to distant areas, particularly the lung and bones. In general, the prognosis is better in younger patients than in those over 50 years of age.

What Is the Treatment of Well-Differentiated Thyroid Cancer?

The primary therapy for all forms of thyroid cancer is surgery. For more aggressive papillary and follicular cancers, the generally accepted approach is to remove the entire thyroid gland, or as much of it as can be safely removed. For intrathyroidal papillary cancer and minimally invasive follicular thyroid cancer, surgeons and endocrinologists continue to debate the merits of total thyroid removal versus the removal of just one lobe and the tissue connecting the two thyroid lobes, known as the isthmus.

Since the outlook is so good for intrathyroidal papillary cancer and minimally invasive follicular cancer, independent of the extent of surgery, it has been difficult to prove which off the two surgical approaches is preferable. Therefore there are no absolute rules for the management of these cancers. Although the general characteristics of tumor behavior are understood, in any particular patient the choice of treatment is best made by physicians skilled in the management of patients with thyroid cancer.

Radioiodine Therapy

Once papillary or follicular cancer has spread through the blood stream into the surrounding tissues or to distant sites (especially lungs and bones), the usual therapy is to administer a radioactive form of iodine (I^{131}) to try to destroy the tumor. To understand this treatment, it is important to know the relationship between iodine and the thyroid gland.

The thyroid gland normally concentrates iodine from the bloodstream, and this process is stimulated by TSH (thyroid stimulating hormone) from the pituitary gland. The iodine is subsequently used to produce thyroid hormone (thyroxine, T4). Thyroid cancers or metastases from thyroid cancer take up only tiny amounts of iodine (or radioactive iodine) under normal conditions. However, under the influence of large amounts of TSH, some thyroid cancer or their metastases can be stimulated to take up significant amounts of iodine. This delivers a large dose of radiation directly to the cancer, without damage to surrounding tissues. If the thyroid gland is present and produces a normal amount of thyroid hormone, the production of TSH by the pituitary remains relatively low. But if the entire thyroid gland is removed or destroyed, and the level of thyroid hormone is allowed to fall, the pituitary gland will increase TSH secretion dramatically. In turn, this will stimulate the thyroid cancer to take up the radioactive iodine.

To undergo radioactive iodine therapy for thyroid cancer that has spread, the entire thyroid gland must almost completely be surgically removed and any remnant tissue then destroyed by a treatment with radioactive iodine. Once that has been done, patients with a residual tumor in the neck or known distant metastases can then undergo a scan with a test amount of radioactive iodine (usually about 2 to 10 millicuries), provided the level of TSH is sufficiently high. If a significant amount of iodine is concentrated in the areas of thyroid cancer, a larger therapeutic dose of radioactive iodine (usually 150-200 millicuries) can be administered in an attempt to destroy the tumor.

A patient who receives treatment with large doses of radioactive iodine must stay several days in the hospital until the amount of radioactivity in the body falls to levels which will not be hazardous to other people. However, this treatment has proved to be safe and well tolerated and has even been able to cure cases of well-differentiated thyroid cancer after the tumor has spread to the lungs.

Because of the safety and effectiveness of radioactive iodine in patients with more aggressive thyroid cancer, many physicians also use it routinely in patients with less aggressive papillary and follicular cancers. In this situation, radioactive iodine is used to destroy tiny remnants of thyroid tissue still present after surgery. This may improve the outlook and makes it easier to monitor patients for tumor recurrence using a blood test for thyroglobulin (see below).

If well-differentiated thyroid cancer continues to spread, even after surgery and the administration of radioactive iodine, then external radiation therapy may be helpful. Chemotherapy is usually not very effective in this situation.

How Are Thyroid Cancer Patients Followed?

Periodic follow-up examinations are essential for patients who have had surgery for papillary or follicular thyroid cancer, because recurrences sometimes occur many years after apparently successful surgery.

These follow-up visits should include a careful history and physical examination, with particular attention to the neck area as well as periodic chest x-rays. Neck ultrasound examination and radioactive iodine scanning to obtain images of the neck and whole body may also be useful.

It is also helpful from time to time after surgery to measure the blood level of thyroglobulin. This substance is released by normal thyroid tissue and also by well-differentiated thyroid cancer cells. The blood level of thyroglobulin is very low after total thyroid gland removal, and in most patients who are taking thyroid hormone after thyroid surgery. An elevated or rising level of thyroglobulin generally implies persistent or growing thyroid cancer, but does not necessarily imply a poor prognosis. A high thyroglobulin level found in a follow-up examination alerts the physician to the possibility that other tests may be needed to be sure the tumor is not recurring. Unfortunately, in some thyroid cancer patients the presence of interfering antibodies in the blood may prevent accurate thyroglobulin measurement.

What About Thyroid Hormone Treatment?

Naturally, if the thyroid gland has been mostly or completely removed, thyroid hormone must be taken for the body to remain normal. Even if part of the thyroid remains, therapy with thyroxine is an important part of the follow-up care in thyroid cancer patients, since studies have shown that cancer is more likely to recur in those patients who do not take this medication. The thyroid hormone should be administered in sufficient quantities to suppress TSH levels to subnormal values, except when medically contraindicated. New, sensitive TSH measurements are extremely useful for monitoring TSH concentrations and confirming that the serum TSH is just below normal in patients at low risk of cancer recurrence. Patients with more aggressive forms of papillary or follicular cancer probably should take larger doses of thyroxine in order to suppress TSH to undetectable levels.

About The Thyroid Foundation of America, Inc.

The Thyroid Foundation of America is a nonprofit organization which was created in 1986 to provide health education and support for thyroid patients and health professionals, to increase public awareness about thyroid problems, and to raise and distribute funds for thyroid research. We prepare educational brochures and a quarterly newsletter for thyroid patients and health professionals with up-to-date reviews of important thyroid topics, reports on TFA Chapter activities, and notices about books and meetings of interest to thyroid patients and health professionals.

For further information, call or write:

The Thyroid Foundation of America, Inc.
Ruth Sleeper Hall, RSL 350
40 Parkman Street
Boston, MA 02114-2698
1-800-832-8321 (Outside MA)
1-617-726-8500 (Inside MA)

Chapter 48

Are All Thyroid Nodules Cancerous?

How Common Is Thyroid Cancer?

Thyroid cancer is found in only about 8,000 people each year and causes about 1,000 deaths per year. The most common form (papillary cancer) moves very slowly, and treatment is almost always successful when the cancer is detected early. A less common form (follicular cancer) also moves relatively slowly. Two less frequent forms of thyroid cancer (undifferentiated, or anaplastic, and medullary) are more serious.

Who Can Get Thyroid Cancer?

Anyone can get thyroid cancer. However, one group in particular has a higher risk: people who have had radiation to the head or neck. From the 1920s to the 1960s, x-ray treatments were used for an enlarged thymus gland, inflamed tonsils and adenoids, ringworm, acne, and many chest conditions.

At that time, doctors thought the x-rays were safe. About 1 million Americans received the treatment, and some of these people will get thyroid cancer up to 40 or more years after receiving the treatment. We now know that radiation therapy to the head or neck increases the chance of developing thyroid cancer later in life. (Radioactive iodine treatments and x-rays used for testing do not increase the risk of cancer.)

Others at risk include a child or elderly person with a new thyroid nodule. If a man has a thyroid nodule, it is more likely to be cancerous than if a woman has one.

What Are Hot and Cold Nodules?

Thyroid nodules do not function like normal thyroid tissue. A thyroid image (scan) done with a radioactive chemical shows the size, shape, and function of the gland and of thyroid nodules. A nodule that takes up more of the radioactive material than the rest of the gland is called a hot nodule.

A nodule that takes up less radioactive material is a cold nodule. Hot nodules are seldom cancerous, but less than 10% of all nodules are hot. Cold nodules may or may not be cancerous. All lumps should be checked by your doctor.

How Do Doctors Test Nodules for Cancer?

Your doctor can use several tests to find out whether or not a thyroid lump is cancerous.

- A thyroid image or scan shows the size, shape, and function of the gland. It uses a tiny amount of a radioactive chemical, usually iodine or technetium, which the thyroid absorbs from the blood. A special camera then creates a picture, showing how much iodine was absorbed by each part of the gland.

- In needle aspiration biopsy, a small needle is inserted into the nodule in an effort to suck out (aspirate) cells. If the nodule is a fluid-filled cyst, the aspiration often removes some or all of the fluid. If the nodule is solid, several small samples are removed for examination under the microscope. In over 90% of all cases, this testing tells the doctor whether the lump is benign or malignant.

- Ultrasound uses high-pitch sound waves to find out whether a nodule is solid or filled with fluid. About 10% of lumps are fluid-filled cysts, and they are usually not cancerous. Ultrasound may also detect other nodules that are not easily felt by the doctor. The presence of multiple nodules reduces the likelihood of cancer.

How Are Nodules Treated?

Nodules that are thought to be benign are usually observed at regular intervals. Some patients may be advised to take thyroid hormone pills. In certain instances, the nodule may be surgically removed because of continuing growth, pressure symptoms in the neck, or for cosmetic reasons. Fluid-filled cysts that come back after several aspirations may need to be removed.

If the testing shows a nodule that is, or might be, malignant, your doctor will recommend surgery. (You should discuss special situations, such as pregnancy, with your doctor.) The goal of surgery is to remove as much of the cancerous tissue as possible. If the cancer is found in the early stages when it is still confined to the thyroid gland, the surgery is almost always successful. With papillary cancer, patients usually do well after treatment, even if the cancer has spread to the lymph nodes in the neck.

The surgeon starts by removing one lobe of the thyroid. This section is tested during surgery (frozen section) to tell the surgeon whether it is benign or malignant. If it is malignant, most or all of the thyroid is removed. If the cancer has spread, lymph nodes in the neck may also have to be removed. In addition, radioactive iodine therapy may be needed six weeks after surgery to destroy any remaining cancerous tissue.

What Happens after Surgery?

After surgery, patients must stay in the hospital for two to four days. They may also need to take some time off from work (one to two weeks for a desk job; three to four weeks for physical labor). Most patients do not have any trouble speaking or swallowing, and they report minimal pain after the surgery. In patients with thyroid cancer, a scan may be done approximately six weeks after surgery to detect any residual thyroid tissue that needs to be treated with radioactive iodine.

Patients with thyroid cancer will need to take thyroid hormone their entire lives. Some patients who have had a noncancerous nodule removed will also be advised to take thyroid hormone pills. These may prevent new nodules from forming in the remaining portion of the thyroid gland.

What Is the Thyroid?

The thyroid is a small, butterfly-shaped gland just below the Adam's apple. This gland plays a very important role in controlling the body's metabolism, that is, how the body functions. It does this by producing thyroid hormones, chemicals that travel through the blood to every part of the body. Thyroid hormones tell the body how fast to work and use energy.

Are All Thyroid Lumps Cancerous?

Thyroid lumps (also called nodules) are growths in or on the thyroid gland. They occur in 4%-7% of the population. More than 90% of these lumps are benign (not cancerous) and usually do not need to be removed. However, about 5%-10% of thyroid nodules are malignant (cancerous).

What Is The Thyroid Society for Education and Research?

The Thyroid Society for Education and Research is a national, not-for-profit organization whose mission is to pursue the prevention, treatment, and cure of thyroid disease. To accomplish this mission, The Thyroid Society participates in, and raises funds for, patient and community education programs, professional education, and scientific research. The work of The Thyroid Society is supported by various grants and by individual contributions.

For more information, call or write:

The Thyroid Society
7515 South Main Street, Suite 545
Houston, TX 77030
1-800-THYROID (1-800-849-7643)
(713) 799-9909

Chapter 49

Hyperparathyroidism

Primary hyperparathyroidism is a disorder of the parathyroid glands. Most people with this disorder have one or more enlarged, overactive parathyroid glands that secrete too much parathyroid hormone. In secondary hyperparathyroidism, a problem such as kidney failure makes the body resistant to the action of parathyroid hormone. This fact sheet focuses on primary hyperparathyroidism.

What Are the Parathyroid Glands?

The parathyroid glands are four pea-sized glands located on the thyroid gland in the neck. Occasionally, a person is born with one or more of the parathyroid glands embedded in the thyroid, the thymus, or elsewhere in the chest. In most such cases, however, the glands function normally.

Though their names are similar, the thyroid and parathyroid glands are entirely separate glands, each producing distinct hormones with specific functions. The parathyroid glands secrete parathyroid hormone (PTH), a substance that helps maintain the correct balance of calcium and phosphorous in the body. PTH regulates release of the calcium from bone, absorption of calcium in the intestine, and excretion of calcium in the urine.

When the amount of calcium in the blood falls too low, the parathyroid glands secrete just enough PTH to restore the balance.

NIH Publication No. 95–3425, February 1995.

What Is Hyperparathyroidism?

If the glands secrete too much hormone, as in hyperparathyroidism, the balance is disrupted: blood calcium rises. This condition of excessive calcium in the blood, called hypercalcemia, is what usually signals the doctor that something may be wrong with the parathyroid glands. In 85 percent of people with this disorder, a benign tumor (adenoma) has formed on one of the parathyroid glands, causing it to become overactive. In most other cases, the excess hormone comes from two or more enlarged parathyroid glands, a condition called hyperplasia. Very rarely, hyperparathyroidism is caused by cancer of a parathyroid gland.

This excess PTH triggers the release of too much calcium into the bloodstream. The bones may lose calcium, and too much calcium may be absorbed from food. The levels of calcium may increase in the urine, causing kidney stones. PTH also acts to lower blood phosphorous levels by increasing excretion of phosphorus in the urine.

Why Are Calcium and Phosphorous So Important?

Calcium is essential for good health. It plays an important role in bone and tooth development and in maintaining bone strength. It is also important in nerve transmission and muscle contraction. Phosphorous is found in every body tissue. Combined with calcium, it gives strength and rigidity to your bones and teeth.

What Causes Hyperparathyroidism?

In most cases doctors don't know the cause. The vast majority of cases occur in people with no family history of the disorder. Only about 3 to 5 percent of cases can be linked to an inherited problem. Familial endocrine neoplasia type I is one rare inherited syndrome that affects the parathyroids as well as the pancreas and the pituitary gland. Another rare genetic disorder, familial hypocalciuric hypercalcemia, is sometimes confused with typical hyperparathyroidism.

How Common Is Hyperparathyroidism?

In the U.S., about 100,000 people develop the disorder each year. Women outnumber men by 2 to 1, and risk increases with age. In women 60 years and older, 2 out of 1,000 will get hyperparathyroidism.

What Are the Symptoms of Hyperparathyroidism?

A person with hyperparathyroidism may have severe symptoms, subtle ones, or none at all. Increasingly, routine blood tests that screen for a wide range of conditions including high calcium levels are alerting doctors to people who, though symptom-free, have mild forms of the disorder.

When symptoms do appear, they are often mild and nonspecific, such as a feeling of weakness and fatigue, depression, or aches and pains. With more severe disease, a person may have a loss of appetite, nausea, vomiting, constipation, confusion or impaired thinking and memory, and increased thirst and urination. Patients may have thinning of the bones without symptoms, but with risk of fractures. Increased calcium and phosphorous excretion in the urine may cause kidney stones. Patients with hyperparathyroidism may be more likely to develop peptic ulcers, high blood pressure, and pancreatitis.

How Is Hyperparathyroidism Diagnosed?

Hyperparathyroidism is diagnosed when tests show that blood levels of calcium as well as parathyroid hormone are too high. Other diseases can cause high blood calcium levels, but only in hyperparathyroidism is the elevated calcium the result of too much parathyroid hormone. A blood test that accurately measures the amount of parathyroid hormone has simplified the diagnosis of hyperparathyroidism.

Once the diagnosis is established, other tests may be done to assess complications. Because high PTH levels can cause bones to weaken from calcium loss, a measurement of bone density may be done to assess bone loss and the risk of fractures. Abdominal radiographs may reveal the presence of kidney stones and a 24-hour urine collection may provide information on kidney damage and the risk of stone formation.

How Is Hyperparathyroidism Treated?

Surgery to remove the enlarged gland (or glands) is the only treatment for the disorder and cures it in 95 percent of cases. However, some patients who have mild disease may not need immediate treatment, according to a panel of experts convened by the National Institutes of Health in 1990. Patients who are symptom-free, whose blood calcium is only slightly elevated, and whose kidneys and bones are normal, may wish to talk to their doctor about long-term monitoring.

In the panel's recommendation, monitoring would consist of clinical evaluation and measurement of calcium levels and kidney function every 6 months, annual abdominal x-ray, and bone mass measurement after 1 to 2 years. If the disease shows no signs of worsening after 1 to 3 years, the interval between exams may be lengthened. If the patient and doctor choose long-term follow-up, the patient should try to drink lots of water, get plenty of exercise, and avoid certain diuretics, such as the thiazides. Immobilization and gastrointestinal illness with vomiting or diarrhea can cause calcium levels to rise, and if these conditions develop, patients with hyperparathyroidism should seek medical attention.

Are There Any Complications Associated with Parathyroid Surgery?

Surgery for hyperparathyroidism is highly successful with a low complication rate when performed by surgeons experienced with this condition. About 1 percent of patients undergoing surgery have damage to the nerves controlling the vocal cords, which can affect speech. One to five percent of patients develop chronic low calcium levels, which may require treatment with calcium and/or vitamin D. The complication rate is slightly higher for hyperplasia than it is for adenoma since more extensive surgery is needed.

Are Parathyroid Imaging Tests Needed Before Surgery?

The NIH panel recommended against the use of expensive imaging tests to locate benign tumors before initial surgery. Research shows that such tests do not improve the success rate of surgery, which is about 95 percent when performed by experienced surgeons. Localization tests are useful in patients having a second operation for recurrent or persistent hyperparathyroidism.

Which Doctors Specialize in Treating Hyperparathyroidism?

Endocrinologists (doctors who specialize in hormonal problems), nephrologists (doctors who specialize in kidney and mineral disorders), and surgeons who are experienced in endocrine surgery. A listing of medical specialists and members of the American Association of Endocrine Surgeons, the American Society of Clinical Endocrinologists, and the American Society of Bone and Mineral Research is available at a public library.

Additional Resources

The Paget Foundation
For Paget's Disease of Bone and Related Disorders
200 Varick St., Suite 1004
New York, NY 10014-4810
800-23-PAGET or (212) 229-1502

Further Reading

Bilezikian, John P. *et al. The Parathyroids: Basic and Clinical Concepts*. New York: Raven Press, 1994.

Parisien, May, et al. "Bone Disease in Primary Hyperparathyroidism," *Endocrinology and Metabolism Clinics of North America*. Vol. 19, No. 1, March, 1990.

Potts, John T., Jr. "Management of Asymptomatic Hyperparathyroidism," *Journal of Endocrinology and Metabolism* Vol. 70, No. 6, 1990. 1489–1493.

National Institutes of Health. "Diagnosis and Management of Asymptomatic Primary Hyperparathyroidism: Consensus Development Conference Statement," *Annals of Internal Medicine* Vol. 114, No. 7, April 1, 1991. 593–596. Reprints are also available from:

Office of Medical Applications of Research (OMAR)
Consensus Program Clearinghouse
P.O. Box 2577
Kensington, MD 20891
1-800-NIH-OMAR

Chapter 50

Diagnosis and Management of Asymptomatic Primary Hyperparathyroidism

Abstract

The National Institutes of Health Consensus Development Conference on Diagnosis and Management of Asymptomatic Primary Hyperparathyroidism brought together endocrinologists, surgeons, radiologists, epidemiologists, and primary health care providers as well as the public to address indications for surgery in asymptomatic patients with hyperparathyroidism (HPT) and how patients not operated on should be monitored and managed to minimize the risk of complications of HPT. Following 1½ days of presentations by experts and discussion by the audience, a consensus panel weighed the evidence and prepared their consensus statement.

Among their findings, the panel concluded that (1) a diagnosis of HPT is established by demonstrating persistent hypercalcemia together with an elevated serum parathyroid hormone concentration; (2) current and acceptable treatment for HPT is surgery to cure the condition; (3) the diagnosis of HPT in an asymptomatic patient does not in all cases mandate referral for surgery; conscientious surveillance may be justified in patients whose calcium levels are only mildly elevated and whose renal and bone status are close to normal; and (4) preoperative localization in patients without prior neck operation is rarely indicated and not proven to be cost-effective.

The full text of the consensus panel's statement follows.

Consensus Statement, NIH Consensus Development Conference, October 29-31, 1990, Volume 8, Number 7.

Introduction

Hyperparathyroidism is increasingly being recognized as a result of the detection of hypercalcemia by widespread use of multiphasic screening. Women are affected twice as often as men, and the incidence of hyperparathyroidism increases with age. Approximately 100,000 new cases occur each year in the United States. Because the disease is now known to be more common than previously appreciated, physicians are increasingly interested in the correct diagnosis and proper management of patients with hyperparathyroidism.

The increased recognition of hyperparathyroidism by screening tests has disclosed a population of patients in whom symptoms are subtle or absent. A new clinical profile of hyperparathyroidism that is characterized by mild hypercalcemia has emerged. Presentation with bone disease that is evident on standard radiographs, nephrolithiasis, or other complications is now uncommon, yet it is not clear that incidentally discovered hyperparathyroidism is benign.

Studies of the natural history of hyperparathyroidism are yielding information about how often and over what time course the mild syndrome remains benign. Silent loss of bone mass and changes in skeletal architecture in this asymptomatic population are being assessed with sensitive new techniques. The clinical significance of changes in bone density is uncertain, but it seems likely that progressive parathyroid-dependent bone loss is an additional risk factor for fractures. The potential for mild hyperparathyroidism to cause or accelerate hypertension, renal deterioration, peptic ulcer disease, and psychiatric symptoms also is being evaluated.

Parathyroidectomy is a highly successful treatment when performed by experienced surgeons. As there is evidence that some patients with asymptomatic primary hyperparathyroidism may have a prolonged benign course, it is possible that such patients can be managed without operative intervention. If patients are not operated on, they must be monitored to detect progression of the disease. For these patients, the principal issue is how this can best be accomplished, balancing the need to identify skeletal, renal, or other complications that are indications for operation against the burdens and expense of long-term monitoring.

Evaluation of the long-term consequences of asymptomatic hyperparathyroidism with and without surgical treatment will answer questions about optimal management of this condition. Predictive factors, if they can be discerned, would help to distinguish subpopulations of patients who will develop adverse effects from those who tolerate mild hyperparathyroidism without complications. Identification of such factors would have a significant impact on the justification for operative or nonoperative management.

To address these issues, on October 29-31, 1990, the National Institute of Diabetes and Digestive and Kidney Diseases, together with the Office of Medical Applications of Research of the National Institutes of Health, convened a Consensus Development Conference on Diagnosis and Management of Asymptomatic Primary Hyperparathyroidism. Following a day and a half of presentations by experts in the relevant fields and discussion from the audience, a consensus panel comprising specialists and generalists from the medical and other related scientific disciplines considered the evidence and formulated a consensus statement in response to the following six previously stated questions:

- What is the most accurate, cost-effective method of diagnosing hyperparathyroidism?

- Are there patients with asymptomatic hyperparathyroidism who can safely be followed? Should they be?

- If not operated on, how should asymptomatic patients be monitored and managed?

- What are the indications for surgery in patients with asymptomatic hyperparathyroidism?

- What is the role of gland localization technology in management of patients with hyperparathyroidism?

- What research should be done to clarify issues in diagnosis and management of hyperparathyroidism?

What Is the Most Accurate, Cost-Effective Method of Diagnosing Hyperparathyroidism?

The diagnosis of primary hyperparathyroidism (HPT) can best be established by demonstrating persistent hypercalcemia together with an elevated serum parathyroid hormone (PTH) concentration.

Measurement of total serum calcium concentration is a sensitive and cost-effective method for screening for primary HPT. When an elevated total serum calcium concentration is encountered, the clinician should first confirm this finding under conditions that minimize the likelihood of false positive values. The repeat blood sample should be obtained with minimal venous occlusion and preferably with the patient fasting. Drugs such as thiazide diuretics that can increase serum calcium concentration should be discontinued for several days.

Because small elevations in serum calcium may be clinically significant, clinicians should know the stated normal range for the laboratories used. Total calcium measurements may be misleading in patients with decreased serum albumin, a problem that can be resolved by the use of an ionized serum calcium determination.

Additional pertinent data may be available from multiphasic screening results. Low serum phosphorous, high chloride, low bicarbonate, and high alkaline phosphatase concentrations are consistent with primary HPT but are not diagnostic; urea nitrogen and creatinine help in evaluating renal function.

Immunoassays for intact PTH using double antibody methods represent a major advance in diagnosis. The majority of patients with primary HPT have unequivocal elevations with these assays; the remainder have minimally elevated or high normal values. Patients with hypercalcemia due to other causes such as malignancy and sarcoidosis have low normal or suppressed PTH values. Because only rare instances of true ectopic secretion of PTH by malignant tumors have been reported, this possibility need only be considered in patients with elevated PTH and evidence of malignancy or in whom neck exploration for primary HPT is unsuccessful.

Borderline elevations or high normal values for intact PTH may be found in familial hypocalciuric hypercalcemia (FHH), an uncommon, benign condition in which neck exploration is contraindicated. In this syndrome, hypercalcemia often is detected at an early age and is associated with low urinary calcium excretion. Definitive diagnosis of FHH can be made by measuring serum and urine calcium in family members. Family studies also are important for detecting kindreds with multiple endocrine neoplasia (MEN) and familial HPT.

Are There Patients with Asymptomatic Hyperparathyroidism Who Can Safely Be Followed? Should They Be?

The consensus panel agrees that there may be a subgroup of patients with primary HPT that can be safely followed. All primary HPT patients should be considered candidates for surgery. Some uncomplicated asymptomatic patients, however, may be considered for judicious nonsurgical medical monitoring. To identify those patients who qualify for such management, physicians must have a clear under-standing of "asymptomatic" primary HPT and undertake a rigorous evaluation and selection process to identify candidates who can be followed without surgical therapy.

We use "asymptomatic primary HPT" to describe the clinical pro-file of patients with documented primary HPT without symptoms or signs commonly attributable to the disease. These patients are usu-ally detected incidentally by multiphasic screening. Some patients may have one or several vague symptoms that cannot be definitively attributed to primary HPT but may instead be nonspecific or arise from a coexisting condition. Nevertheless, for purposes of this confer-ence, such patients were considered "asymptomatic." In contrast, patients who present significant bone, renal, gastrointestinal or neu-romuscular symptoms typical of primary HPT are defined as "symp-tomatic" and require surgery.

Our uncertainty regarding the natural history of asymptomatic primary HPT can be likened to the understanding of hypertension or hypercholesterolemia before large-scale epidemiological and clinical studies. There are no clinical signs or absolute laboratory criteria that can be used to identify patients who are likely to develop complica-tions. Decisions regarding surgical or medical management must re-main founded on clinical judgment on a case-by-case basis. The only acceptable treatment for these patients other than surgery is consci-entious long-term medical surveillance.

Indications for Medical Monitoring

To qualify for nonsurgical management, a patient must have a se-rum calcium that is only mildly elevated, no previous episodes of life-threatening hypercalcemia, and normal renal and bone status.

Indications for Surgical Treatment

Conversely, some asymptomatic patients will have objective mani-festations of primary HPT that are indications for surgery:

- Markedly elevated serum calcium
- History of an episode of life-threatening hypercalcemia
- Reduced creatinine clearance
- Presence of kidney stone(s) detected by abdominal radiograph
- Markedly elevated 24-hour urinary calcium excretion
- Substantially reduced bone mass as determined by direct mea-surement

The mean bone density often is below normal in patients with primary HPT. This diminished bone mass is most consistently observed at sites of cortical bone. Sparse long-term data are available regarding bone loss in asymptomatic primary HPT patients. Furthermore, no published data or study presented to the conference had the requisite power, in terms of numbers of patients or duration of followup, to compare fracture rates in patients with asymptomatic primary HPT to normals. Because low bone mass in postmenopausal women is associated with increased risk of fracture, we assumed that this relationship is likely to be valid in patients with primary HPT, although this assumption remains to be established.

The data were not sufficient to justify precise quantitative recommendations for surgery for any of the above listed tests. Nevertheless, panel members felt some examples should be offered as possible guidelines. The values mentioned below are ones that panel members perceived as warranting operation. It is clear, however, that many physicians will recommend for less prominent elevations than we cite below. Examples of values on which there was consensus regarding need for operation include serum calcium elevations 1 to 1.6 mg/dL (0.25 to 0.4 mmol/L) above the accepted normal range, i.e. 11.4 to 12 mg/dL (2.85 to 3.0 mmol/L), given a normal range of 8.8 to 10.4 mg/dL (2.2-2.6 mmol/L); creatinine clearance reduced by 30 percent compared with age-matched normals; confirmed 24-hour urine calcium excretion > 400 mg; and bone mass more than two standard deviations below age-, gender-, and race-matched controls.

In addition, surgery is indicated in those patients in whom medical surveillance is neither desirable nor suitable:

- Patient requests surgery
- Consistent followup is unlikely
- Coexistent illness complicates management
- Patient is young (< 50 years old)

Surgery is recommended for younger patients because the outcome of several decades of primary HPT is not known. In addition, for such patients, long-term compliance may be inadequate to ensure a safe outcome, and the cumulative expense and time invested in rigorous monitoring greatly outweigh the expense and time of an operation. Care should be taken to avoid surgery in FHH; in such patients, surgery is inappropriate.

Despite this outline for management, some patients will decline recommended surgery. They should be followed at least as intensively as uncomplicated asymptomatic patients in the manner described in the next section.

If Not Operated On, How Should Asymptomatic Patients Be Monitored and Managed?

Monitoring Procedures

When it is decided to follow a patient with asymptomatic hyperparathyroidism, that patient must understand that a decision to forgo parathyroid surgery is considered safe only if the patient and the physician remain committed to conscientious long-term monitoring. The goals of such followup include the early recognition of worsening hypercalcemia, the deterioration of bone, renal impairment, or the appearance or growth of renal stones.

The patient should be seen at least semiannually until the lack of progression of the disease has been established. Once stability of the various parameters has been established over 1 to 3 years, the intervals between these various observations can be safely extended. The patient should be specifically queried regarding neuromuscular weakness, depression, and symptoms related to the skeletal, gastrointestinal, and renal systems, and the following determinations are recommended at each visit:

- Blood pressure
- Serum calcium
- Serum creatinine and creatinine clearance

In addition, we recommend the following:

- Abdominal radiographs annually
- 24-hour urinary calcium in selected patients
- Repeat bone mass measurement after 1 to 2 years

The panel suggests that a second determination of bone mass be sought after an interval of time that is adequate to assess whether there has been significant loss of bone. The appropriate interval will depend on the precision of the instrument available. It is acknowledged that there is inadequate information identifying the ideal methodology for monitoring changes in bone mass in patients with asymptomatic HPT. There is some indication that measurement of the forearm bone density with single photon absorptiometry may be useful

435

to monitor changes in bone density. The development of alternative densitometric methodology such as dual energy x-ray absorptiometry may soon become preferable to identify subtle changes in cortical bone. Although a recommendation for a change to surgical therapy can be made solely on the basis of an abnormally low value of bone density, such a decision remains controversial in asymptomatic HPT.

Management During Surveillance

There are certain aspects of management that should be advised for all patients being followed; the patients should avoid dehydration, immobilization, and a diet with restricted or excess calcium. Loop or thiazide diuretics should be used with caution. Because of the risk of a hypercalcemic crisis, patients should be advised to seek immediate medical care with the appearance of a medical illness that may produce dehydration (e.g., vomiting, diarrhea, etc.). There should be adequate treatment of hypertension, even when it is mild.

Many physicians prescribe estrogen therapy for postmenopausal women because of the beneficial actions of estrogens on postmenopausal osteoporosis and cardiovascular risk factors. While there is evidence that estrogen therapy can reduce the action of PTH on bone and lower serum calcium without causing PTH levels to rise, there are limited data on long-term therapy with estrogens in postmenopausal patients with asymptomatic hyperparathyroidism.

Other drugs such as the bisphosphonates, oral phosphate, calcitonin, or mithramycin, which modify the PTH-induced stimulation of bone resorption, are not presently indicated in patients with asymptomatic HPT. However, bisphosphonates or oral phosphate may be considered in the rare patient with symptomatic hyperparathyroidism who is not a surgical candidate because of severe concurrent diseases.

What Are the Indications for Surgery in Patients With Asymptomatic Hyperparathyroidism?

During monitoring of asymptomatic patients, the following developments may warrant consideration for operative intervention:

- Typical parathyroid-related symptoms involving skeletal, renal, or gastrointestinal systems

- Sustained increase in serum calcium of greater than 1.0 to 1.6 mg/dL (0.25-0.4 mmol/L) above the normal range

- Significant decline in renal function

- Nephrolithiasis or worsening calciuria

- Significant decline in bone mass

- Significant neuromuscular or psychologic symptoms without other obvious cause

- The inability or unwillingness of the patient to continue under medical supervision

In addition to the absolute level of serum calcium, clinicians need to take into account the magnitude of the changes over time.

Assessment of renal function should be made by measurement of creatinine clearance. Although the panel could not define precise values, a confirmed decrease of more than 30 percent was considered significant.

The significance of declining bone mass is controversial and a decrease to two standard deviations below the mean for age-, sex-, and race-matched controls was considered sufficient to warrant operation, as already discussed.

The relationship of psychologic symptoms to hyperparathyroidism is uncertain. All investigators have suggested that neuromuscular symptoms are frequent and often reversed by successful parathyroidectomy while other less specific somatic symptoms are rarely improved by operation.

What Is the Role of Gland Localization Technology in Management of Patients With Hyperparathyroidism?

Imaging of the parathyroid glands before an initial neck exploration is not necessary.

In the past 4 years, extensive experience has been acquired in nonoperative methods for localization of abnormal parathyroid glands. Both noninvasive methods (ultrasound, computed tomography, thallium-technetium scanning, magnetic resonance imaging) and invasive methods (arteriography, venous sampling, needle aspiration) are available. Such methods may be useful when a previous operation has failed. However, because of their potential risks, invasive imaging techniques should never be employed before a first neck exploration.

The use of noninvasive imaging procedures before a first operation is controversial. Some surgeons never use these techniques, while others find them helpful in planning the sequence of an operation.

The usefulness of all noninvasive imaging methods is diminished by their unreliability (about 15 percent false positives and only 60 percent true positives). By comparison, operative exploration of the neck by experienced surgeons has a demonstrated success rate of 95 percent. There is no evidence that preoperative imaging can significantly improve surgical therapy by: (1) shortening the time of operation or decreasing its cost, (2) decreasing complications of an operation, or (3) preventing failed operations. The results of imaging studies should seldom, if ever, be used as the basis of selecting patients for operative or nonoperative manage meet.

What Research Should Be Done to Clarify Issues in Diagnosis and Management of Hyperparathyroidism?

Ultimately, the ability to predict outcomes in asymptomatic HPT and decide on operative versus nonoperative management will require a multicenter, randomized, controlled trial of sufficient size and duration to assess the long-term incidence and progression of complications. However, many specific issues were identified during the conference that need to be resolved before such a trial can be designed. In particular, it is important to define the neuromuscular, psychological, cardiovascular, and gastrointestinal effects of primary HPT. The effects of asymptomatic HPT on bone mass and structure are being defined in ongoing studies, but effects on bone strength and susceptibility to fracture also should be addressed.

The case-control method might be a feasible initial approach. Objective analysis could be carried out in patients with HPT before and after surgery and in carefully matched controls undergoing other elective surgical procedures such as thyroidectomy. Epidemiologic studies using existing databases such as the National Health and Nutrition Examination Survey might identify conditions associated with primary HPT, because the majority of subjects identified with hypercalcemia would have HPT. In addition, it may be desirable to organize and collect available data on fracture, change in bone mass and histomorphometry, and other complications from patients currently being followed in specialized centers.

A preliminary clinical trial comparing bone mass outcomes and biochemical measures of bone turnover in postmenopausal women with HPT randomly assigned to estrogen plus surgery versus estrogen alone for a limited time might establish feasibility and provide guidance for the design of a large multicenter trial. Such a trial would permit analysis of the effects of HPT without the confounding effects of estrogen deficiency yet provide access to the patient population with the highest incidence of HPT.

Basic studies are needed on the etiology of hyperparathyroidism and its molecular and cellular pathophysiology. Identification of the gene locus on the long arm of chromosome 11 for the MEN I gene, discovery of reciprocal translocations in parathyroid adenomas involving the parathyroid hormone gene, and evidence for deletions of one or both copies of the MEN I gene in hyperplasia and adenomas (suggesting the MEN I gene is an antioncogene) all provide an exciting opportunity to explore abnormal parathyroid function. Insight into pathogenesis and complications also could be achieved by developing animal models of hyperparathyroidism.

Recent clinical studies using calcitriol and its analogs to treat secondary hyperparathyroidism suggest that parathyroid gland function may be controlled pharmacologically. Development of antagonists of PTH synthesis, secretion, and end organ effect would substantially increase therapeutic options for HPT and influence the design of clinical trials.

Conclusions and Recommendations

- The diagnosis of primary HPT is established by demonstrating persistent hypercalcemia together with an elevated serum parathyroid hormone concentration.

- Current and acceptable treatment following the diagnosis of primary HPT is operative intervention for cure.

- The diagnosis of primary HPT in the asymptomatic patient, however, does not in all cases mandate referral for imminent operative intervention; conscientious surveillance may be justified in patients whose calcium levels are only mildly elevated and whose renal and bone status are close to normal.

- During the long-term medical and nonoperative followup of these patients, a schedule of monitoring has been devised with assessment of specific symptoms, biochemical parameters, and measurement of bone mineral content. Management guidelines are devised to minimize the risk of deterioration of renal, skeletal, or gastrointestinal complications of HPT.

- Changes that may warrant operative intervention during monitoring include rising serum calcium, deterioration of renal function, decline in bone mass, and onset of parathyroid-related symptoms.

- Preoperative localization in patients without prior neck operation is rarely indicated and not proven to be cost-effective.

- A randomized multicenter clinical trial is needed to compare operative versus nonoperative management of asymptomatic HPT. Pilot studies would be useful to define the multi-system effects of HPT. Further basic research is required to understand the pathogenesis and develop pharmacologic therapy for HPT.

Part Six

Other Disorders of Endocrine and Metabolic Functioning

Chapter 51

Alkaptonuria and Ochronosis

Alkaptonuria is a rare disease in which the body does not have enough of an enzyme called homogentisic acid oxidase (HGAO). It is a genetic disease, meaning that it is inherited from a family member. Because normal amounts of the HGAO enzyme are missing, homogentisic acid (HGA) is not used and builds up in the body. Some is eliminated in the urine, and the rest is deposited in body tissues where it is toxic. The result is ochronosis, a blue-black discoloration of connective tissue including bone, cartilage, and skin caused by deposits of ochre-colored pigment.

Patients with alkaptonuria are usually not aware of the disease until about age 40 when symptoms are present. Dark staining of the diapers sometimes can indicate the disease in infants, but usually no symptoms are present until much later in life.

Alkaptonuria and ochronosis affect many body systems, as described below:

- *Skeletal* (bones and cartilage)—The knees, shoulders, and hips are most affected; arthropathy (diseased joints) is common. Deposits of pigment cause cartilage to become brittle and eventually to fragment (break apart).

- *Cardiovascular* (heart and blood vessels)—The aortic and mitral heart valves are most affected. Ochronotic granules can

---

An undated fact sheet produced by the National Heart, Lung, and Blood Institute (NHLBI).

443

cause valves to calcify or harden. Pigment deposits also can lead to the formation of atherosclerotic plaques (hard spots in arteries) containing cholesterol and fat.

- *Genitourinary* (genital and urinary systems and organs)—In men, the prostate is most commonly affected. Pigment deposits can form stones in the prostate.

- *Respiratory* (organs and structures involved in breathing)—Heavy pigment deposits in the cartilage of the larynx (voice box), the trachea (windpipe), and the bronchi (air passages to the lungs) are common.

- *Ocular* (eyes)—Vision is not usually affected, but pigmentation in the white part of the eye is evident in most patients by their early forties.

- *Cutaneous* (skin)—Effects are most noticeable in areas where the body is exposed to the sun and where sweat glands are located. Skin takes on a blue-black speckled discoloration. Sweat can actually stain clothes brown.

- *Other*—The teeth, central nervous system (brain and spinal cord), and endocrine organs (which make hormones) also may be affected.

Arthropathy (joint disease characterized by swelling and enlarged bones) and discoloration of the skin cause the greatest disability.

Usually a physician can diagnose alkaptonuria based on symptoms of joint discomfort and skin discoloration. The diagnosis is confirmed by verifying family history of the disease, examining skin cells, and testing the urine. Urine left standing for several hours will turn brownish black if a patient has alkaptonuria.

Diets low in protein—especially in amino acids, phenylalanine (found in aspartame), and tyrosine—help reduce the levels of HGA, thereby lessening the amount of pigment deposited in body tissues. Symptoms of alkaptonuria (e.g., arthropathy, cardiovascular disease) are treated when possible. Unfortunately, the course of the disease remains unchanged, and no cure is available. However, patients tend to have a normal life span and die of causes comparable to those of the general population.

Resource

For more information, contact:

Information Center
National Heart, Lung and Blood Institute
P.O.Box 30105
Bethesda, MD 20824-0105
(301) 251-1222
(301) 251-1223 Fax

This information was provided as a public service of the National Heart, Lung, and Blood Institute (NHLBI). The NHLBI supports and conducts research related to the causes, prevention, diagnosis, and treatment of heart, vascular, lung, and blood diseases. This information is not meant to substitute for individual medical diagnosis or treatment. Only a physician, with knowledge of the patients current condition and medical history, can provide appropriate advice.

Chapter 52

Galactosemia

Introduction

Galactosemia, a term that denotes the presence of galactose [a milk sugar] in the blood, has been used to name the rare inborn error of galactose metabolism due to a deficiency of the enzyme galactose-1-phosphate uridyl transferase (GALT). [Enzymes assist in the chemical processes of metabolism.] GALT catalyzes the exchange of galactose-1-phosphate (gal-1-p) for the glucose-1-phosphate (glc-1-p) in uridine diphosphate glucose (UDPGlc) to form uridine diphosphate galactose (UDPGal). Accumulation of metabolites [substances created by metabolic processes] of galactose, particularly gal-1-p, resulting from the enzymatic block are presumed to be injurious to cells and responsible for the clinical manifestations. Galactosemia as a clinical entity has been known for decades and although dietary management has been effective in reversing the acute manifestations, the long-term results have not met expectations.

This chapter will briefly touch upon the chronology of galactosemia, the natural history of the disease, the effectiveness of treatment, and the future directions of basic and clinical research that may have the potential of yielding improved clinical outcomes in patients with galactosemia.

Donnell, George N. M.D. "Clinical Aspects and Historical Perspectives of Galactosemia," *Galactosemia: New Frontiers in Research*, National Institute of Child Health and Human Development, NIH Pub. No. 93-3438, February 1993. Bracketed comments have been added to assist the layreader.

Historical Highlights

von Reuss, in a 1908 publication entitled, "Sugar Excretion in Infancy," reported on a breast-fed infant with failure to thrive, hepatosplenomegaly [a condition in which the liver and spleen are enlarged], and galactosuria [galactose in the urine]. Urinary galactose excretion ceased when milk products were removed from the diet. The infant, however, did not survive and at autopsy marked cirrhosis of the liver was found. Because there was suspicion that tea laced with cognac had been given this newborn in the first few days of life the author speculated, based upon a report by Bauer, that the cirrhosis and secondary galactosuria were due to alcohol ingestion. Though confirmation of the diagnosis was not possible at that time, it has generally been accepted that von Reuss was the first to report on a patient with galactosemia.

In 1917, Goeppert observed galactosuria in an infant with hepatomegaly [enlarged liver] and mental retardation. Similar involvement in siblings pointed to a heritable basis for this disorder. The first American publication was that of Mason and Turner, who coined the term "chronic galactemia" to describe a patient with failure to thrive, hepatomegaly, proteinuria, and galactosuria—features of which were reversed by removal of milk from the diet. There followed many clinical reports documenting the natural history of the disease and the clinical response to dietary restriction of galactose.

Clinicians from the outset recognized galactosemia as an inherited disorder, but it remained for Schwarz and coworkers to first suggest the site of the metabolic block, with the demonstration that gal-1-p accumulated in blood cells of patients with galactosemia. His hypothesis was shown to be correct when Isselbacher and his associates demonstrated that activity of transferase [a type of enzyme] was deficient in cells of patients with galactosemia.

The most recent chapter in the continuing saga of galactosemia has been written by Reichardt and Berg, with the successful cloning and characterization of the gene encoding the human GALT enzyme. This important contribution will provide the means of addressing many of the fundamental questions still remaining on the genetics and pathogenesis [disease development] of galactosemia.

Biochemistry

Galactose is a constituent of many foods of animal and plant origin, but the principal dietary source of the sugar is lactose in mammalian milks. Ingested lactose is enzymatically hydrolyzed [broken down in conjunction with water] in the intestine to its constituents, galactose and glucose which, following absorption, provide sources of energy and the means for the synthesis of a number of necessary cellular components. Galactose also can be derived endogenously [developed inside the body] from turnover in the cells of galactose-containing compounds.

Galactose is metabolized in three sequential enzymatic steps. The first entails the phosphorylation of galactose by a specific galactokinase [an enzyme] to form gal-1-p. The second step mediated by GALT results in an exchange of gal-1-p for the glc-1-p moiety [part] of UDPGlc to form UDPGal. In the third step, UDPGal is transformed to UDPGlc by the enzyme UDPGal-4'-epimerase (epimerase). It is in this last step that galactose actually is converted to glucose. The epimerase reaction has important theoretical implications on the dietary management of galactosemia. Galactose is not considered to be an essential nutrient because the synthesis of many galactose-containing compounds can be accomplished endogenously by reversal of the epimerase reaction.

Several accessory metabolic pathways also are known to exist, but their significance in the disposition of galactose still is not clear. One of these, with a bearing on the pathogenesis of galactosemia, involves reduction of free galactose by aldose reductase (AR) [an enzyme] to the sugar alcohol, galactitol. This compound has been implicated in the development of both lenticular [lens] cataract formation and cerebral edema [brain swelling].

Another reaction of particular interest is the reversible pyrophosphorylase [an enzyme] reaction that produces UDPGal from gal-1-p. Gitzelmann and associates have proposed that the persistent elevations found in erythrocyte [blood cell] gal-1-p of treated galactose patients result from this reaction.

Clinical Manifestations

Most untreated patients with the transferase deficiency exhibit significant clinical manifestations early in life, requiring prompt medical intervention.

The affected infant usually appears normal at birth and the signs and symptoms of galactosemia do not develop until a few days after milk feedings have been initiated. The earliest manifestations include feeding difficulties, lethargy, hypotonia [diminished muscle tone], jaundice, hepatomegaly, and increased intracranial pressure, and susceptibility to bacterial infection, particularly to *E. coli* (Table 52.1).

The cause of the increased susceptibility to infection is not known, but has been ascribed to impaired white cell function secondary to the accumulation of galactose metabolites. Lenticular cataracts and delayed physical and mental development become evident as the illness progresses. The mortality rate has been high in untreated neonates [newborns].

Table 52.1. Presenting findings in 43 symptomatic galactosemic patients.

Type	Signs & Symptoms	% Affected
General	Anorexia and weight loss (failure to thrive)	53
	Pallor and/or cyanosis	14
Hepatic	Hepatomegaly	91
	Jaundice	79
	Splenomegaly	14
	Ascites and/or edema	16
Gastrointestinal	Vomiting	40
	Abdominal distention	21
	Diarrhea	7
Ophthalmological	Cataracts	62
Blood	Hemorrhagic phenomenon	7
Central Nervous System	Lethargy	16
	Bulging anterior fontanel	9
Infection	Sepsis	12

Genetic and Clinical Diversity

Involvement of siblings of both sexes born to clinically normal parents suggested an autosomal recessive pattern of inheritance for galactosemia. Oral galactose tolerance tests used to examine family members often did not establish the genotype [genetic makeup] of a particular individual because of overlapping values between the carriers and normal individuals. Enzymatic methods now in use can with accuracy both confirm the diagnosis of galactosemia and identify the heterozygous [possessing different copies of the affected gene] individual.

It has become apparent, over time, that clinical expression of the disease is quite variable. Although galactosemia often presents as a fulminant [appearing suddenly] life-threatening disorder in the very young, there are individuals in whom the clinical picture is less severe and the diagnosis may not be recognized for weeks or even months. In milder cases, signs and symptoms have included vague digestive difficulties, retarded physical and mental development, hepatic enlargement, cataracts, and perhaps intolerance to milk. In these individuals, accompanying mellituria [sugar in the urine] and proteinuria [excess protein in the urine] should include galactosemia in the differential diagnosis. The urinary findings, however, are dependent upon ingestion of galactose and may be absent if milk products have been withheld for even a few days. It also is known that outcome cannot be predicted on the basis of the severity of the presenting symptoms or the degree of compliancy to treatment.

How much of the differences in clinical expression is due to individual variability and how much to genetic heterogeneity is not known. Genetic biochemical diversity in galactosemia is more common than had originally been anticipated. Ng and colleagues have stated that about 15 percent of the patients identified through newborn screening appear to be variants of galactosemia based upon quantitative measurements of red cell enzyme activity and/or patterns of transferase migration on gel electrophoresis [a type of test that examines the movement of particles, conducted in a gel medium, such as agar]. Ng defined classical galactosemia as a condition in which no erythrocyte enzyme activity could be demonstrated by methods employed in his laboratory, while variants exhibited some degree of enzyme activity ranging from 0.05 percent to 10 percent of the normal values. Ng intentionally excluded from his calculations the commonly encountered Duarte/galactosemia compound heterozygotes in this report; otherwise, the incidence of variants would have been even higher.

Patients with small amounts of enzyme activity (variants) appear to follow milder clinical courses than patients with no demonstrable activity. By way of examples are individuals of Afro-American descent reported by Segal to have the capacity to oxidize galactose *in vivo* [in the body] and the variant patients reported by Kaufman who appear to be less likely to develop ovarian insufficiency.

More data on galactosemia genotypes and their corresponding phenotypes [kinds distinguished by their characteristics] would be helpful in sorting out the extent of the contribution of clinical variability and genetic diversity to the clinical picture. It also has been assumed that the clinical manifestations of galactosemia are due to accumulation and/or deficiency of metabolites secondary to the enzymatic block. It is also possible that the gene defect has a more direct role in the expression of the disease.

Diagnosis

The signs and symptoms associated with transferase deficiency are not exclusive to galactosemia and should serve only to raise the suspicion of the diagnosis.

Galactosuria is not a confirmatory test. Measurable amounts of galactose can be found in urine of normal newborns and of sick infants. Loading an infant or child with galactose (galactose tolerance test) originally was employed to establish the diagnosis of galactosemia, but it has been replaced by enzymatic methods (Beutler test) that are more specific and less hazardous to the patient. Erythrocytes of affected individuals exhibit little or no enzyme activity, but it must be recognized that improper handling of samples may result in some loss of transferase activity and thus lead to false diagnoses. Conversely, patients with galactosemia who have received recent blood transfusions can be missed because they will have falsely high enzyme values reflecting the enzyme activity of the donor cells. A presumptive diagnosis in a patient suspected to have galactosemia under these circumstances can be made by the finding of elevated erythrocyte gal-1-p values in the patient's blood and by demonstrating that both parents have GALT values consistent with the carrier state.

However, the finding of half-normal erythrocyte GALT activity is not always indicative of the heterozygous state for galactosemia because there are other low activity GALT variants. As an example, the Duarte variant homozygote exhibits about one-half of the normal red cell activity, a value similar to that for the galactosemia heterozygote. The frequency of occurrence of the Duarte variant/normal heterozygote is high among Caucasians (about 12 percent). Lower incidences are reported for blacks and Asians. Fortunately, the Duarte variant GALT can be distinguished by its faster mobility than normal GALT on gel electrophoresis.

Pathogenesis

A direct toxic effect of galactose or its metabolites on tissues has been the most widely accepted explanation for the clinical manifestations in galactosemia. There is considerable evidence that gal-1-p

452

plays a principal role in the pathogenesis of galactosemia. *In vitro* [in a laboratory test situation] studies have shown that high concentrations of gal-1-p inhibit cellular enzymes such as phosphoglucomutase, glucose-6phosphatase, and UDPGlc pyrophosphorylase.

Galactose and its metabolites accumulate in affected fetuses. Analysis of tissues from a 20-week-old affected fetus obtained after elective termination of pregnancy revealed unusually high values of galactose, gal-1 -p and galactitol. Lenticular cataracts presumably due to accumulation of galactose metabolite were found at postmortem examination of this particular fetus. Infants have been delivered with mild or even severe manifestations of galactosemia, suggesting onset of the disease process *in utero*.

Additional evidence of abnormal utilization of galactose by the fetus is provided by cord blood gal-1-p measurements. The gal-1-p values have been elevated in all affected newborns tested despite varying degrees of maternal galactose restriction during pregnancy. The values of gal-1-p in cord blood, however, are considerably lower than the gal-1-p levels in red blood cells of affected neonates who have been on milk feedings for a few days, indicating a lower degree of metabolite exposure prenatally than postnatally (six- to ten-fold or less). Galactitol, another metabolite of galactose presumably cleared by the fetal kidney, has been found to be elevated in amniotic fluid of affected pregnancies. As with gal-1-p, galactitol concentrations in amniotic fluid do not change substantially when maternal ingestion of galactose is restricted during pregnancy.

The observations that galactose and its metabolites accumulate in affected fetuses during gestation provide an attractive hypothesis to explain the variable outcome of treated galactosemic children. To investigate the assumption that the intrauterine environment is damaging to galactosemic fetuses, the group in Los Angeles compared galactosemic sib pairs—one of which was treated from birth. It was hypothesized that if the intrauterine environment was not damaging, the younger children who ostensively had not been exposed to galactose postnatally would have better test results than their older sibs. On the other hand, the test results among the sibs would not be dissimilar if the intrauterine environment was equally detrimental to galactosemic fetuses.

The retrospective study involved 13 sib pairs. The index cases were diagnosed after birth (average of 2.1 months) while the younger sibs with one exception were started on treatment from birth. The mean IQ scores were higher for the patients (101 *vs* 96) who were treated at a younger age, but the difference was not statistically significant.

In all but two of the sib pairs, the earlier-treated sibling had a higher IQ score. The younger siblings also had a lower percentage of abnormal visual-perceptual tests and of abnormal EEGs, although neither difference was found to be statistically significant. These findings suggest that postnatal exposure to galactose is the important factor.

Unfortunately, the study does not provide conclusive answers, due in great part to the small sample size and also to the methodologies used in estimating differences in outcome. The younger children as a group outperformed their sibs in all of the areas tested, but not sufficiently so to be of statistical significance. This finding, and the knowledge that early treatment is not synonymous with good results, continue to support the hypothesis that both prenatal and postnatal factors exert an influence on clinical outcome. More clinical data in siblings would be useful in determining the influence of the intrauterine environment on galactosemic fetuses. Relevant factors such as the quality of postnatal treatment, the ability of the fetus to metabolize galactose, the concentrations achieved of the presumably toxic compounds, the degrees of sensitivity of developing fetal tissues to galactose metabolites, and possibly others also must be considered.

Treatment

Laboratory test results may be slow in reaching the clinician, and treatment of patients suspected of galactosemia should not await confirmation of the diagnosis. Restriction of galactose to avoid the accumulation of toxic metabolites has been the mainstay of therapy. Because the major source of this sugar is the disaccharide lactose, milk and its products must be withheld from the infant's diet. In addition, antibiotics and supportive measures may be required, as indicated by the patient's clinical status.

Proprietary milk substitutes essentially free of lactose have been available for many years. Casein hydrolysates [milk protein] with the lactose removed have been used routinely to treat patients with galactosemia in the United States, despite the knowledge that a small amount of lactose was present.

The hydrolysates have been effective in reversing the acute clinical manifestations in neonates, but it is not known whether using preparations containing small amounts of galactose have an adverse effect on outcome. Casein hydrolysates have for the most part been supplanted by lactose-free soy bean preparations. The latter are readily available, easy to use, and less costly. Soy bean formulas, however, do contain varying amounts of galactose as complex sugars, and

454

their suitability as a food for galactosemia has been questioned. Soy bean is now considered by many, but not all, clinicians to be an acceptable food for galactosemia, based upon reports indicating that alpha-linked galactose-containing oligosaccharides are not digested to any extent by the human intestine.

As the children mature, careful scrutiny of labels, review of published lists of acceptable foods, and contacting the product source should be undertaken to ensure that unrecognized sources of galactose are not ingested by patients.

A strict adherence to a galactose-restricted diet has been generally accepted as the treatment regimen of choice for infants with galactosemia, but opinion has been divided as to the necessity of rigid control of galactose intake in the older child. The question of how long the dietary restriction should be maintained also has not been answered. In the past, many centers have had the tendency to ignore intake of small amounts of galactose in school-aged children and adults for reasons of compliance and because a galactose-free diet is difficult to achieve. Although it has not been recommended that this diet be discontinued at a particular age, this has occurred in many patients by their own decision. There have been no reports of significant deterioration in health status of these patients.

It had been speculated that in time children would adapt to galactose intake through development of alternative pathways of galactose metabolism. It also has been the impression that adults with galactosemia tolerate a regular diet better than children. The UDPGal pyrophosphorylase reaction, the oxidative path of galactose to xylulose [a sugar compound], and the formation of galactonic acid and galactitol have been proposed as potential routes of disposal of galactose in the absence of the transferase enzyme. It appears, however, that these alternative pathways, either alone or in combination, have not been equal to the task of handling substantial amounts of galactose.

The apparent improved tolerance to galactose in the adult can be ascribed to the smaller intake of galactose relative to his/her body size and metabolic capabilities as compared to the infant and child, rather than to an adaptive process. About 40 percent of the caloric intake in the newborn comes from lactose as compared to only 3-4 percent in the adult on liberal milk intake. The pattern of disposal of large loads of galactose was evaluated in one patient, at different ages, to determine if there was improvement in the patient with increasing age. No change was found over time to indicate improved tolerance for galactose.

Counseling of families is necessary for proper patient care in galactosemia. Parents should be fully informed about the clinical aspects of the disease, its mode of inheritance, treatment that is available, and prognosis. Prenatal diagnosis is feasible in galactosemia, providing pregnancy options to families at risk and a means of determining the need for maternal restriction of galactose intake during pregnancy.

Monitoring the Diet

Management of galactosemia, as with other disorders requiring controlled diets, must include attention to compliance and to methods for the evaluation of the response to treatment. Assessment of clinical progress, nutritional status, dietary history, and periodic measurements of erythrocyte gal-1-p have been methods employed to document a patient's response to treatment. Measurement of erythrocyte gal-1-p as an objective measure of galactose intake has a number of shortcomings. The test is dependent upon the elevation of erythrocyte gal-1-p values persisting between the ingestion of galactose and when the blood for testing is collected. Gal-1-p values tend to fall rapidly after ingestion of galactose, and intake of this sugar will not be reflected in gal-1-p values unless the deviations from the prescribed diet are both large and repetitive.

It has been shown that children on treatment irrespective of the degree of compliance have at all times measurable amounts of gal-1-p in their erythrocytes. Each patient tends to maintain his/her own pattern of erythrocyte gal-1-p levels. Undoubtedly, ingestion of galactose both suspected and unsuspected is one explanation. However, it appears that even under rigid control of galactose intake, measurable amounts of gal-1-p can still be found in erythrocytes of all patients. The source of the gal-1-p in the absence of galactose intake is not dear. Proposed mechanisms for the accumulation of this metabolite have included endogenous turnover of galactose-containing compounds and action of pyrophosphorylase on UDPGal to yield gal-1-p.

Diet Devoid of Galactose

Galactose is not an essential nutrient, since the donor molecule (UDPGal) required for the biosynthesis of galactose-containing compounds can be derived from UDPGal through reversal of the epimerase reaction. The diets prescribed (usually under supervision of a nutritionist) have been considered nutritionally adequate. No harmful effects of a restricted diet have been described in patients on treatment.

Results of Treatment

By now there has been more than four decades of experience with the dietary management of transferase-deficiency galactosemia. There have been only a few published reports of results in the treatment of galactosemia of a sufficient magnitude to be meaningful. The immediate effects of dietary restriction of galactose usually are dramatic. There is rapid improvement with reversal of the acute manifestations within a few days after initiation of therapy. Over the long term, however, results have been less gratifying.

Treated patients in general have had good health and normal physical development. A slow pattern of growth has been reported in some patients, but the ultimate heights reached in adults have been satisfactory. The marked susceptibility to gram negative infections encountered in untreated newborns with galactosemia does not persist into later life. The response of older patients to infection is similar to that of their unaffected siblings.

One important aspect of the prognosis in galactosemia is the intellectual progress of treated patients. Patients with galactosemia as a group have had intelligence quotient scores in the low end of the normal range. The spread of scores among individuals is wide and the distribution of intelligence quotient scores of treated galactosemics tends to be skewed toward the lower end of the scale.

Manis recently studied a group of patients from Los Angeles utilizing a more sophisticated battery of tests (Woodcock-Johnson). These tests are newer and more comprehensive in their scope than traditional instruments that have been employed in the past. More than 30 patients (age ranges 4 to 38 years) have been so tested. Results of his studies have reaffirmed and extended the earlier findings. The overall scores for all ages fell between the 3rd and 7th percentile of normal. The scores of cognitive functioning were lowest in the areas of expressive vocabulary, visual-motor integration, writing, and mathematical achievement.

In general, school performance for children with galactosemia has been variable. Some have needed placement in special classes and/or have required personal tutoring. Visual-perceptual problems are a common finding and undoubtedly have contributed to their learning difficulties. Earlier recognition and active treatment of the visual-perceptive problems have helped to improve school performance to some degree.

It has been assumed that patients started on treatment earlier in life would have improved outcomes, but this has not invariably been the case. Some children diagnosed late have done as well as, if not better than, others treated much earlier in life. Furthermore, there appears to be no relationship between the age at which treatment is started and outcome. If there were advantages to the early institution of galactose restriction, the patients identified through newborn screening should have improved prognoses. The hope that newborn screening would result in specific treatment prior to development of symptoms has not been realized. A recent international survey has reported that a majority of newborns identified through screening had developed signs and symptoms of galactosemia by the time treatment was begun. The median age at which treatment was started in the screened group was 9 days as compared to a median age of 1 day for patients suspected on the basis of a positive family history. The turn-around time between sampling of the patient and the reporting of results to the clinician was sufficiently long to allow for the development of the clinical picture. Shortening of turn-around times remains an important challenge for screening centers.

This type of information has provoked debate regarding the value of newborn screening for galactosemia. Detractors argue that the low frequency of the disorder, the questionable benefits of early treatment,

Table 52.2. Intellectual status of parents and unaffected siblings of galactosemic patients.

Subjects	Number	IQ Range	Mean
Fathers	33	87-138	110 ± 12.7
Mothers	33	70-127	106 ± 14.2
Normal Siblings			
Brothers	5	92-114	103 ± 8.9
Sisters	9	82-116	101 ± 12.5
Heterozygote Siblings			
Brothers	13	91-123	105 ± 11.3
Sisters	13	86-125	105 ± 11.1
Homozygote Patients	59	50-125	95 ± 16.0

and the fact that sequelae of the disorder are not prevented do not justify the costs of universal screening. The supporters counter that lives are saved and that the financial and psychological burden of families is markedly lessened. Furthermore, they add that the methods now in use are specific, easily implemented, and low in cost if incorporated into existing programs.

Most children with galactosemia manifest psychological problems. The younger patients tend to be shy, sensitive, and sometimes withdrawn. In later life, this is often reflected in dependency upon the family. In a study of a group of galactosemia subjects with ages ranging from 18-35 years, Fishler stated that of those not attending school, about one-half were gainfully employed and of these only a few had white collar positions. It is not possible on the basis of the information at hand to implicate any single factor as being of particular importance in the social adaptation of children with galactosemia. The variables such as parental attitudes, the burden of dietary restriction, and the effects of being a subject in continuing studies all need to be considered.

The neuropsychological problems are not the only long-term clinical manifestations of concern. Other bothersome sequelae are commonly encountered in patients with galactosemia. More than one-half of the children have had speech difficulties. It has been reported that no correlation was found for speech defects with age at diagnosis, severity of symptoms, or degree of biochemical control.

Minor neurologic abnormalities such as tremors with onset in early childhood have been described with some frequency, but only a few patients have had more severe neurological defects including ataxia [uncoordinated muscular movement], seizures, dysarthria [difficulty with muscular movement resulting in diminished ability to articulate words], diminished IQ and difficulties with visual spacial discrimination. Some of these patients have been on treatment since birth, suggesting that the neurologic findings were not related to the time when treatment was started or to the degree of gal-1-p elevation in infancy.

Based on the few reports of successful childbearing of normal offspring in galactosemic women, it had been assumed that fertility was not adversely affected by their inborn error of metabolism. Kaufman et al.'s report of a high frequency of ovarian failure in galactosemic patients came as a surprise. The ovarian damage in her patient was manifested clinically by partial or complete failure of secondary sexual development and primary amenorrhea, by post-pubertal occurrence of oligomenorrhea, or by secondary amenorrhea.

The hypergonadotropic hypogonadism [diminished sexual development] in females with galactosemia, as with the other complications of galactosemia, could not be correlated with time of diagnosis, severity of presenting symptoms, or dietary compliance. Interestingly, males do not appear to be at risk for reproductive complications.

While postnatal management of galactosemia has received much attention, there is still no uniform opinion regarding the long-term benefits of dietary treatment.

It has been said without supporting evidence that the earlier the treatment is started, the better are the results. It is certain that lack of treatment is detrimental to the patient, but evidence that treatment beginning in the first weeks of life has special benefits is only circumstantial. We have attempted to answer the question by reviewing the outcome in 75 patients under our care. For this study, patients have been divided into three groups according to the age at which treatment was begun: before 2 weeks, between 2 weeks and 3 months, and after 3 months of age. An anticipated lower mean IQ in those patients started on treatment later in infancy was not evident. Although the mean DQ/IQ score of the later-treatment group was lower than that of the earlier groups, the differences were not significant. Interestingly, females in each of the treatment categories had lower mean scores than males. This difference between sexes (97 *vs* 77) was greatest in the group of patients begun on treatment after 3 months of age. However, these differences were not statistically significant, perhaps due to the small number of subjects. In addition, information was not available to evaluate other contributing factors with a bearing on outcome such as family intelligence, adequacy of dietary compliance, and the extent of intrauterine exposure to galactose. Consequently, more information is required before it can be said that there is a gender difference in intellectual outcome among treated galactosemia patients. Collection of sufficient data on treated patients necessary for analysis would be possible only through collaborative efforts among a number of centers. Until more is known, it would be prudent to begin treatment as soon as the diagnosis is suspected and to maintain dietary restriction of lactose for as long as possible.

The Future

This overview notes that our expectations with the dietary management of galactosemia have not been achieved. Despite the knowledge of the enzymatic defect for many years and recognition that treatment by dietary restriction of substrate [the substance that acts on an enzyme] can quickly reverse the acute manifestations in the affected infants, it has become apparent that treatment does not prevent handicapping sequelae. Patients have been plagued with cognitive defects, speech abnormalities, and some neurological problems even when those patients were considered to be under good dietary control. In addition, females are at significant risk of ovarian failure. A potential explanation for these complications is that virtually all patients under treatment have persistent elevations of erythrocyte gal-1-p. That is probably unrelated to adherence to the prescribed diet, as suggested by the small elevations of gal-1-p in those patients who totally exclude galactose from the diet. One possible explanation for the persistence of gal-1-p is self-intoxication due to endogenous production of gal-1-p by epimerase and pyrophosphorylase. It is not known whether these small elevations of gal-1-p found in red blood cells of the treated patient are reflected in tissues and whether cell function is affected at these levels. Variants of galactosemia generally fare better clinically than patients with classical galactosemia even though they also exhibit elevations in erythrocyte gal-1-p (though lower than in patients with complete GALT deficiency), suggesting that gal-1-p alone may not be responsible for all of the long-term sequelae.

In this context, several additional questions seem relevant. Does gal-1-p play a role primarily in the acute neonatal stages of galactosemia when it is at its highest level, or does the persistence of gal-1-p even at the relatively low levels found in all patients also affect outcome? Skepticism about gal-1-p as the sole toxic agent has led to examination of both sides of the transferase reaction for an explanation of the pathogenesis of galactosemia. Recently, there have been reports of decreased UDPGal in tissues of patients with galactosemia. UDPGal, the product of the transferase reaction, is central to the synthesis of many galactose-containing compounds in the body; disruption of these synthetic processes with its consequent effects at the cellular level could explain the development of the central nervous system and ovarian complications in galactosemia. For instance, Haberland et al. found both qualitative and quantitative changes in the galactose-containing compounds in brain tissue of a galactosemic adult, a finding consistent with a deficiency of UDPGal.

Uridine has been shown in both *in vitro* and *in vivo* studies to increase the concentration of UDPGal and is currently being evaluated as an adjunct to dietary therapy in galactosemia. However, there is need to be cautious in the use of uridine in galactosemia. Segal has found that uridine inhibits transferase activity in suckling rat liver preparations with accompanying increase in gal-1-p value. Further-more, the levels of uridine-producing inhibition of enzyme activity under his experimental conditions are higher than those achieved in erythrocytes of galactosemic individuals treated with uridine. Galac-tosemic subjects in the uridine study have exhibited no increases in red blood cell gal-1-p while receiving uridine for more than 1 year. Other therapeutic approaches have been suggested by the work of Segal and Rogers, who showed that normal transferase was increased in rats during the newborn period by pharmacologic agents and cer-tain hormones. Based upon these models, he has suggested trials of progesterone and folate in patients with galactosemia to determine whether these metabolites might be beneficial.

As with clinical outcome, evaluation of the effectiveness of any new therapeutic approaches will be difficult in any given center because of the limited number of patients available. Large collaborative stud-ies will be required. In such studies, in view of the extent of clinical variability, attention will need to be given to collection of data on ga-lactosemia genotypes and then corresponding phenotypes. Attention must also be given to the time when the new pharmacological agent should be started for optimal effectiveness. It is likely that older pa-tients will benefit less from alternative approaches, since the patho-logic process may have already progressed too far. Use of any agent in the pregnant woman to provide treatment to the affected fetus will require consideration of safety to both mother and fetus. Specifically, possible teratogenicity [tendency to cause birth defects] of uridine would have to be determined.

No criteria have been established for discontinuation of the dietary restriction of galactose in galactosemia. Recommending a regular diet and monitoring for harmful clinical effects cannot be justified. It is wise to continue dietary control of galactose in affected patients un-til a basis for discontinuation has been determined.

Consideration should be given to cooperative and collaborative ef-forts among centers to increase cohort size. This will greatly increase the knowledge of the natural history of the disease and of evaluating the effectiveness of dietary and other forms of treatment. The PKU collaborative projects past and present are good models for the inter-ested parties to emulate.

Chapter 53

Glycogen Storage Diseases

The Biochemistry of Glycogen Storage Disease

The underlying problem in all the glycogen storage diseases is the use and storage of glycogen. Glycogen is a complex material composed wholly of glucose molecules linked together. This is how the human body stores glucose.

As humans, one of the important sources of energy that we consume is glucose—the basic sugar (see Figure 53.1). The glucose molecule is the fundamental transport form of energy in the blood stream. The body usually maintains a level of glucose in the blood within narrow concentrations: 60-100 units (milligrams per 100 milliliters). To do this the body must be able to perform some rather complex biochemical reactions. The necessity of the biochemical maneuvers is created by the fact that we consume food periodically, in irregular compositions and we use energy in an equally irregular manner.

After we consume large amounts of glucose, the excessive glucose is stored in the liver as glycogen. Glycogen is simply a large molecule made of many glucose molecules linked together in a chain like fashion with many branches off the long chains (see Figure 53.2). I like to think of glycogen as a tree. The branches are very important because

Excerpted from *Glycogen Storage Diseases: A Patient-Parent Handbook*, Department of Pediatrics, University of Texas Health Science Center ©1989; reprinted with permission. [This document provides basic information about glycogen storage diseases and important medical definitions. For up-to-date, individual treatment options, the patient's physician should be consulted.]

these make the glycogen much more soluble in the body. (Plants store glucose as starch; starch is very much like glycogen except it lacks the branch points; most of you know how difficult it is to get starch into solution!).

The glycogen thus stored serves as a reservoir for the glucose when the body's blood sugar drops below normal, or when the muscle exercises vigorously and needs more instantaneous energy. Through hormones in the body signals are sent to the liver that the stored glycogen is needed for glucose. When the glycogen is broken down, it is released as glucose into the blood. In some of the glycogen storage diseases (but not all) maintaining the blood glucose levels is a very central and major problem.

Let's look at some of these regulatory mechanisms. We get glucose in our diet in many ways; common table sugar, sucrose (a disaccharide, two sugar molecules hooked together) is broken down in the intestine to one molecule of glucose and one of fructose (a similar sugar).

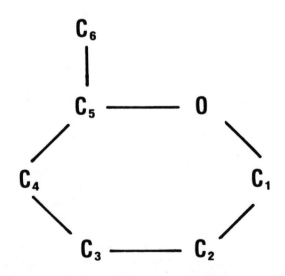

Figure 53.1. *Glucose molecule. C = carbon atom; O = oxygen.*

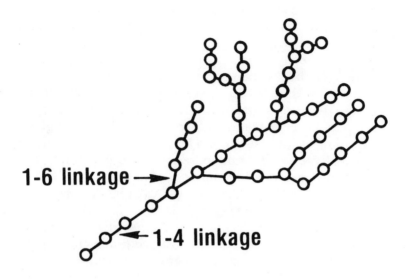

Figure 53.2. *A glycogen molecule is made of many glucose molecules linked together.*

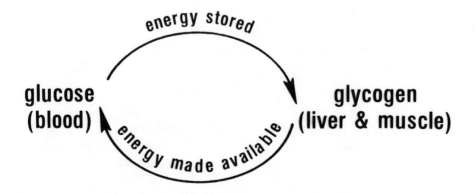

Figure 53.3. *Key chemical reactions in the formation of glycogen from dietary glucose.*

Starches in our diet are broken down by enzymes to glucose; these sugars are taken into the body by the intestine into the large vein from the intestines which is called the portal vein. This large vein goes directly to the liver where the sugars are largely handled; they are either sent to the body tissues (if needed) or stored if hormonal signals tell the liver that is the proper disposition.

When the body is in the fed state insulin, a hormone, is released from the pancreas (an organ near the stomach). Insulin enters the blood stream and exerts its effects by reducing high blood glucose levels. Insulin induces glucose uptake by tissues and glycogen accumulation in the liver (in normal persons insulin cannot cause the accumulation of "excessive" amounts of glycogen as the body's regulatory systems see to that). The accumulation by the liver consists of actual putting together of glycogen molecules. Figure 53.3 illustrates the key chemical reactions in the formation of glycogen from dietary glucose. Glucose is first converted to glucose-6-phosphate (G6P); the 6 refers to the position on the glucose molecule to which the phosphorus (P) is attached. The next step in the sequence is the movement of the phosphorus to the 1 position; although they sound similar there is a world of difference to the body between the 1 and 6 position in glucose; once a molecule of glucose is converted to G1P it can begin the intimate process of building the glycogen molecule. Uridine diphosphoglucose (UDP glucose) is produced from G1P by the addition of a uridine diphosphate molecule.

At this point we will deviate from Figure 53.3 to discuss a topic central to understanding all the glycogen storage diseases. The reactions glucose→G6P→G1P→UDPG require enzymes. Enzymes are protein molecules which expedite chemical reactions to occur in the body without undergoing any change themselves. Without enzymes reactions proceed so slowly that major roadblocks occur. They are usually are written above a chemical reaction thus:

$$\text{enzyme}$$
$$A \rightarrow B \rightarrow C \rightarrow D$$

The enzyme itself is unchanged by the reaction.

Back to Figure 53.3; once we have UDP glucose we can, with the help of the enzyme glycogen synthetase, link the glucose molecules together in a chain-like fashion. As the chains are elongated, an important enzyme enters the picture; about every 8 to 10 links, the brancher enzyme enters the picture and produces a branch point. This branch point is between the 1-6 linkages of glucose molecules.

466

When a person is fasting glycogen is broken down or modified. The long straight portions of glycogen (the 1,4 linkages) are broken by phosphorylase in its active form and yields glucose-1-phosphate which is further utilized. When phosphorylase breaks down glycogen and nears a branch point (a 1,6 linkage) a special enzyme is needed to break this branch, i.e., debranching enzyme. Debranching enzyme releases free glucose. After the debrancher has worked, phosphory-lase (active) can again break down the linear portions of glycogen. If there is no debrancher enzyme, glycogen accumulates short outer branches, limit dextin (like a tree with its branches clipped short).

Important Terms

It is well known that medicine has a language of its own. To understand much of what is written and discussed about your child you will need to know a few basic terms.

Heredity, Chromosomes, and Genes

A very important concept is **heredity.** All of the glycogen storage diseases are inherited, that is they are genetically determined. They do not result from any actions of the parents, but they are encoded in the parents genes. They are passed on to children as a part of their make up.

Every human being has 46 **chromosomes**, consisting of 23 pairs. They reside in the center (the nucleus) of the cell. Half of these chromosomes come from the mother and half from the father. The germ cells, that is the sperm cell and the egg cell, have only ½ of each persons chromosomes, one member of each of the 23 pairs. The chromosomes are rather "big," in that they can be seen under the light microscope with special stains.

Located on the chromosomes are the **genes**. The genes are very small and cannot be seen with the microscope. Man has about 1,000,000 genes arranged on these 23 chromosomes. The gene is the basic biological information unit in which characteristics are passed on to a child such as hair color, eye color, ultimate height potential, and importantly the codes for all the enzyme proteins in the body, including those involved in glycogen synthesis and degradation. One of the 23 pairs of the chromosomes is a special pair, the sex chromosomes; these 2 chromosomes (one pair) carry all the genes which determine whether the child is male or female.

As mentioned, the germ cells each have one member of each chromosome pair. The distribution of the chromosomes, when chromosomes

467

divide, is random. This segregation is necessary to form the germ cells. When the sperm and the egg unite at conception, the maternal chromosomes join with the paternal chromosomes and a typical human cell with 23 pairs, or 46 chromosomes is formed. A remarkable feature of human biology is that each enzyme, except those that are located on the sex chromosomes which are not "matched," are duplicated; that is, there is a spare copy for every enzyme protein. If there is a defective gene on one chromosome, the partner on the other chromosome makes the protein. Although the protein may be in reduced amounts, it is usually more than adequate. Such a situation would be a carrier or **heterozygote**. Each of us is a carrier or heterozygote for at least 6 or 7 serious defects, but we never usually know this unless we by unlikely chance mate with someone who is deficient in exactly the same gene. In this situation an offspring can be produced who is deficient in both genes on both chromosomes and can make no active enzyme.

All but one of the glycogen storage diseases are transmitted from generation to generation in an **autosomal recessive** fashion. Autosomal is the name given to all the chromosomes except the sex chromosomes. Recessive means that both members of a chromosomal pair must carry the gene for the disease to be manifest, as in the manner which is discussed above.

There is no area of medicine that is moving as rapidly as molecular genetics. Although genes are very small, and cannot be seen, impressive new techniques have developed that permit the isolation and characterization of human genes; these human genes can be isolated in the laboratory and copied many times (cloned). As the genes are isolated, they can be studied in the greatest detail and the defects outlined at the molecular level. These techniques will have a very dramatic effect on the diagnosis of the glycogen storage diseases in the next few years; it is also reasonable to hope that there will be important discoveries that will lead to better and more specific treatment. Some treatments might come from new abilities to activate genes that are present but not turned on. Much work is focussed on the insertion of new genetic information when needed within the cell; this will come in time but presents formidable problems to be solved.

Amniocentesis and Chorionic Villus Sampling

The next topic is **amniocentesis**. Amniocentesis is the penetration of the pregnant female womb via the abdomen by a needle to draw out fluid (amniotic fluid) in which the fetus is suspended. This fluid contains some cells washed off the fetus, and can be grown in the laboratory and examined to detect disease states in the unborn. Glycogen storage disease due to alpha-1,4-glucosidase deficiency, debrancher deficiency (not always), brancher deficiency and phosphorylase b kinase deficiency can be detected in this fashion. Glycogen storage disease due to glucose-6-phosphatase deficiency can not be detected in this fashion.

Amniocentesis is usually performed between the 14th and 16th weeks of pregnancy. It takes several weeks to a month for the laboratory to complete the tests. The danger to the fetus is very low, and the accuracy of the test approaches 100% but of course is not perfect.

Your physician can advise you on whether amniocentesis can be performed if you would find this technique suitable for your needs and wishes. It is safe and can be done on an outpatient basis.

Chorionic villus sampling, a technique where a small amount of the chorionic villus (tissues surrounding the fetus) is biopsied, is an additional method of prenatal diagnosis. The advantage is that the test can be done earlier, and the results are ordinarily available sooner. The same glycogen storage diseases can be diagnosed by both techniques; neither will diagnose glucose-6-phosphatase deficiency.

Biopsies

The last topic of general interest in the term **biopsy**. A biopsy is the removal of a small piece of body tissue for laboratory examination. A punch biopsy can be done (needle sized) from both liver and muscle, and is adequate if one is reasonably sure of the diagnosis.

An open biopsy of both liver and muscle is preferred, for then extensive studies can be done; light and electron microscopic studies can be done, as well as extensive biochemical studies. The risk for surgical liver and/or muscle biopsies under proper circumstances is very modest indeed. The removal of the tissue (commonly done in a surgical suite for sterility) does not harm the person, as a small amount of tissue is taken. The tissue is taken or sent out for special studies. The biopsy should always have light and electron microscopy, and be examined fully, preferably before freezing. A full evaluation of a biopsy can take a full week's work in an experienced laboratory. Only a few laboratories in the United States are equipped for a comprehensive study of such biopsies; these few laboratories receive biopsies from all over the world; excellent work, but not the most ideal, can be done on frozen tissue as necessary.

The Glycogen Storage Diseases

Glycogen storage disease is a broad term used to describe conditions which involve genetic enzyme (metabolic) errors that lead to the body being unable to utilize correctly sugars as energy sources. These abnormalities lead to abnormal concentrations of glycogen, or to the storage of glycogen that is abnormal in its structure.

There are at least eight types of abnormalities leading to glycogen storage disease, and in many instances many subtypes in these many groups; they are known by a variety of names and numbers.

The first disease in man in which a specific enzyme was shown to be deficient in liver was glucose-6-phosphatase glycogen storage disease. When this was discovered by the Coris, it was labeled Type I glycogen storage disease. Although this number is consistent world wide, there is some discrepancy in the numbering systems for later diseases; therefore it is more exact to refer to the enzyme that is deficient, i.e. glucose-6-phosphatase deficiency. All forms of glycogen storage disease (GSD) are genetically transmitted, and in virtually all instances the genes responsible are derived from both parents.

Type I Glycogen Storage Disease

Type I glycogen storage disease (Type I GSD) is one of the more common disorders in glycogen metabolism; it is known by a myriad of names:

- Type I Glycogen Storage Disease
- von Gierke's Disease
- Glucose-6-Phosphatase Deficiency Glycogen Storage Disease
- Hepatorenal Glycogenosis

The glucose-6-phosphatase system has several components which are required for proper function. Deficiencies of the glucose-6-phosphatase enzyme system are known as Type Ia glycogen storage disease. Deficiencies of the translocase enzyme, required to move glucose-6-phosphate across the membrane to make it available to the enzyme are termed Type Ib (rare). There is an extremely rare type (Ic) in which there is an additional deficiency in this system. The difference between Types Ia and Ib are not great (Patients with Type Ib tend to have infections due to abnormal functions of the white blood cells). Patients with suspected Type I glycogen storage disease should be referred to a center where the liver biopsy can be assayed fresh (without freezing) so that the most exacting diagnosis can be made.

In this form of the glycogen storage disease, the basic defect is that the patient cannot convert glucose 6 phosphate to free glucose. The immediate problem is low blood sugar; some patients as infants have serious hypoglycemia, but not all. The enzyme is defective in the liver, kidney, and small intestine, where it normally functions. The problem metabolically is centered in the liver.

The liver normally stores glucose as glycogen (usually up to about 5 grams of glycogen per 100 grams of liver tissue). Normally when the blood sugar falls this glycogen is converted to free glucose and keeps the person's blood sugar normal. Since patients with Type I Glycogen Storage Disease (GSD) can store glucose as glycogen but not release it normally, with time the stored glycogen builds up in the liver. Hormones, particularly glucagon are increased in the body's attempt to raise blood sugar but to no avail. Other products, particularly lactic acid (from the attempted breakdown of glycogen to glucose) and fats are markedly increased in the blood. Fats, which are mobilized, are stored in the liver along with the glycogen, and these lead to enlargement of the liver. The liver does its many other functions normally, and there is not usually any evidence of liver failure such as occurs in patients with some kinds of liver disease.

The low level of glucose in the blood (hypoglycemia) of these patients often results in chronic hunger, fatigue and irritability which is especially noticeable in infants. If the blood sugar falls to a low enough point, some patients may experience seizures similar to those seen in epilepsy. Patients with glycogen storage disease are however remarkably tolerant to low blood sugar.

The presence of low blood sugar eventually leads the body to reduce its insulin output; eventually there is significant growth retardation. This slow growth rate is commonly the complaint that brings the child to a physician.

When blood studies are done, it is discovered that there is usually a low blood sugar, elevated blood lactic acid, elevated cholesterol and other fats and elevated uric acid concentration. Treatments should be aimed at correcting all three abnormalities.

It is important that the uric acid concentrations be maintained at a normal level (if the dietary treatment does not correct it, it will be necessary to use a xanthine oxidase (Allopurinol) inhibitor as uricosuric agents do not work). High blood pressure has been seen in a number of patients and when this occurs, appropriate treatment must be given.

In adulthood, several very important areas must be monitored. Most patients as they approach puberty will develop knots (adenomatas)

471

in the liver tissue; the exact reason for these is not known, but their size and distribution must be monitored. On very rare occasions in the past, these nodules have become cancerous; it is my belief (not proven) that these nodules will not become cancerous in patients who are treated carefully; studies by others have shown that they might disappear or become smaller with treatment.

Kidney disease has been recognized in recent years, and functions of the kidney must be monitored carefully.

The diagnosis of Type I glycogen storage disease will always include blood studies, x-rays (including some of kidneys), measurements, ultrasound of the liver and liver biopsy. The only situation in which I would not want a liver biopsy would be when a brother or sister had the same problem and had a liver biopsy performed on one.

The treatments of glycogen storage disease Type I have continued to change over the years. Some time ago portacaval shunts were done; it was a complicated procedure with considerable complications; some of the patients however benefited considerably. It should not be done at the current time. Liver transplants have been done, and may be indicated in certain very selected situations; they will be rarely if ever be indicated at the current time. As complications are reduced they may be used in the future.

Methods aimed at keeping the blood sugar normal are the basis of all current effective treatment. In the early 1970's a group from England reported their results with glucose infusion, using a micro pump in their patients with glycogen storage disease. Greene and his associates, as well as others, have pioneered nutritional treatments.

Currently, it is known that if the blood sugar is maintained at 70 mgm/100 ml or above during the night considerable improvement occurs. This has been done with a variety of methods (Vivonex®, glucose, glucose polymers) and it seems to matter little what is used as long as the blood sugar stays up.

Sidbury and Crigler and their associates have shown that during the day, the blood sugar can be maintained in patients beyond infancy with starch solution: considerable benefit derives from this.

Therefore at the current time, the appropriate treatment for glycogen storage disease is careful monitoring by an expert in the areas of complications and a custom-designed regime that included nocturnal feeds and starch by day. Other medications might be necessary as indicated. The nocturnal feeds which are usually administered by a tube into the stomach are usually accomplished without major difficulty; the patients themselves usually prefer to insert the tube at a rather remarkably young age.

We never restrict activity of patients unless there is some unusual problem. We have never seen any complication from considerable activity; we do however restrict contact sports (football, etc.) as we are concerned that a direct blow, severe, to the liver could be harmful. We have, however, never seen an injured liver in over 25 years of monitoring a large number of patients.

This condition is inherited as an autosomal recessive condition; of necessity, both parents are carriers (heterozygotes); as with other heterozygous conditions, carriers are normal. It is not currently possible to diagnose carriers with accuracy. Patients who are affected with glucose-6-phosphatase deficiency glycogen storage disease will not have affected children unless they marry a carrier, which would be rare unless one was marrying a family member.

The Future. Although glucose-6-phosphatase deficiency glycogen storage disease was the first form of this condition diagnosed, work in the area has been slow. This comes from the fact that the enzyme system is within membranes of the body and very difficult to purify; as it nears purity, its activity is lost. There are some very innovative techniques of molecular genetics that will likely be applied to this area in the future; if they are successful, they will have rather dramatic effects on the diagnosis of this condition, and on the identification of heterozygotes. In the future, such knowledge might be of benefit in specific treatment.

Generalized Glycogenosis

Generalized glycogenosis is also known as Type II glycogen storage disease, and was originally known as Pompe's Disease. Professor Pompe, a Dutch pathologist, described this dramatic condition in the 1930s because at death these infants have characteristically had dramatic enlargement of the heart and liver and significant accumulation of glycogen in the brain and musculature. An interesting aside was that Professor Pompe was killed for his anti-Nazi activities just as the war was ending.

Although this condition was described very early, it was quite late in being elucidated as far as biochemical defects were known. The usual enzymes of glycogen synthesis and degradation are all normal; there is an enormous accumulation of glycogen of normal structure in all the tissues. It has now been recognized that the defect is due to a deficiency of a lysosomal enzyme, alpha-1,4-glucosidase. This enzyme works best at acid pH and is also known as acid maltase (the sugar maltose can be used in the assay in the laboratory, hence the name maltase). In the absence of this lysosomal enzyme, the glycogen that accumulates within the lysozyme during tissue degradation accumulates to very large concentrations, and produces actual mechanical damage. The lysozyme is composed of membranes so the glycogen within the lysozyme is not able to be broken down by the enzymes which are present in solution in the cell.

Currently we recognize at least three forms of this disease; the most common being the infantile form of the disease. The infants present during early infancy with weakness and floppiness; they are unable to hold up their heads and cannot do other motor tasks common for their age. The muscles do not appear wasted. The liver is enlarged and the heart is usually very large. The very large heart is usually the most important clue; electrical studies of the heart (EKG) show changes which are quite characteristic. The profound weakness, which also involves the muscles of respiration, and the heart involvement usually leads to death in early infancy (the average age of death is about 5½ months).

In a second group of patients the disease has a later onset, in infancy or early childhood, and progresses more slowly than the infantile form. Organ involvement varies among the individual patients but muscle weakness is generally seen. The life expectancy for this group is better than for the first, but there have not been reports of patients surviving beyond 19 years.

The third group of patients, with the adult form of the disease, do not usually show signs of organ enlargement but are marked by muscular weakness mimicking other chronic muscle diseases; they usually carry a diagnosis of another myopathy. Some of these patients have presented with pulmonary (lung) insufficiency due to muscle weakness and this remains a very important clinical area. Many of these patients are in mid adult life and clearly will live a long life span, although likely reduced. Heart involvement does not appear to be a significant feature.

The biochemical finding in patients with these disorders appears similar; there is a deficiency of lysosomal alpha-1,4-glucosidase. This deficiency can be shown with leukocytes (care must be taken to correct for other enzymes in the assay), cultured skin cells and biopsies of muscle and/or liver. Tissues such as muscle biopsies will show a great increase of glycogen or normal structure; electron microscopic studies on these biopsies (these should always be done) show increased glycogen which is enclosed within membrane lined structures (lysosomes).

There are no curative treatments; high protein diets have been recommended to produce clinical improvement. Older patients, in particular, must have a well established plan to follow in the event that pulmonary (lung) infections occur. We recommend that adults with this disorder obtain baseline pulmonary function studies.

Since alpha-1,4-glucosidase appears in cells which can be cultured from amniotic fluid cells, this condition can be (and has been) diagnosed reliably prenatally.

Anyone with a positive family history of alpha-1,4-glucosidase deficiency would be strongly advised to consult their physician concerning their carrier state and a possible amniocentesis in the event of pregnancy if this is desired.

The acute infantile form can be readily diagnosed prenatally in families where the condition is known to occur. Prenatal diagnosis is reliable, and accurate. This technique discussed above, has been applied more commonly in Type II (alpha-1,4-glucosidase deficiency) glycogen storage disease than in any other type.

The Future. This enzyme has been purified and considerable progress has been made on the molecular biology of the gene. This information will likely be of use first in diagnostic areas; it is likely to present long term therapeutic opportunities.

Debrancher Deficiency Glycogen Storage Disease

Debrancher deficiency glycogen storage disease is also known as type III glycogen storage disease, Cori's Disease and limit dextrinosis. If you refer back to the biochemistry section, you will recall that the debrancher enzyme is required to break the branch points when glycogen is being broken down (another enzyme, the brancher enzyme makes these same branch points when glycogen is being made). When this debrancher enzyme is not present, the glycogen that accumulates has many short branch points and therefore has an abnormal structure. The accumulation of glycogen with short outer branches (limit dextrin) and the failure to break down glycogen to glucose is what causes most of the symptoms that are seen.

The symptoms of debrancher deficiency are a lot like those that were outlined for glucose-6-phosphatase deficiency glycogen storage disease; however the usual patient with debrancher deficiency usually has a milder course. Patients will have a large liver, suffer severe growth retardation, and have low blood sugar levels. Muscle wasting and weakness is present commonly in childhood and can at times be severe. For reasons that are not clear, many of us have seen the liver return to normal size at puberty, although the enzyme defect persists.

Depending on the assay used, there have been observed a variety of subtypes of this disorder; there appears to be considerable variation in the tissues affected by the defect (such as white blood cells, muscle, liver, and so forth). Chemical findings on the blood usually show low blood sugar, elevated glycogen content in red blood cells, elevated levels of fat, but uric acid and lactic acid are usually normal. Enzymes derived from liver (such as serum glutamic pyruvate transaminase) are elevated. Biopsy of the liver shows inflammatory changes, but I have never seen this continue to the severe scarring of cirrhosis seen in other conditions. The liver biopsy shows great elevations of glycogen content with short outer branches; there is a deficiency of the brancher enzyme and usually a modest, and we feel clinically insignificant, reduction of glucose-6-phosphatase activity. Biopsy of muscle shows accumulation of glycogen (abnormal structured also) and deficiency of debrancher activity also.

Since this disease cannot be reliably distinguished from the other glycogen storage diseases, we feel it important to have biopsy material for enzyme analysis. In addition to liver and muscle biopsies, commonly red blood cells and cultured skin fibroblasts are studied.

Treatment for this disease consists of frequent feedings and a high protein diet. Continuous nasogastric feedings and the starch regimes outlined under glucose-6-phosphatase deficiency are useful.

Since cultured amniotic fluid cells only sometimes express the genetic defect, they have been used for prenatal diagnosis. Since the defect is not always expressed in fibroblasts the usefulness of this technique has to be individualized.

Persons with debrancher deficiency have lived well into late adulthood; muscle disorders seem to be an increasing problem with age. We have studies on adults with this disorder who developed heart disease; on biopsy of the heart, glycogen infiltration was seen and debrancher deficiency was demonstrated. The frequency of this is not known.

The Future. This enzyme has been purified and considerable progress has been made towards characterizing this gene. This information will likely be of first use in diagnostic areas, but in the long term we hope will have considerable therapeutic usefulness.

Brancher Deficiency Glycogen Storage Disease

This rare form of the glycogen storage diseases is also known as amylopectinosis, Andersen's disease, and Type IV glycogen storage disease. Unlike all the other glycogen storage diseases which we will discuss, this disorder does not demonstrate an increased amount of glycogen in the tissues; the glycogen which accumulates has very long outer branches, as there is a genetic deficiency of the branching enzyme. The glycogen which accumulates is very much like starch, and is very much less soluble than is normal glycogen. Skilled pathologists have recognized that it stains a different color with the dyes that they use, and appears to be "out of solution," rather clumped in the middle of the cell. This structural abnormality of glycogen is thought to trigger the body's immune system; it attacks the glycogen and the tissues in which it is stored; this results in tremendous cirrhosis (scarring) of the liver as well as other organs, such as muscle. The typical symptomatology of this disease is the result of the scarring process.

A baby with the typical brancher deficiency appears to be normal at birth. The first indication of a problem is a "failure to thrive." The rate of growth and mental progress of the baby stops at a certain point and does not continue normally. There is little weight gain, lack of muscle tone, and the liver and spleen continue to enlarge. The course of the disease is one of progressive cirrhosis and the problems associated with this. Death occurs typically within the second year. The central problem is consistently that of liver failure.

Recently, there have been older patients with brancher deficiency who have been very different from this typical, rare patient. A 7½ year-old-girl has been seen with severe muscle problems and disease of the heart muscle; in Germany several young children have been seen, and recently a middle aged man with a thirty year history of progressive muscle weakness, and biochemical evidence for the presence of abnormal glycogen of the type associated with brancher deficiency.

Treatment has been aimed at the failing liver, which has been symptomatic. At least one patient has had a liver transplant; however after transplant, muscle disease predictably will then be the problem. It is clear that we will be seeing a variety of other patients who have brancher defects.

The brancher enzyme is present in cultured amniotic fluid cells, and prenatal diagnosis can, and has been, carried out. The disease is transmitted as an autosomal recessive disorder, each parent being a carrier. Carriers can be detected using white blood cells from a peripheral blood sample, as well as cultured skin fibroblasts.

There is no significant progress at the level of molecular genetics at the current time.

Muscle Phosphorylase Deficiency

Muscle phosphorylase deficiency is also known as McArdle's Disease and by some has been called Type V glycogen storage disease.

As you will recall from the section on biochemistry, phosphorylase plays a vital role in the degradation of glycogen. Phosphorylase exists in both active and inactive forms; the enzyme system responsible for activating phosphorylase is called phosphorylase b kinase (the inactive phosphorylase is called phosphorylase b). Because of the complexity of this system, a variety of possibilities exist for genetic deficiencies.

It is important to understand also that the phosphorylase enzyme that exists in human liver and phosphorylase enzyme that exists in muscle are under different genetic control in the body. Although they have the same function, they have several biochemical differences and are clearly different genetically. Therefore, you can have a deficiency of the liver enzyme and not the muscle enzyme, and vice versa.

Many of the tests that are done clinically to examine a patient's ability to break down glycogen function at this important step in glycogen breakdown. For instance, when a person is given epinephrine or glucagon, both these drugs serve to activate phosphorylase. When phosphorylase is activated, glycogen breakdown occurs.

The typical person with muscle phosphorylase deficiency was described clinically by McArdle, whose name is commonly used to describe the findings. The usual person is a young adult male (more males than females are known) who presents with painful muscle cramps after exercise. Commonly these persons are considered to have nonorganic disease because they present in late adolescence (a time for considerable turmoil!) and the tasks that commonly bother them are such things as mowing lawns and the like.

The physical exam is normal; these persons are commonly muscular, do not have hypoglycemia, do not have large livers, and are normal in height.

Frequently these young persons have been very active; I care for one young man who was a competitive long-range runner when he developed painful cramps after a very hard run. He, in typical fashion, developed myoglobinuria which showed up as dark red or red brown urine. The myoglobin in the urine comes from the breakdown of muscle after stress (myoglobin is the red protein in muscle).

These painful cramps arise from the fact that there is a genetic deficiency of phosphorylase in the muscle; when there is extensive exercise, the muscle needs to breakdown glycogen to supply extra energy; when this cannot be done the muscle cramps and this is painful.

Diagnostically, any person with painful cramps after exercise should be evaluated. The test that is done is an anaerobic lactate test. This is carried out in the following manner: The blood flow to the arm is interrupted with a blood pressure cuff and the arm exercised. Since no blood is coming to the arm, the energy for such exercise must come from the glycogen in the muscle. If glycogen cannot be broken down normally, no lactate will be present in the blood from the vein from the working muscle. Also there will be a marked increase in hypoxanthine from the breakdown of stored high energy compounds in the muscle. A muscle biopsy must be done to confirm the diagnosis. The muscle will show increased concentrations of glycogen, and a deficiency on assay of the enzyme phosphorylase. A rare patient has been described whose enzyme deficiency will be phosphofructokinase; these patients are virtually identical to the phosphorylase deficient patients and will not be considered separately except briefly.

The liver phosphorylase activity is normal. There is no hypoglycemia, and responses to injected glucagon and epinephrine are normal (because of the normal liver phosphorylase activity).

The patient described above is by far the most common and usual; however, as in all of the glycogen storage diseases, variations are well known. A infant has been described with a fatal infantile myopathy due to muscle phosphorylase deficiency; at the other end of the spectrum, a patient with phosphorylase deficiency has been recognized who presented with muscle weakness in the seventh decade of life.

There is no specific treatment for this disorder. It is very important to exercise moderately for extensive exercise can cause considerable muscle breakdown and a great deal of myoglobin in the urine. This large amount of myoglobin has been know to precipitate (come out of solution) in the kidneys and cause at least temporary kidney failure.

The outlook for these patients long term is good; however some patients have developed significant muscle problems (myopathies) in old age. Some persons report improved exercise tolerance after high carbohydrate intake; this makes sense as more energy would be available to the muscle from the blood going to these tissues. It is possible that some of the drugs which increase blood flow to the muscles might be of benefit.

There has been some very interesting research in this area in recent years. It is possible to measure high energy materials within muscles using an important new technology known as nuclear magnetic resonance (MRI). This could be very helpful in testing the usefulness of new drugs or diet, since you could measure changes in high energy phosphates in muscle without invasive techniques.

The gene for muscle phosphorylase has been isolated using molecular genetic techniques; the messenger mRNA in the cells is copied and a complimentary DNA (cDNA) for the enzyme is prepared. These studies have shown that in patients with muscle phosphorylase deficiency there is no mRNA in some patients and low levels in others; other studies also show that there are either no enzyme protein or low levels of enzyme protein. This means that abnormal proteins are not made, but either no protein or low levels of a normal enzyme protein are made.

Recent studies have also shown that the gene for muscle phosphorylase is located on chromosome number 11.

Liver Phosphorylase Deficiency

Glycogen storage disease resulting from a deficiency of liver phosphorylase has also been called Her's disease as well as Type VI glycogen storage disease. As we have discussed previously in the section on muscle phosphorylase deficiency, the liver and muscle phosphorylase enzymes are different and are under different genetic control. This condition appears to be quite rare in the United States; since phosphorylase is such a key enzyme, total deficiencies of this enzyme activity would not likely be compatible with life. Therefore, all the patients reported with deficiencies of this enzyme very likely have only partial deficiencies due to genetic modifications in the enzyme protein.

Phosphorylase is the enzyme which acts on liver glycogen to cleave off glucose units as glucose 1 phosphate. With a deficiency of this enzyme, glycogen cannot be broken down to glucose and the accumulating glycogen results in an enlarged liver.

Clinically, this form of glycogen disease appears to be similar to, but usually considerably milder than glucose-6-phosphatase deficiency glycogen storage disease (Type I glycogen storage disease). Extreme enlargement of the liver, growth retardation, and mild hypoglycemia are seen, but children can certainly present with few symptoms and be able to lead normal lives.

The diagnosis of the disease is based on liver biopsy material; assays must be done for glycogen content (which is increased) as well as for phosphorylase activity. Phosphorylase activity is present but reduced. It is essential that these studies be done in a very experienced laboratory as reductions of phosphorylase and other enzyme activities can result from improper collection and storage of the material.

The genetics of phosphorylase deficiency usually show an autosomal recessive inheritance. There have been reports also of autosomal dominant inheritance; such autosomal dominant inheritance is extremely unusual for inherited enzyme deficiencies in man.

Due to the mildness of the clinical findings, treatment is usually not required; should hypoglycemia and growth failure be a major problem, these patients should receive the same nutritional management that has been effective in glucose-6-phosphatase and debrancher deficiency glycogen storage disease.

The enzyme liver phosphorylase, because of its central importance in human metabolism has been widely studied for many years. It has been purified to homogeneity and recently the cDNA has been isolated and considerable work done to characterize the gene. The gene has been located on chromosome number 14. Recent studies have identified certain properties of the gene products that will be quite helpful in diagnosis and in family studies. Studies of the gene products have demonstrated restriction fragment polymorphisms which will be helpful in family studies, as well as in predicting whether fetuses are affected with this disorder. These are molecular genetic techniques which demonstrate differences as the gene level.

Phosphofructokinase Deficiency Glycogen Storage Disease

As we have mentioned before, the deficiency of phosphofructokinase presents clinically almost identically to the deficiency of muscle phosphorylase deficiency. This condition has also been called Type VII glycogen storage disease and Tarui's Disease.

Phosphofructokinase is the enzyme that catalyzes the conversion of fructose-6-phosphate to fructose-1,6-phosphate which is the controlling step in the breakdown of glucose into energy via glycolysis. If deficient in muscle, effective glycogen breakdown (glycolysis) during muscle stress cannot be accomplished and pain and cramping in the exercising muscles result.

The diagnostic studies and biopsy procedures are the same as for muscle phosphorylase deficiency (McArdle's Disease). In this condition, red blood cell phosphofructokinase is reduced to about half normal activity, because of the loss of the muscle form of the enzyme in the red blood cells.

Treatment approaches would be similar to phosphorylase deficiency.

Phosphorylase b Kinase Deficiency Glycogen Storage Disease

Phosphorylase b kinase deficiency glycogen storage disease has also been called Type IX glycogen storage disease; a series of subtypes have been described. These subtypes, when numbered, are only confusing and this terminology should be discouraged.

The enzyme phosphorylase b kinase is a complicated one indeed; there are four enzyme subunits (labeled in the Greek form of alpha, beta, gamma, and delta). The enzyme as it is active consists of two each of these subunits. The enzyme also requires a metal ion. To make things even more complicated, it is now clear that some of these subunits function in other systems, not apparently related to glycogen metabolism.

There has been an enormous amount of molecular biologic research on this enzyme system, and some of these findings will be relevant to the glycogen storage diseases.

There is clearly none of the glycogen storage diseases that have such a broad spectrum of clinical presentations; we will describe what has been the 'typical' patient and then some of the more recently recognized variants of this condition.

Phosphorylase kinase is the enzyme system responsible for converting inactive phosphorylase (phosphorylase b) to the active form (phosphorylase a). We have commented about the important function of phosphorylase in biological systems. For reasons that are clear, some patients who lack phosphorylase b kinase have been called phosphorylase deficiency, since their phosphorylase, although present would be inactive.

The usual patient with hepatic phosphorylase b kinase deficiency would present with significant hepatic enlargement during the course of a routine physical examination. The spleen is sometimes also modestly enlarged. The patient is usually short for his age, although in virtually all instances, catch up growth occurs at puberty (which is delayed) and the patient ends up in adulthood with a normal height. Blood studies are usually normal, except for modest elevations of transaminases from the liver.

Biopsy of the liver shows very large increases in glycogen (the largest we see) which is normal in structure. The liver shows some fibrosis, minimal inflammatory changes, but not true or frank cirrhosis (severe fibrous changes of the liver). The vast majority of patients of this type are male, and the disease appears to be inherited in an X-linked recessive pattern. This means that the recessive gene for this form of phosphorylase b kinase deficiency is carried on one of the sex chromosomes. A sex chromosome is that chromosome which is involved in the sexual identity of a child, i.e., male vs. female. A female has two X chromosomes; a male has one X chromosome received from the mother and one Y chromosome from the father. Because of this inheritance pattern, it is only possible to conceive a child with this form of glycogen storage disease if the child is female with both X chromosomes carrying the recessive gene (most unlikely!) or if the child is male and his one X chromosome has the recessive gene. Because of this, this presentation is seen only in males.

Much work is going on in molecular genetics in this field; the genes for two of the subunits have been isolated and characterized; both of them are on autosomes (i.e. not the sex chromosomes). That means that we will expect, and we certainly are aware of, patients who have deficiencies of this enzyme who are inherited in both the X-linked and the autosomal recessive pattern.

As more and more studies have been done in this area, we have seen an array of findings associated with phosphorylase b kinase deficiency. In addition to the patient type described above, some patients have been described (particularly as infants) with a profound and striking myopathy; a typical floppy infant. Recent work has described a patient with heart failure and apparently severe lack of phosphorylase b kinase activity in the heart (the heart is usually unaffected). In this patient, only the phosphorylase b kinase in the heart was affected.

The important conclusion is that there is a vast array of clinical and biochemical variations in phosphorylase b kinase deficiency. The complexity of the enzyme system, with location of subunits on a variety of chromosomes leads to this.

Diagnostic studies include assays of leukocytes, erythrocytes (very commonly show the deficiency) in addition to muscle, liver, fibroblasts or other tissues suspected to being involved.

The lack of severe symptoms (except in those involving muscle) leads to no specific treatment at the current time. The work in molecular genetics in this area will undoubtedly lead to new and very helpful diagnostic techniques. There are young animals who also lack phosphorylase b kinase activity; interestingly enough these animals show a considerable increase in phosphorylase b kinase activity with age. It is at least conceivable that the improvement that has been seen with some persons could be due to the same phenomena. This has not been shown.

Parent, Family, and Patient Involvement

Coping with glycogen storage disease for all concerned must go beyond gaining a knowledge of the biochemistry and medical results of the condition.

Everybody in the family unit will at some time need support in dealing with the emotional stress which a chronic condition such as glycogen storage disease can produce.

This section reviews some of the common concerns created by GSD. One must realize that in no way should this brief discussion be expected to answer all your questions about dealing with GSD, and there is no substitute for good question and answer sessions over the years, which includes emotional reaction to problems, with your doctor. Also everyone's experience with chronic illness is different, and since GSD has many forms, ranging from a relatively mild muscle ailment to severe and fatal forms, this discussion must be rather general.

The first phase in dealing with GAD is often denial; there is a strong wish and hope that things were "right." There is often "shopping" for physicians who will tell you things are okay, and that the persons who had made the diagnosis were in error. Very commonly, because of the rarity of these conditions and the highly technical studies required for a diagnosis, families are referred to physicians who are new to them, and in whom confidence must develop with time. The denial reaction is common, and requires emotional support from family, friends, church, medical staff, and frequently discussions with other families of persons with glycogen storage disease. Knowledge and time can help reduce the denial reaction, which has part of its base in a fear of the condition which can be reduced by understanding and information.

Another problem experienced by many parents is a feeling of guilt; every parent will at some time ask, "Am I to blame; am I the one responsible?" There is no way, or need to, assign blame or responsibility in this situation, as there is no guilty party. These situations are natural events, and we know of no act (alcohol, drugs, etc.) that the parents may have been involved in that contributed to this disorder.

Many couples find that the strength of their marriage is placed under stress by these emotional factors as well as financial demands. Recognizing that these problems will and do occur can commonly help everybody in dealing with them.

The major goal of the parents (and friends) of persons with glycogen storage disease is helping the patient understand the disease and to support that person in achieving the development of a realistic and positive self-image and an adequate sense of self-esteem. The child will have a good deal of self-doubt and questioning when he or she begins to recognize that he is "different." Children will wonder: am I weird? A parent should attempt to answer the child's questions frankly and not avoid them. Your child will recognize the fact that you are reluctant to discuss his or her questions, and this can serve to heighten his anxiety. Instead answer the questions as clearly as possible with appropriate vocabulary and with proper concern. For example a child with GSD might ask, "Why is my tummy so big?" or "Why can't I eat that?" The parents' answer might include the idea that the child's body is special and that it works differently from others and as a result they must do special things to be healthy. As a child's curiosity develops it is very important to begin to let him be a part of his own treatment; this helps him develop an understanding of his condition and some sense of independence and control. As the child grows older more detail will of course be included in conversations. It is somewhat surprising to many of us how early some children begin inserting their nasogastric tubes at night and taking a major role in their care; this is to be encouraged, but not unduly forced.

Lastly, it should be pointed out that there will be times when a parent will feel defeated and ready to give up. The stress of hospitalization, finances, emotional drains, treatment demands, and various aspects of coping with a chronic illness will at times seem insurmountable. When this occurs seek support from sources that have been mentioned. It is also strongly recommended that you attempt to contact other parents of children with GSD. They, more than any others, will understand your situation and may have answers to many of your questions.

The only thing different about your child with glycogen storage disease is a metabolic imbalance; your child will still have the natural wants, desires, and love of any child. The child must grow up learning the usual rules and demands that are made on everybody; the expectations should not be modified except in the few objective ways that are necessary due to the disease condition. It will always be important to focus on the special talents of the child and the special abilities and to minimize the few areas in which unusual restrictions must take place.

Where to Get More Information

The most important source of information about the patient with glycogen storage disease is the patient's physician. As we have outlined, there are many types of glycogen storage disease and each patient is

485

unique with respect to the situations which he presents. Each person has in the range of 1,000,000 genes; the defective gene is only one of these. This defective gene functions in a unique environment of other genes, and produces a very special person.

Because of the rarity of this diagnosis, the individual doctor might not be fully aware of all the current research and treatment of the glycogen storage diseases. The ideal situation is to develop a relationship with a group of specialists whom your personal physician recommends, and together they can form the team to provide the best diagnosis and treatment program. It is essential to have a physician who sees the patient on a regular basis and provides all the care needed, in addition to the special needs.

You will want to avail yourself of other sources of information. We have included some suggestions; be cautious about out of date medical materials; books that are more than 5 years old are likely to be very much out of date; the field is moving so rapidly that a few years usually dates material. Be sure to show the material to your physician. Libraries will be of little help except those of a large college or medical school facility.

Be aware of word of mouth, old wives tales, and testimonies from nonprofessionals involved in GSD treatment and research.

Major textbooks of internal medicine will have brief, accurate descriptions of the glycogen storage diseases; the most widely accepted textbook is *Cecil's Textbook of Internal Medicine*, edited by Wyngaarden and Smith; published usually every 3-4 years; don't rely on old editions.

Pediatric medical textbooks such as *Nelson's Textbook of Pediatrics* (edited by Behrmann and Vaughn) published by W. B. Saunders, and *Rudolph's Textbook of Pediatrics* (Appleton-Century, Crofts, New York) may be helpful. A medical dictionary and patience will be required by the nonprofessional reader for these texts.

The most detailed and comprehensive review of all aspects of the glycogen storage diseases is published in *The Metabolic Basis of Inherited Disease*, Wyngaarden, Stanbury, Fredrickson, Brown and Goldstein, Editors. This is very technical and complex and will be useful to only rare nonprofessional readers.

The Ray, Newsletter for the Association for Glycogen Storage Diseases, P.O. Box 46, Stockton, IA 52769 is a publication that is a must for parents and persons with glycogen storage disease. The newsletter is filled with helpful, authoritative and current information. The group itself is parent oriented and is advised by a national, experienced group of professionals.

Questions and Answers

A small group of parents have prepared a list of questions which they feel have been of significant interest to them; and which they have been asked by other parents and friends of persons associated and not associated with glycogen storage disease.

Many of the questions do not have a clear, single, correct answer but the response given is based on the currently available best information about the disease.

Why does the size of the liver shrink or stop growing larger when on the nasogastric tube treatment? The liver has been observed to shrink while on nasogastric feedings. This is related to the fact that the body chemistries are returned much more toward normal, particularly the blood sugar. But with the more normal blood sugar, there is less mobilization of fat, and the fat in the liver is reduced; this accounts for the reduction in the size of the liver. The glycogen concentration in the liver is not changed during the nasogastric feeding. In glucose-6-phosphatase glycogen storage disease, the liver enlargement is due largely to fat present, but is also contributed to by the excessive amount of glycogen present.

Does the liver release any stored glycogen as a waste into the system? Glycogen itself is not released from the liver into the body. Glycogen is a very large molecule and cannot pass through cell walls. Even in patients with glycogen storage disease, however, the glycogen is constantly being made and broken down to some considerable extent to glucose and/or lactic acid.

Does glycogen store in any organs other than the liver with glucose-6-phosphatase deficiency glycogen storage disease (Type I)? Glucose-6-phosphatase deficiency glycogen storage disease is also known as hepatorenal glycogen storage disease. This comes from the fact that there is storage of glycogen within the kidney as well as the liver. This leads to enlargement of the kidneys, but usually does not directly affect renal (kidney) function. Some patients do develop high blood pressure but it is unclear what the cause of this is.

Do many children have convulsions when their blood sugar drops? Some children with glucose-6-phosphatase deficiency and debrancher deficiency who have serious manifestations do rarely have convulsions related to low blood sugar. It would appear that most children, however, gradually change the metabolism within their brain to use other energy sources and do not have convulsions even when blood sugar is low.

Are there different kinds of convulsions, seizures, or spells they can have? Patients with glucose-6-phosphatase deficiency (Type I) glycogen storage disease and low blood sugar have a variety of different types of spells. These may be a direct loss of consciousness so that the patient lies motionless or drops motionless to the floor. At other times there are generalized jerking movements, chewing movements, and seizures not unlike those seen in epilepsy.

Is a high protein diet important to these children? We have noted above that there appears to be considerable benefit to persons with alpha-1,4-glucosidase deficiency (Type II) and debrancher deficiency (Type III) when a high protein diet is used. In patients with glucose-6-phosphatase deficiency protein cannot be converted to glucose, due to a deficiency of this key enzyme. It is helpful to maintain a relatively low carbohydrate diet in order to maintain a steady insulin output and a more steady blood sugar. It is felt at the current time that relatively low fat diets have benefit to all persons. Since lipid (fat) levels tend to be high in several of the liver forms of the glycogen storage diseases, good judgement would indicate a diet low in saturated fats, and in cholesterol.

Does it do much harm or throw their systems off if they were to eat candy, or foods that are restricted? The important thing is to eat a well balanced nutritious diet. Occasional indiscretions are not likely to produce serious problems. There is little clear benefit to a very restricted diet.

Does the nasogastric tube contribute to sore throats and ear infections? The nasogastric tube goes through the back of the nose, mouth and the throat, and also along the base of where the ears drain into the back of the nose. This makes the children have a bit more problem with sore throats and they are somewhat more prone to ear infections.

Is there a possibility that a time released capsule could be swallowed to replace the tube and drip? The starch (suspension) that is in common use does essentially this; the starch consists of glucose residues in long linkage; they are gradually degraded by the body and absorbed as free glucose.

488

When children get very sick with vomiting and nothing stays down, even glucose, what is the best solution? Children with glycogen storage diseases associated with a low blood sugar, and who have significant and continued vomiting might well require fluids by vein. Your doctor can best assess this but experienced parents are good judges. You should make plans for this in advance (have your doctor write instructions for a local 24 hour facility, either an emergency room or other emergency facility). If traveling out of your area, it is worthwhile having your physician provide written materials so this can be handled in a strange city.

Is there any kind of test that our other children without glycogen storage disease can have to find out of they are carriers? At the current time there are no reliable carrier tests for glucose-6-phosphatase deficiency; this will change when the gene for the enzyme is cloned and characterized. Currently tests are available (various degrees of reliability in different families) for alpha-1,4-glucosidase deficiency, debrancher deficiency, brancher deficiency. and phosphorylase b kinase deficiency.

What are the chances of a child with glycogen storage disease having children of their own? Many adults with glucose-6-phosphatase deficiency, debrancher deficiency, alpha-1,4-glucosidase deficiency, phosphorylase b kinase deficiency and muscle phosphorylase deficiency have children of their own. As more patients live into adulthood with better care, these numbers will likely even be larger.

At what age can a child start to be weaned off glucose? Is there anything to take after puberty? One of the major clinical effects of nasogastric feeding is enhanced growth. Certain patients, however, who are fully grown continue on nasogastric feeding because of the considerable improvement in their feeling of well being.

If two children at age 4 years had liver biopsies (one who has been on nasogastric feedings and other with no special treatment) could you see a difference in their livers? The liver biopsy of the patient who had been well controlled on nasogastric feeding would show less fat deposit. The glycogen concentration would not be significantly changed and the enzyme defect (glucose-6-phosphatase deficiency) would persist.

What is the life expectancy of a person with glycogen storage disease? The life expectancy of persons with glucose-6-phosphatase deficiency, debrancher deficiency, and with liver phosphorylase deficiency is probably somewhat reduced although many do quite well. The big risks are kidney disease and high blood pressure. The usual patient with alpha-1,4-glucosidase deficiency and brancher deficiency dies in early childhood. Patients with muscle phosphorylase deficiency (McArdle's Disease) and usual forms of phosphorylase b Kinase deficiency probably have a usual life expectancy.

Is a child with glycogen storage disease really helped by the nasogastric tube feeding, the gastrostomy, and special diets? The benefits of special diets other than those mentioned in this text are questionable. Nasogastric feeding and starch feeding, when carefully controlled and carefully carried out are generally of substantial benefit. These benefits are usually increased growth, shrinkage of the abdomen due to shrinkage of the liver, and a considerable improvement in well being and increased activity. A gastrostomy is simply an opening through the wall of the abdomen that goes through the skin and in through the stomach. In some very small infants gastrostomies have been done to provide feeding similar to that which is used with the nasogastric tube. Gastrostomies are rarely necessary except in very small infants. Nasogastric feedings, do not of course, cure the basic problem.

Does the tube hurt the child when it is put down or while its in place? The usual child, when first beginning on nasogastric feedings will find the insertion of the tube uncomfortable, and will be aware of its presence while in. After being accustomed to the tube it's usually not painful to insert and does not create undue awareness of its presence. The tube is not painful while in place.

With nasogastric feedings is it necessary to maintain a restricted diet? With nasogastric feedings it is important to calculate the caloric value of the nasogastric feedings along with the rest of the total diet. It is important that there no be excessive carbohydrates in order to avoid obesity; a low fat content is felt to be prudent and a goodly protein intake. The values of high protein diets have been reviewed above.

Will the liver ever be a normal size in proportion to the body size? The liver in glucose-6-phosphatase deficiency will never be normal in size; however as the person grows taller, the liver 'fits' better and the abdomen is considerably less prominent. The liver in debrancher deficiency does get smaller following puberty; this is also possibly the case in phosphorylase b kinase deficiency, but not well established.

Will my child outgrow glycogen storage disease? One never outgrows glycogen storage disease; this is a genetic defect which is permanently encoded in the genetic makeup of the person.

How does glycogen storage disease affect other body functions, i.e. immunity to diseases, bleeding and mentality? There are many answers to this question; some patients with glucose-6-phosphatase deficiency related to a translocase defect (Type Ib) have increased infections due to abnormal white blood cell function. There is an increased tendency to bleeding in all persons with glucose-6-phosphatase deficiency, but not serious uncontrollable bleeding. Mentality is normal in most of the glycogen storage diseases; the infantile alpha-1,4-glucosidase deficiencies would be an exception.

How much larger is his liver than normal? Will it decrease or continue to grow? The liver of a patient with glucose-6-phosphatase deficiency glycogen storage disease (Type I) is roughly twice normal size. It will continue to grow but less rapidly than the body grows, and generally 'fits' the body much better at the older age. It does not decrease with age.

How tall can he be? Children with most of the glycogen storage diseases are shorter than their parents or unaffected siblings. There is significant improvement with nasogastric feedings. There is considerable catch up growth at puberty (which is delayed) particularly in debrancher deficiency and phosphorylase b kinase deficiency.

Are our other children still able to have it? No. Children are either born with or without glycogen storage disease; they cannot acquire the condition after birth.

Why doesn't our child walk? He is over a year old and our other children walked at 9 months. Children with glycogen storage disease that leads to an enlarged liver are slow to walk, simply by reason of the difficulties in balance that takes more time to master.

Is research being done for a cure? There is a great deal of work being done in the glycogen storage diseases. Several of the key enzymes have been purified, and in some the gene has been isolated and characterized.

Glucose-6-phosphatase, whose deficiency causes Type I glycogen storage disease has been particularly tricky to study; this enzyme is within the endoplasmic reticulum (membranes) and loses activity when attempts to purify the enzyme are made. The rapid advances in molecular genetics, however, will impact the area of glycogen storage disease quite positively. Much of this work is being supported by the National Institutes of Health; those forms of glycogen storage disease which affect the muscles (and as you recall there are several) are being studied by scientists receiving funding from the Muscular Dystrophy Association.

How many patients are there? Each of the 8 or 9 kinds of glycogen storage disease occurs in about one in 50,000 to 100,000 births. That means that there are several thousand such persons in the United States. Some patients might die before diagnosis with severe infantile forms; some milder forms might go unrecognized.

Is this disease restrictive to one nationality? No. All nationalities are affected with about the same frequencies. There are some interesting frequencies, such as glucose-6-phosphatase deficiency glycogen storage disease is extremely uncommon in Israel, while debrancher deficiency is relatively common among the non-Ashkenazi Jews in Israel.

Where do you go for treatment? Where are the best or most knowledgeable clinics? Children and adults with very complicated illnesses such as the glycogen storage diseases are usually best handled at the regional university medical centers and teaching hospitals, in conjunction with the local personal physician, a vital link. At the current time there are only a few places in the United States where biopsy material is analyzed biochemically; frequently material is sent to these places from all over the world. Biochemical studies are preferable on fresh, unfrozen material.

What type of diagnosis is most correct, blood or biopsy? Currently, glucose-6-phosphatase deficiency requires a liver biopsy for absolute diagnosis. This can at times be done with a needle biopsy but is ordinarily done on the surgical (open) biopsy. Muscle phosphorylase deficiency requires a muscle biopsy; certain of the conditions (alpha-1,4-glucosidase deficiency, phosphorylase b kinase deficiency) can at times reliably be diagnosed with leukocytes, red blood cells and cultured skin cells (fibroblasts).

Would a liver transplant help a child with glycogen storage disease? Liver transplants have been done in the glycogen storage diseases with some very good results. Liver transplants are extremely complex and risky, and would be done now only in life-threatening problems. If done in glucose-6-phosphatase deficiency it can be expected to have good results. However, liver transplants today have major complications, and should not be considered except in exceptional circumstances. In brancher deficiency where liver failure is prominent, transplanting the liver would produce survival from liver disease, but would be supplanted in time with muscle failure.

Is it possible to produce a synthetic enzyme to replace the missing one? Certain of the enzymes deficient in the glycogen storage diseases have been purified highly. The problems are in obtaining a large enough supply of enzyme and getting it into the correct location in the body. Several years ago, very interesting studies were done in Australia with cattle who have a disease similar to infantile alpha-1,4-glucosidase deficiency. There was an attempt to put a certain receptor on purified enzyme that would help it go to the correct place in the cell (the lysosome in this case). Unfortunately these studies were not successful.

It is likely that the introduction of proper genes in the cell will be the mechanism which is successful; although this is an area of very active research, we would not expect useful results in the near future.

Can we talk to anyone who will understand? Are there other parents and patients? Yes. The Association for Glycogen Storage Disease is a parents/patients group. Their address:

Association for Glycogen Storage Disease
Box 896
Durant, IA 52747

Summary of Terms Related to Glycogen Storage Disease

Glycogen: A polysaccharide (this means many glucoses) is basically a group of glucose molecules attached in a linear fashion, with branch points. The body stores glucose in this way, and uses glycogen breakdown to elevate blood sugar.

493

Types of Glycogen Storage Disease

Glucose-6-phosphatase deficiency: Hepatorenal glycogen storage disease, von Gierke's Disease, and Type I glycogen storage disease. Type Ia, Ib, and Ic have complex chemical differences but affect the patient similarly.

Alpha-1,4-glucosidase deficiency: Type II glycogen storage disease, acid maltase deficiency, Pompe's Disease. There are at least three types, by age of onset and severity: infantile, juvenile, and adult.

Amylo-1,6-glucosidase deficiency: Type III glycogen storage disease; also known as Debrancher deficiency, Cori's Disease, and Limit Dextrinosis.

Alpha-1,4-Glucan: alpha-1,4-Glucan 6 glucosyl transferase Deficiency: Type IV glycogen storage disease; also known as Andersen's Disease, or Brancher Deficiency, amylopectinosis.

Muscle Phosphorylase Deficiency: Type V glycogen storage disease; also known as McArdle's Disease. A very similar clinical picture is seen with deficiency of muscle phosphofructokinase, known as Tarui's Disease (Sometimes called type VII glycogen storage disease).

Hepatic Phosphorylase Deficiency: Type VI Glycogen storage disease; also known as Her's Disease.

Phosphorylase b kinase deficiency: Type VIII Glycogen storage disease. There are several subtypes that affect muscle, liver, heart and brain; would not recommend numbering or naming the subtypes at the current time.

—text edited by R. Rodney Howell, MD,
Department of Pediatrics,
University of Texas
Health Science Center,
Houston, Texas;
currently at
Department of Pediatrics,
University of Miami
School of Medicine,
Miami, FL 33101

Chapter 54

Hurler Syndrome

Description

Hurler syndrome (mucopolysaccharidosis type I—MPS I) appears in 3 forms of varying severity. Hurler syndrome (MPS I-II) is the most severe; Scheie syndrome (MPS I-S) is milder; and Hurler/Scheie syndrome (MPS I-H/S) is considered to be the intermediate form.

Synonyms

Mucopolysaccharidosis Type I

Signs and Symptoms

Newborns with Hurler syndrome (MPS I-II) usually appear normal, although inguinal and umbilical hernias may be present. Onset of symptoms occurs from 6 months to 2 years of age. Craniofacial abnormalities occurring at this time include coarse facial features, a prominent forehead, macroglossia, misaligned teeth, and clouding of the cornea. Also evident are recurrent upper respiratory infections, noisy breathing, and a persistent nasal discharge. Hydrocephalus appears after 2 to 3 years of age. Developmental delay becomes apparent from 1 to 2 years of age. The child is short of stature, and mental retardation is progressive thereafter. Joint stiffness is severe, resulting in claw hand, and kyphoscoliosis and hepatomegaly may develop.

Hurler/Scheie syndrome (MPS I-H/S), the intermediate form, is characterized by normal intelligence but progressive physical involvement that is milder than in Hurler syndrome. Corneal clouding, joint stiffness, deafness, and valvular heart disease can develop by the early to mid teens.

In Scheie syndrome (MPS I-S), the mild form, stature, intelligence and life expectancy are normal. Onset of symptoms such as stiff joints, clouding of the cornea, and aortic valvular disease and/or stenosis usually occurs after 5 years of age, but diagnosis often is not made until the patient is 10 to 20 years.

Diagnosis can be made prenatally.

Etiology

The three forms of Hurler syndrome described above are autosomal recessive, and all are due to alpha-L-iduronidase deficiency.

Epidemiology

Males and females tend to be affected equally. Incidence is approximately 1:100,000 live births.

Related Disorders

The mucolipidoses are a family of similar disorders, producing symptoms very much like those of MPS. Mucolipidoses II resembles Hurler syndrome; the two disorders are very difficult to distinguish.

Treatment

Standard

Treatment is symptomatic and supportive. Physical therapy and medical and genetic counseling services may be useful to patient and family.

Investigational

Treatment approaches for checking early development of MPS are under study. These include enzyme replacement therapy and bone marrow transplantation.

Please contact the agencies listed below for the most current information.

Resources

For more information on Hurler syndrome contact:

National Organization for Rare Disorders (NORD)
PO Box 8923
New Fairfield, CT 06812-8923
(203) 746-6518

National MPS Society
17 Kraemer Street
Hicksville, NY 11801-4321
(516) 931-6338

National Institute of Diabetes, Digestive & Kidney Diseases
Information Clearinghouse
One Information Way
Bethesda, MD 20892-3560

For genetic information and genetic counseling referrals:

March of Dimes Birth Defects Foundation
1275 Mamoroneck Avenue
White Plains, NY 10605
(914) 428-7100

National Center for Education in Maternal and Child Health (NCEMCH)
2000 15th Street N, Suite 701
Arlington, VA 22201-2617
(703) 524-7802

Reference

The Metabolic Basis of Inherited Disease, 6th ed. C.R. Scriver, et al., eds.; McGraw-Hill, 1989. pp. 1573–1574.

Chapter 55

Hypercalcemia

Management of Acute Hypercalcemia

Hypercalcemia is a relatively frequent medical problem. Among its many causes (Table 55.1), by far the most common are cancer and primary hyperparathyroidism. Hypercalcemia requiring urgent attention is most often caused by the former, but it can be caused by the latter (parathyroid crisis) or, rarely, by the other disorders listed in Table 55.1. Distinguishing between cancer-related hypercalcemia and primary hyperparathyroidism is usually not difficult, and the diagnosis is readily confirmed by measurements of serum parathyroid hormone. Most patients with primary hyperparathyroidism have elevated serum concentrations of parathyroid hormone, whereas virtually all patients with cancer-associated hypercalcemia have low concentrations. Hypercalcemia in patients with cancer is usually due to secretion of parathyroid hormone-related protein by the tumor. Less often, it is caused by the secretion of other bone-resorbing substances by the tumor, the conversion of 25-hydroxyvitamin D to 1,25-dihydroxyvitamin D by the tumor, or the local effects of osteolytic bone metastases. Assays for parathyroid hormone-related protein are now available, so the presence of this cause of cancer-related hypercalcemia can be confirmed. Although parathyroid tissue also contains parathyroid hormone-related protein, serum concentrations of the substance are not elevated in primary hyperparathyroidism.

New England Journal of Medicine, Vol. 326, No. 18, April 30, 1992; copyright © 1992 Massachusetts Medical Society. All rights reserved.

This review deals with the care of patients with hypercalcemia who require immediate treatment in the hospital. When hypercalcemia is severe, the immediate steps are similar in all patients and are independent of the cause of the hypercalcemia.

Table 55.1. Causes of Hypercalcemia

Primary Hyperparathyroidism

Cancer
        Parathyroid hormone—related protein
        Ectopic production of 1.25-dihydroxyvitamin D
        Other factors produced ectopically
        Lytic bond metastases

Nonparathyroid endocrine disorders
        Thyrotoxicosis
        Pheochromocytoma
        Adrenal insufficiency
        Vasoactive intestinal polypeptide hormone—producing tumor

Granulomatous diseases (1,25-dihydroxyvitamin D excess)
        Sarcoidosis
        Tuberculosis
        Histoplasmosis
        Coccidioidomycosis
        Leprosy

Medications
        Thiazide diuretics
        Lithium
        Estrogens and antiestrogens

Milk—alkali syndrome

Vitamin A intoxication

Vitamin D intoxication

Familial hypocalciuric hypercalcemia

Immobilization

Parenteral nutrition

Acute and chronic renal insufficiency

Pathophysiologic Mechanisms of Acute Hypercalcemia

The process leading to severe hypercalcemia is initiated by accelerated bone resorption caused by the activation of osteoclasts, which are multinucleated, calcium-resorbing bone cells. These cells are activated by various substances such as parathyroid hormone related protein and parathyroid hormone, and their activation underlies virtually all cases of marked hypercalcemia. Excessive absorption of calcium from the gastrointestinal tract is usually not an important cause of hypercalcemia, although it can contribute to hypercalcemia caused by an excess of vitamin D. Hypercalcemia develops when the entry of calcium from bone into the extracellular space overwhelms the normal mechanisms that maintain normocalcemia. One of these mechanisms—the suppression of parathyroid hormone secretion by calcium—is obviously negated when the cause of accelerated bone resorption is parathyroid hormone. In cancer-associated hypercalcemia, the secretion of parathyroid hormone is suppressed, but the humoral factors that activate osteoclasts (e.g., parathyroid hormone-related protein) are secreted autonomously. In the setting of accelerated bone resorption, the kidney becomes the principal defense against hypercalcemia. When renal function is normal, the tendency for the serum calcium level to rise is attenuated by increased urinary excretion of calcium.

A cascade of events is responsible for the development of severe hypercalcemia, which is defined as a serum calcium concentration greater than 3.50 mmol per liter (14 mg per deciliter), a level usually associated with symptoms of hypercalcemia. First, the factors that induce osteoclast-mediated bone resorption, such as parathyroid hormone or parathyroid hormone-related protein, also stimulate renal tubular reabsorption of calcium, impairing the ability of the kidneys to excrete the increased filtered load of calcium. Second, the hypercalcemic state interferes with the renal mechanisms for the reabsorption of sodium and water, leading to polyuria. This polyuria may not be matched by a commensurate oral intake of fluid because of anorexia and nausea, frequent symptoms of hypercalcemia. The result is a depletion in the volume of extracellular fluid and a reduction in the glomerular filtration rate, which further increases the serum calcium concentration. Hypercalcemia may be exacerbated by immobilization, another stimulus for the loss of bone-related calcium, in severely ill patients. To a greater or lesser extent, these pathophysiologic mechanisms are operative in virtually all patients with severe hypercalcemia.

501

The Decision to Treat

The magnitude of the hypercalcemia is a key consideration in determining the need for immediate, aggressive therapy. If the serum total calcium concentration is greater than 3.50 mmol per liter (the upper limit of normal varies among laboratories but is generally about 2.60 mmol per liter [10.5 mg per deciliter]), immediate treatment is indicated, regardless of symptoms. The value of 3.50 mmol per liter is based on the assumption that the serum albumin concentration is normal, but in patients with severe hypercalcemia the serum albumin concentration may be elevated because of dehydration or reduced because of chronic illness. A convenient rule of thumb is to adjust the serum total calcium concentration by 0.20 mmol per liter (0.8 mg per deciliter) for each 10 g by which the serum albumin level is above or below 40 g per liter (each 1 g above or below 4.0 g per deciliter). If the serum albumin concentration is elevated, the serum total calcium concentration should be adjusted downward; if the serum albumin concentration is reduced, the serum total calcium concentration should be adjusted upward. When the serum calcium concentration is only moderately elevated (3.00 to 3.50 mmol per liter [12 to 14 mg per deciliter]), the clinical manifestations of hypercalcemia should serve as a guide to the type of therapy necessary and the dispatch with which it should be administered.

The clinical manifestations of hypercalcemia reflect disturbances in gastrointestinal, cardiovascular, renal, and central nervous system function. The gastrointestinal symptoms include anorexia, nausea and vomiting, constipation, and rarely, acute pancreatitis. The cardiovascular symptoms include hypertension if intravascular volume is maintained, a shortened QT interval on the electrocardiogram, and enhanced sensitivity to digitalis. The symptoms of renal dysfunction are polyuria, polydipsia, and occasionally nephrocalcinosis. The central nervous system symptoms are cognitive difficulties and apathy, drowsiness, obtundation, or even coma. Few patients have all these symptoms, and some may have none at all. The great variability in the symptoms of hypercalcemia is due in part to the age of the patient, the presence of concurrent medical conditions, the duration of the hypercalcemia, and the rate of increase in the serum calcium concentration. With moderate hypercalcemia, therapeutic decisions should therefore be based not only on the serum calcium concentration but also on the symptoms. The underlying condition, if known, is also a factor that must be considered. When the patient has an incurable, widely disseminated cancer for which no specific therapy is

502

contemplated, less aggressive or even no specific antihypercalcemic treatment may be appropriate.

A particularly difficult issue is presented by patients whose hypercalcemia is in the range one would not usually treat aggressively (less than 3.00 mmol per liter) but who have central nervous system symptoms. It can be exceedingly difficult to ascertain that changes in the sensorium are due to hypercalcemia, not only in older patients whose hypercalcemia is not severe, but also in younger patients, in whom hypercalcemia is likely to be tolerated better. In this setting, it is important to seek other causes of altered central nervous system function before attributing them to hypercalcemia. On the other hand, when the serum calcium level is moderately elevated (3.00 to 3.50 mmol per liter), it is entirely reasonable to suspect that altered central nervous system function is due to hypercalcemia. Reversal of the hypercalcemia should reverse the altered central nervous system function if the conditions are related to each other.

Treatment of Hypercalcemia

There are four basic goals of therapy of hypercalcemia: to correct dehydration, enhance the renal excretion of calcium, inhibit accelerated bone resorption, and treat the underlying disorder.

General Measures

Hydration. The intravenous administration of isotonic saline is the first step in the management of severe hypercalcemia. When the depleted intravascular volume is restored to normal, the serum calcium concentration should decline, at least by the degree to which dehydration raised it. This reduction usually amounts to 0.40 to 0.60 mmol per liter (1.6 to 2.4 mg per deciliter), but hydration alone rarely leads to normalization of the serum calcium concentration in patients with severe hypercalcemia. The expansion of intravascular volume is also helpful because it increases renal calcium clearance. First, the increase in the glomerular filtration rate leads to increased filtration of calcium. Second, proximal tubular sodium and calcium reabsorption, which is increased initially, decreases as the glomerular filtration rate increases. Third, as more sodium and water are presented to distal renal tubular sites, an obligatory calciuresis ensues. The rate of administration of saline should be based on the severity of the hypercalcemia, the extent of dehydration, and the tolerance of the cardiovascular system for volume expansion. A widely used regimen is to administer 2.5 to 4 liters of isotonic saline daily, recognizing the need to adjust the rate of fluid administration or to administer a diuretic agent if symptoms and signs of fluid overload appear.

Loop Diuretic Agents (Furosemide). In addition to hydration with saline, adjunctive therapy with a loop diuretic drug may be indicated. There are two reasons to consider the use of such a drug in the management of hypercalcemia. The first is to facilitate urinary excretion of calcium. Loop diuretics, such as furosemide and ethacrynic acid, enhance the calciuric effects of volume expansion by inhibiting calcium reabsorption in the thick ascending limb of the loop of Henle. Thiazide diuretics should never be used in this situation because they enhance distal tubular reabsorption of calcium and thus may actually exacerbate hypercalcemia. Volume expansion must precede the administration of furosemide, because the drug's effect depends on the delivery of calcium to the ascending limb. Intensive administration of furosemide (80 to 100 mg intravenously every one to two hours) with fluid and electrolyte replacement based on urinary losses is a problematic but effective regimen for the treatment of hypercalcemia. This aggressive approach will lead to marked hypercalciuria, but it requires frequent measurement of water and electrolyte excretion. The condition of patients who are already marginally compensated can be destabilized further if losses of fluid and electrolytes, except calcium, are not matched by adequate replacement therapy. Such intensive therapy with furosemide is not necessary in most patients.

The second reason for considering a loop diuretic is to guard against the volume overload that may accompany the administration of saline. Concern about volume overload is particularly relevant in older patients whose cardiovascular function may be marginal. In this situation, it is reasonable to administer moderate doses of furosemide (for example, 10 to 20 mg intravenously every 6 to 12 hours, depending on the patient's capacity to handle the volume load). If fluid tolerance is not a major concern, furosemide should not be used; it should be held in reserve in case signs of fluid overload become apparent.

Specific Management of Hypercalcemia

The serum calcium concentration will decline appreciably when patients are hydrated with saline. However, the use of saline, with or without furosemide, does not affect the principal pathophysiologic feature of hypercalcemia, which is the excessive mobilization of calcium from bone. Thus, along with the general measures described above, specific therapy to inhibit osteoclast-mediated bone resorption should be instituted in patients who have severe symptoms of hypercalcemia or whose serum calcium concentrations remain moderately or markedly elevated after volume expansion. Such specific therapy is thus indicated in symptomatic patients whose initial serum calcium concentrations are 3.50 mmol per liter or higher. It is also usually indicated in patients who remain symptomatic and have serum calcium levels of more than 3.00 mmol per liter after the administration of saline.

Many of the published studies of osteoclast inhibitors are difficult to interpret because the extent of previous saline and diuretic therapy is not stated. In addition, most studies have involved patients with hypercalcemia caused by cancer or, much less often, primary hyperparathyroidism. Presumably, patients with hypercalcemia caused by other disorders would respond similarly. Finally, it is self-evident that treatment that inhibits osteoclast-mediated bone resorption is not specific treatment of the cause of the hypercalcemia. Treatment of hypercalcemia should not interdict the treatment of its cause.

Bisphosphonates. The bisphosphonates are compounds structurally related to pyrophosphate, which is a normal product of metabolism. Unlike the phosphorus-oxygen-phosphorus bond in pyrophosphate, the phosphorus-carbon-phosphorus bond in the bisphosphonates is a backbone that renders them resistant to phosphatases. They bind to hydroxyapatite in bone and inhibit the dissolution of crystals. Their great affinity for bone and their resistance to degradation account for their extremely long half-life in bone. They are excreted unchanged by the kidney. The chief property shared by all bisphosphonates is their inhibitory effect on osteoclasts; not only can they inhibit osteoclast function, but they can also decrease osteoclast viability. Each bisphosphonate appears to have its own mechanism of osteoclast inhibition. The absorption of these compounds from the gastrointestinal tract is generally poor, averaging less than 10 percent, and it is particularly poor when they are given with food. The intravenous administration of bisphosphonates has proved to be effective therapy for acute hypercalcemia.

There are three bisphosphonates available worldwide: etidronate (1-hydroxyethylidene-1, 1-bisphosphonate, or EHDP), pamidronate (3-amino-1-hydroxypropylidene-1, 1-bisphosphonate, or APD), and clodronate (dichloromethylenebisphosphonate, or Cl_2MBP). Etidronate and pamidronate are available at this time in the United States. In addition to these three compounds, a new generation of bisphos-phonates is currently under investigation.

Etidronate is administered in a dose of 7.5 mg per kilogram of body weight intravenously over a four-hour period daily for three to seven days. The serum calcium concentration begins to decrease within two days after the first dose and reaches its nadir within seven days. The nadir is within the normal range in 60 to 100 percent of patients. The response is better in patients who are well hydrated before etidronate is given. Whether etidronate should be given for seven days depends on the level of hypercalcemia after hydration and on the patient's sensitivity to the drug. Interrupting therapy is reasonable if the patient's serum calcium concentration declines after the first two or three doses by more than 0.50 to 0.75 mmol per liter (2 to 3 mg per deciliter) or if the level is nearly normal. Continuing to administer etidronate until the serum calcium concentration has normalized could lead to a subsequent period of hypocalcemia.

The action of etidronate (and other bisphosphonates) in inhibiting bone resorption is confirmed by the decreases in urinary excretion of calcium and hydroxyproline that accompany the reduction in the serum calcium level. The duration of action of etidronate varies according to the rate of underlying bone resorption. In patients in whom the intravenous administration of etidronate lowered serum calcium concentrations, oral administration has been used in an attempt to prevent recurrent hypercalcemia, but the evidence that it does so is not conclusive.

The treatment of hypercalcemia with etidronate is safe, the only reported adverse effects being transient increases in serum creatinine and phosphate concentrations. Although long-term administration of etidronate can impair bone formation and cause osteomalacia, short-term use does not. This adverse effect of etidronate is not shared by any of the other bisphosphonates currently available or under investigation in the dosages used.

Pamidronate, a much more potent bisphosphonate than etidronate, has also proved to be effective therapy for hypercalcemia. Three different regimens have been used: a slow intravenous infusion of 15 to 45 mg daily for up to six days; a single 24-hour intravenous infusion of up to 90 mg; or the oral administration of 1200 mg daily for up to five days. The time course of the decrease in serum calcium levels is similar to that in patients treated with etidronate. It is difficult to evaluate the studies that have attempted to compare pamidronate and etidronate or the three regimens of pamidronate. The single-dose regimen has been reported to lead to the normalization of serum calcium concentrations in 70 to 100 percent of patients. The intravenous route is preferred in view of the limited gastrointestinal tolerance of many patients with hypercalcemia and the gastrointestinal side effects that may be associated with oral administration of the drug. Oral pamidronate has also been used to prevent hypercalcemia in patients with cancer and bone metastases. The adverse effects of parenteral pamidronate are limited to a mild, transient increase in temperature (less than 2°C), transient leukopenia, and a small reduction in serum phosphate levels.

Clodronate was one of the first bisphosphonates used to treat patients with cancer-related hypercalcemia. It can be administered either as an intravenous infusion in a dose of 4 to 6 mg per kilogram given over a period of two to five hours daily for three to five days or as a single intravenous infusion given over a two-to-nine-hour period. Daily infusion may be associated with more prolonged normocalcemia. Oral clodronate has been reported to be effective, but the intravenous route is preferred in patients with acute hypercalcemia. With intravenous administration, the serum calcium concentration declines at a rate that is typical for the bisphosphonates, the initial substantial decrease occurring after two days and normalization after seven days. Like pamidronate, clodronate has the potential to reduce the progression of metastases and to prevent hypercalcemia in patients with cancer. Clodronate is well tolerated. Potential nephrotoxicity can be avoided by slow infusion over a period of at least two hours. Concern that the drug might be associated with leukemia has not been substantiated.

Plicamycin (Mithramycin). Plicamycin, an inhibitor of RNA synthesis in osteoclasts, is an effective treatment for hypercalcemia. It is given intravenously in a dose of 25 μg per kilogram over a period of four to six hours. The dose can be repeated several times at intervals of 24 to 48 hours, although a single dose may be sufficient to normalize the serum calcium concentration. The serum calcium concentration begins to decrease as early as 12 hours after the administration of the drug, and the maximal reduction occurs in 48 to 72 hours. The duration of normocalcemia after the administration of plicamycin ranges from a few days to several weeks, depending on the extent of on going bone resorption. Recurrent hypercalcemia can be retreated with plicamycin, but toxicity can limit its usefulness in this regard.

Plicamycin has several side effects. Nausea can be minimized by slow intravenous infusion. Care should be taken to avoid extravasation of the drug, because it can cause local irritation and cellulitis.

Hepatic toxicity, most often manifested as transiently elevated serum aminotransferase concentrations, occurs in approximately 20 percent of patients. Nephrotoxicity (an increased serum creatinine concentration and proteinuria) and thrombocytopenia are possible, the latter especially in patients who have previously received chemotherapy or radiotherapy. These adverse effects are infrequent when plicamycin is given in the usual dosage at intervals of several days or more, but are more likely if the interval is shorter and if more than three or four doses are given. Because of the concern over side effects, the use of plicamycin has decreased as other agents have become available that are as effective but do not have the same potential for adverse consequences. Contraindications to the use of plicamycin are overt hepatic or renal dysfunction, thrombocytopenia, or any coagulopathy.

Calcitonin. A naturally occurring peptide hormone, calcitonin, would appear to be an ideal therapy for hypercalcemia because it inhibits bone resorption and also increases renal excretion of calcium. It is usually administered subcutaneously or intramuscularly in the form of salmon calcitonin, in a dosage of 4 units per kilogram every 12 hours, although doses as high as 8 units per kilogram every 6 hours have been used. Among the major anticalcemic agents available, calcitonin has the most rapid onset of action. The serum calcium concentration may decline within a few hours after therapy is initiated. This early effect is likely to be related to the drug's hypercalciuric action. The nadir of the serum calcium concentration is reached within 12 to 24 hours, but it often rebounds despite continued calcitonin administration. Unlike the bisphosphonates and plicamycin, calcitonin is a relatively weak agent, and the maximal reduction in serum calcium associated with its use rarely exceeds 0.5 mmol per liter. Thus, unless the patient has mild hypercalcemia or is unusually responsive to the drug, the serum calcium level is unlikely to become normal (or remain normal should it become so) with calcitonin alone.

The relatively weak and short-lived effect of calcitonin has led to trials of combinations of calcitonin and other agents in an effort to amplify and prolong its lowering of serum calcium. Whether glucocorticoids enhance and prolong the action of calcitonin is controversial. This combination was not more effective than pamidronate or plicamycin in one study. Combination therapy with calcitonin and pamidronate or etidronate has been reported to cause a more rapid decrease in serum calcium than therapy with the diphosphonate alone. Combination chemotherapy is not more effective than the additive effect of each agent alone.

Calcitonin is safe. It occasionally causes mild, transient nausea, abdominal cramps, and flushing. Allergic reactions to salmon calcitonin, the preparation that has been used most widely, are unusual, although an initial skin test with 1 unit of salmon calcitonin is recommended before therapy is initiated. Human calcitonin, which is not as potent as salmon calcitonin, is not likely to offer a great advantage over salmon calcitonin.

Despite the fact that calcitonin is a relatively short acting and only moderately effective agent, it has a role in the treatment of hypercalcemia. When hypercalcemia is severe and the need to lower the serum calcium concentration is urgent, calcitonin will induce the most rapid, albeit moderate, decrease in the serum calcium level. In such a setting, it is reasonable to administer one or two doses of calcitonin while therapy with more long-lasting, more potent, but slower acting agents such as plicamycin, bisphosphonate, or gallium nitrate is being considered. In addition to its calcium-lowering action, calcitonin has potent analgesic properties and can therefore provide impressive relief of pain in some patients with metastatic skeletal disease.

Gallium Nitrate. Gallium nitrate has been approved by the Food and Drug Administration for the parenteral therapy of hypercalcemia. It appears to inhibit bone resorption by adsorbing to and reducing the solubility of hydroxyapatite crystals. Gallium nitrate does not alter the histologic features of bone cells, and there is no evidence that it impairs osteoclast function directly. Clinically, its use is accompanied by reductions in the urinary excretion of calcium and hydroxyproline, confirming its action as an inhibitor of bone resorption. Gallium nitrate is administered as a continuous intravenous infusion (200 mg per square meter of body surface area in 1 liter of fluid daily) for five days. In a controlled, double-blind study comparing calcitonin with gallium nitrate, the serum calcium concentration fell to normal more frequently with gallium nitrate (75 percent vs. 31 percent) and for a longer period (six days vs. one day). The decrease in the serum calcium concentration, however, was slower in the patients treated with gallium nitrate; their serum calcium concentrations did not reach normal until the five-day infusion was completed, and the nadir was not reached until three days later. In a study comparing gallium nitrate and etidronate, the serum calcium concentration fell to normal in 82 percent of the patients who received gallium and 43 percent of those who received etidronate. In that study, however, the rate of response to therapy with etidronate was unusually low in comparison with that in most other published reports.

A major side effect of gallium nitrate is nephrotoxicity, manifested by an increase in the serum creatinine concentration. Other potential nephrotoxic agents, such as aminoglycosides, should not be administered to patients receiving gallium nitrate therapy. Careful attention to the patient's state of hydration is required. The drug should not be given to patients with renal insufficiency. Other reported side effects are hypophosphatemia and a small reduction in the hemoglobin concentration. Although gallium nitrate is a promising therapeutic agent for hypercalcemia, clinical experience with it is still quite limited.

Glucocorticoids. Under certain circumstances, glucocorticoids can be effective calcium-lowering agents. For this purpose, 200 to 300 mg of hydrocortisone, or its equivalent, is given intravenously every day for three to five days. The actions of glucocorticoids in inhibiting the growth of neoplastic lymphoid tissue account for their beneficial effects in some patients with hematologic cancers such as lymphoma and multiple myeloma. Their actions in counteracting the effects of vitamin D account for their efficacy in patients with hypercalcemia caused by excess vitamin D, as in vitamin D intoxication or granulomatous diseases. In general, patients with nonhematologic cancers do not respond to glucocorticoids, nor do those with primary hyperparathyroidism.

Phosphate. The serum calcium concentration can be lowered rapidly and profoundly by intravenous administration of sodium phosphate. This treatment, however, is very dangerous because of the risk that calcium-phosphate complexes will be deposited in blood vessels, lungs, and kidneys. Precipitation of these complexes can lead to severe organ damage and even fatal hypotension. The use of intravenous phosphate should therefore be restricted to patients with extreme, life-threatening hypercalcemia in whom all other measures have failed. Oral phosphate is of little value in the therapy of severe hypercalcemia because its calcium lowering activity is limited and because amounts of more than 2 g a day are often associated with diarrhea. Hyperphosphatemia and azotemia are contraindications to phosphate therapy.

Other Therapies. Prostaglandins have been implicated as local mediators of osteolysis in some patients with cancer-related hypercalcemia. Despite a sound rationale and encouraging early reports, the efficacy of prostaglandin synthetase inhibitors in such patients

510

is very limited. Amifostine (WR-2721) is a chemoprotective agent that showed early promise as a useful anticalcemic. It inhibits parathyroid hormone secretion and bone resorption and facilitates the urinary excretion of calcium. This drug, however, has not proved very useful in the setting of acute hypercalcemia because its effects are rather limited and very transient. Moreover, it frequently causes nausea vomiting, somnolence, and hypotension. Dialysis is very effective in lowering the serum calcium concentration. Either peritoneal dialysis or hemodialysis using a low-calcium bath can be particularly effective in patients with renal failure. Ambulation should be encouraged in any patient with hypercalcemia to prevent the mobilization of skeletal calcium associated with the loss of weight bearing.

Choice of Agent

No one regimen for the therapy of acute hypercalcemia is applicable to all clinical settings. Variations in the cause of hypercalcemia, in the extent to which hypercalcemia is a clinical problem and therefore in the urgency of the need to reduce it, and in the actions and side effects of the different treatments all argue for the importance of tailoring the therapy to the individual patient. When hypercalcemia is mild (serum calcium level, <3.00 mmol per liter), hydration with saline is often adequate, and most patients do not require drug therapy. Even when hypercalcemia is more severe, hydration with saline is the first step in management. However, if time is of the essence because hypercalcemia is life-threatening (serum calcium level, >4.00 mmol per liter [16 mg per deciliter]), unequivocally symptomatic, or both, more specific therapy is required in addition to saline. In this situation, the most rapid-acting osteoclast inhibitor, calcitonin, becomes a first-line drug. Since calcitonin alone is unlikely to reduce the serum calcium concentration to normal, however, additional therapy should be considered. If there are no contraindications, such as renal or hepatic dysfunction, thrombocytopenia, or coagulopathy, plicamycin is a good choice. It has the advantage of being relatively rapid-acting and is given in a single dose. Alternatively, a bisphosphonate can be used. If the hypercalcemic state is likely to be sensitive to steroids, the concurrent administration of calcitonin and glucocorticoids is worthy of consideration.

There are times when, despite the presence of marked hypercalcemia, there is less need for an urgent reduction in serum calcium. For example, in a patient whose serum calcium level is high (>3.50 mmol per liter) but who has only moderate symptoms of hypercalcemia and whose condition is otherwise stable, one might use a bisphosphonate along with saline (with or without furosemide), rather than calcitonin or plicamycin. A bisphosphonate would be preferred for such a patient because it is more potent than calcitonin and less toxic than plicamycin. The indications for the use of gallium nitrate are not yet clear, because clinical experience with the drug is still quite limited. It appears, however, that gallium nitrate is similar to plicamycin and the bisphosphonates in potency and in rapidity of action. The side effects of gallium nitrate preclude its use when renal function is impaired or when potentially nephrotoxic antibiotics are being used. Finally, in rare patients the serum calcium concentration may be higher than 5.00 mmol per liter (20 mg per deciliter). Such patients require the most aggressive approach and should be treated with calcitonin, plicamycin, and perhaps hydrocortisone as well. A bisphosphonate could be substituted for plicamycin, especially if hepatic or renal dysfunction is apparent.

Therapy of the Underlying Disorder

The actions of the measures described to reduce the serum calcium concentration quickly are temporary. Patients whose serum calcium levels have been normalized by treatment are still subject to the same pathophysiologic events that initially led to the hypercalcemic state, and hypercalcemia can thus recur. It may be possible to keep the serum calcium level normal or nearly normal by vigorous oral hydration; oral bisphosphonates may be useful for this purpose. Definitive therapy of hypercalcemia, however, requires treatment of the underlying disorder. For example, successful parathyroidectomy will prevent the recurrence of parathyroid crisis if acute hyperparathyroidism was the cause of the hypercalcemia. A more difficult task is the management of a cancer causing hypercalcemia, because it is usually advanced by the time the hypercalcemia develops. Regardless of cause, successfully managing acute hypercalcemia provides time to plan for the management of the underlying disease.

— by John P. Bilezikian, M.D.,
Departments of Medicine and Pharmacology,
College of Physicians and Surgeons,
Columbia University, New York;
supported in part by a grant (DK32333)
from the NIH.

Chapter 56

Neuroendocrine Manifestations of Acquired Immune Deficiency Syndrome AIDS

Over one million persons in the United States are infected with the HIV virus. In its later stages, the Acquired Immune Deficiency Syndrome (AIDS) is characterized by progressive immune dysfunction and unexplained weight loss. Recent observations suggest that neuroendocrine dysfunction is frequent in patients with HIV disease and may contribute to the wasting syndrome. The endocrine systems most commonly affected in patients with AIDS include the adrenal, gonadal and growth hormone axes. Adrenal insufficiency and hypogonadism most commonly result from disturbed hypothalamic and pituitary regulation of ACTH and gonadotropin secretion, but primary disease of the adrenals and gonads has been well described in this population. In addition, many of the medications now used to treat HIV disease and its associated opportunistic infections, including megesterol acetate (Megace), are known to affect pituitary function. In this article, the neuroendocrine manifestations of AIDS will be reviewed. In addition, recent advances in our understanding of potential endocrine mechanisms of the wasting syndrome and anabolic strategies to reverse weight loss in this population will be discussed.

The adrenal axis is commonly affected in HIV disease: adrenal insufficiency is seen in 4% and abnormal Cosyntropin tests in 17% of hospitalized patients with AIDS. Primary adrenal insufficiency is most commonly due to destruction of adrenal tissue by cytomegalovirus

From *Neuroendocrine Center Bulletin*, Vol. 1, Issue 2, Summer 1996, Massachusetts General Hospital, 55 Fruit Street, BUL 457B, Boston, MA 02114-2696; reprinted with permission.

(CMV), which is frequently seen at autopsy. Because destruction of adrenal tissue must be extensive for this to occur, adrenal insufficiency secondary to CMV adrenalitis is still relatively rare. Primary adrenal disease has also been described as a result of infection with typical and atypical tuberculosis. Finally, adrenal insufficiency may be caused by hypothalamic or pituitary disease from opportunistic infection or idiopathic inflammation and tissue destruction. Panhypopituitarism related to toxoplasmosis and CMV have been well described in patients with AIDS, and idiopathic pituitary necrosis was recently described in 11% of patients at autopsy, suggesting that HIV may have a direct effect on pituitary tissue. In addition to overt adrenal insufficiency, which is life threatening, patients with AIDS may have more subtle impairments in adrenal function which may manifest as exaggerated ACTH responses to CRH and decreased adrenal androgen production.

Elevated cortisol levels without associated symptoms of cortisol excess have also been described in patients with early and late stage HIV disease and may relate to stress, abnormalities in cortisol binding globulin (CBG) and/or a newly defined glucocorticoid resistance syndrome. Evaluation of the cortisol axis should proceed as in other patients with suspected adrenal dysfunction. Cosyntropin testing is usually an adequate first step, except in those patients in whom hypothalamic or pituitary insufficiency of recent onset is suspected. In patients with clinical symptoms of adrenal insufficiency and elevated cortisol levels, cortisol resistance may be present. In addition, use of CRH testing may be a new strategy to detect early primary adrenal insufficiency in this population. It is important to remember that Megace, a potent synthetic progestational agent, also impairs adrenal function.

Gonadal dysfunction is common among patients with AIDS. Thirty to fifty percent of men with AIDS exhibit hypogonadism and low serum levels of testosterone. Less is known of gonadal function in women with AIDS, but preliminary data demonstrate oligoamenorrhea in approximately 25%. The mechanism of hypogonadism in these patients is unknown but appears to be central in the majority of cases. Potential mechanisms include severe illness and cytokine effects, elevated cortisol levels and/or severe under-nutrition. In addition, Megace may also affect gonadal function in this population. Of note, a primary defect in gonadal function is seen in 25-35% of cases and may relate to testicular destruction by opportunistic infection. More often, only nonspecific inflammation is seen and a direct role of HIV and/or paracrine effects of local cytokines has been postulated but not proven. Because sex hormone binding globulin levels may be significantly increased in up to 50% of men with AIDS, assessment of gonadal function must include measurement of free testosterone levels. The significance of hypogonadism in this population may relate to the pathogenesis of the wasting syndrome and the disproportionate loss of lean body and muscle mass with advancing HIV disease.

Abnormalities in the GH-IGF-I axis have also been reported recently in patients with AIDS, with decreased serum levels of IGF-I and increased GH levels. Resistance to endogenous GH has been suggested based on evidence of abnormal IGF-I responses to GH administration. Preliminary work investigating the effects of rhGH in patients with AIDS suggests that GH may be efficacious in altering body composition. However, large pharmacologic doses of GH may be necessary to overcome endogenous GH resistance and long-term benefits have not been established. Further work is needed to characterize GH secretory dynamics, regulation of binding proteins, production of IGF-I and the anabolic responses to GH in this population.

The potential contribution of neuroendocrine dysfunction to the wasting syndrome in AIDS has recently become a major focus of research interest at the Massachusetts General Hospital and at other centers around the country. The AIDS Wasting Syndrome affects over 75% of men with AIDS who have lost more than 10% of their initial body weight. More importantly, the weight loss is characterized by a disproportionate loss of lean body and muscle mass, which may contribute to the fatigue and inanition characteristic of late stage disease. The mechanisms of the wasting syndrome have not yet been elucidated, but may relate to the loss of the potent anabolic hormone, testosterone, which is deficient in 30-50% of all men with AIDS. Because testosterone is known to be a critical hormone in the maintenance of lean body and muscle mass in aging men and other populations with acquired gonadal dysfunction, clinical studies are now underway in the Neuroendocrine Unit to determine the mechanisms of gonadal dysfunction in men and women with AIDS and the potential use of testosterone and other anabolic factors to reduce weight loss and increase lean body mass in this population.

Selected References

1. Croxson TS, Chapman WE, Miller LK, Levit CD, Senie R, and Zumoff B. 1989. Changes in the hypothalamic-pituitary-gonadal axis in human immunodeficiency virus-infected homosexual men. *J Clin Endocrinol Metab* 68:317-21.

2. Findling J, Buggy B, Gilson IH, Brummitt C, Bernstein B, and Raff H. 1994. Longitudinal Evaluation of Adrenocortical Function in Patients Infected with the Human Immunodeficiency Virus. *J Clin Endocrinol Metab* 79:1091-1096.

3. Grinspoon SK, and Bilezikian JB. 1992. HIV Disease and the Endocrine System. N Engl J Med. 327:1360-1365.

4. Krentz AJ, Koster FT, Crist DM, Finn K, Johnson LZ, Boyle PJ, and Schade DS.1993.Anthropometric, metabolic, and immunological effects of recombinant human growth hormone in AIDS and AIDS-related complex. *J Acquir Immune Defic Syndr* 6:245-51.

5. Membreno L, Irony I, Dere W, et al. 1987. Adrenocortical Function in Acquired Immunodeficiency Syndrome. *J Clin Endocrinol Metab* 65:482-487.

—*by Steven Grinspoon, M.D.*

Chapter 57

Phenylketonuria (PKU)

Introduction

Phenylketonuria, called PKU for short, is an inherited condition which prevents the affected individual from normally metabolizing— or using—phenylalanine (phe), one of the essential amino acids found in all protein foods. Unless the condition is detected and treatment is initiated soon after birth, this hereditary biochemical abnormality prevents normal brain development and usually results in severe mental retardation. Other manifestations such as skin rash, seizures, excessive restlessness, irritable behavior and a musty body odor may also be present.

Fortunately, detection of the condition shortly after birth through the use of a routine blood screening procedure has become standard practice in every state and Canadian province since 1991. Placing the baby on a phenylalanine-restricted diet within the first weeks of life, and maintaining good diet control thereafter, is effective in preventing the damaging effects of PKU. Treatment requires elimination of foods naturally high in protein. Special care must be taken to maintain enough—but not too much—phe in the child's diet. Such a balance is obtained only through careful nutritional, biochemical and medical supervision, and considerable effort by the parents.

This chapter contains excerpts from the National Institute of Child Health and Human Development, "The Mental Retardation and Developmental Disabilities Branch Report to Council," January 1993 and NIH Pub. No. 92-3318, "Education of Students with Phenylketonuria (PKU)."

Beginning at an early age, most children with PKU learn to discriminate between foods that are allowed on their diet from those that are not. However, maintaining the diet may become more difficult when a child with PKU enrolls in school. "Swapping" lunch items may be a temptation; or students may try a diet soft drink which uses the artificial sweetener, *NutraSweet* (a product containing phe).

Benefits of Treatment

Untreated or late-treated persons with PKU usually develop mild to severe mental retardation. Therefore, it is imperative that the diagnosis of PKU be established within the first days of life, before the onset of mental damage. All states and Canadian provinces have blood screening programs to detect PKU shortly after birth, and similar programs are in place in many other countries.

The Collaborative Study of Children Treated for Phenylketonuria has demonstrated the value of the phe-restricted diet in preventing mental retardation without affecting physical growth and development (Williamson et al., 1981). When treatment is instituted within the first few days of life, and the diet is maintained as prescribed by a PKU treatment center, normal development can be anticipated (Holtzman et al., 1986).

Like other children, those with PKU contract the usual childhood illnesses, and during periods of high fever, the child's blood phe levels may rise dramatically. It is the general consensus that these deviations from optimal phe levels are best ignored; they are transient, have not proven detrimental, and should not be the source of parental anxiety. Of greater significance are the long-term effects of persistently high blood phe levels due to chronic poor dietary control.

At this time, early treated children with PKU are enrolled in public schools, and many cannot be distinguished from non-PKU children, except by their adherence to a special diet (Azen et al., 1991). However, a number of early and well-treated children with PKU have some discrete mild to moderate learning disabilities despite normal IQs. These problems are often in the mathematics area and may be complicated by distractibility and short attention span. The exact number of these learning disabled children with PKU is not yet clear. It is important that these difficulties be identified early so that remedial steps can be taken and the inevitable frustration and subsequent behavior problems be avoided or minimized. Some of the oldest individuals identified by newborn screening, and compliant to long-term phenylalanine restrictions, have graduated from high school and are successfully pursuing college educations (Koch et al., 1985; Fishler, et al., 1987; Fishler et al., 1989).

During the 1960s and 70s, it was common practice to discontinue diet therapy during childhood. In the 1980s, data suggested that there were IQ changes in children in the Collaborative Study of Children Treated for Phenylketonuria who had discontinued the phe-restricted diet (Koch et al., 1987). Therefore, it is now believed that the continued use of the phe-restricted diet is indicated throughout school and indefinitely. It has been established that women with PKU who are not on the diet will have babies with birth defects and mental retardation (Lenke and Levy, 1980). The Maternal PKU Collaborative Study is locating young women with PKU reaching child-bearing age to inform them of this problem and to encourage them to stay on (or to return to) a restricted-phe diet, and thus reduce the possibility of damage to their unborn child (American Academy of Pediatrics, 1985; Koch et al., 1991).

Screening, Diagnosis and Incidence

After its discovery in 1934 by Dr. A. Folling in Norway, and until the early 1960s, PKU was detected with a urine "wet diaper" test. This method has many disadvantages, and since 1964 has been replaced by a blood test which can be administered with great accuracy as early as the first few days of life. Infants initially screened before 24 hours of age should be rescreened by three weeks of age (American Academy of Pediatrics, 1982). When the baby has higher than normal levels of phe in the blood, confirmatory tests must be performed, and if the diagnosis is established, diet treatment begins as soon as possible. Results from the Collaborative Study of Children Treated for Phenylketonuria clearly indicate a loss in IQ scores if the baby is not put on the diet within the first 20 days of life and kept in good dietary control.

Approximately five children with PKU are born in the United States each week. This means an estimated incidence of one baby with PKU born in about 15,000 live births.

Diet Management

Proper diet management is essential in the treatment of PKU. This involves severely limiting the child's intake of all foods containing protein. Protein contains the amino acid, phenylalanine (phe), which the child cannot effectively utilize. Milk and other dairy products, meat, fish, eggs, dried beans and peas, and nuts are concentrated sources of phe; fruits, vegetables, and cereals contain smaller amounts. The only foods that do not contain phe are sugar, oil, pure starch and water; and products made with these ingredients such as hard candy and soft drinks. Special medical foods which provide protein and important nutrients are an essential part of the food intake pattern of individuals with PKU. Special low protein foods and baking ingredients are available from several companies.

Normally, the body uses a small part of the phe from dietary protein for growth and repair of body tissue, and changes part of the phe into other useful chemical compounds such as tyrosine. Tyrosine is another amino acid and is needed to make proteins, hormones and neurotransmitters which control brain functions. Tyrosine also helps to make pigments for skin and hair coloring. The enzyme necessary to convert excess phe into tyrosine does not work effectively in the person with PKU. The absence of tyrosine combined with the excess phe and abnormal compounds circulating in the body leads to brain damage. This is particularly true in the first few years of life when dietary compliance is critical to prevent damage and to insure normal growth and development.

Even after reaching school age, continued use of a restricted-phe diet is indicated. The Collaborative Study of Children Treated for Phenylketonuria found that children with PKU who were taken off diet began to show a drop in I.Q. scores and poorer school performance (Williamson et al., 1981).

The special PKU diet is designed to give each individual the exact amount of phe required for adequate growth and to prevent buildup of harmful amounts. This delicate balance, unique to each person, is achieved by careful measuring of all food and calculating the phe intake on a daily basis. Nutritionists and parents have developed cookbooks and food lists to assist in this exacting task. Frequent blood tests are necessary to monitor the blood phe levels and to determine dietary effectiveness.

In order to supply the other essential elements of protein needed for normal growth and development, a special protein source is necessary. These sources of protein, called medical foods, contain all the amino acids except that most or all of the phe has been removed. Some of the products have added fat and carbohydrates, while all have been fortified with vitamins and minerals. These medical foods are generally taken as a liquid beverage. The medical food plus carefully selected foods low in protein provide a balanced diet for the child. Often the student with PKU will take the product before or after school, rather than bring it to school.

Special diet management problems may occur at school. For example, young children with PKU cannot have a high protein snack. Special events, such as a birthday, may involve a cake containing forbidden high-phe food ingredients. Because the child with PKU should not eat these foods, he/she may be identified as "different." Parents commonly provide alternatives for their child. However, teachers and administrators must be aware of potential problems and help the child with PKU to participate maximally in all activities, including snacktime and parties by notifying parents to send substitutes.

If a school lunch program is provided, some foods can be safely eaten by the child with PKU. It is often helpful to send the week's menu home so the parents can indicate which items (and in what quantity) are allowed, and which must be avoided, and return the menu to the teacher. By the time children with PKU reach middle school, and often earlier, they themselves will be able to identify foods that are on their diet. However, they may still require help in determining the appropriate quantity. The ability of children with PKU to participate in the same lunchroom program as their classmates, if appropriate, will lessen the feelings of being different, and thus contribute to the student's healthy social and emotional growth.

Role of School Personnel

As children treated for PKU reach school age, like all children, they move out from the protective environment of their home to a more complex school situation. The child with PKU may wish to experiment with foods that other children are eating. The teacher and other school personnel need to be aware of the potential danger that such innocent food-swapping holds for the child with PKU. While an occasional dietary indiscretion will not cause serious harm, frequent variations—especially when not reported to the parents—could lead to problems which will affect school performance and behavior. An important role for school personnel, therefore, is to work effectively with the parents in maintaining good dietary control.

Children who have been diagnosed early and maintained on an appropriate PKU diet are subject to the same problems, likes and dislikes as other school children of the same age. Variations in height, weight or other physical aspects are probably unrelated to the existence of PKU, or to dietary treatment. The Collaborative Study of Children Treated for Phenylketonuria found that children who have been identified early and satisfactorily treated for PKU have normal growth and development. Likewise, the average IQ scores of children in the study were near the mean score of 100 (Koch et al., 1984). An evaluation of psycho-educational measures, such as the Illinois Test of Psycholinguistic Abilities, the Frostig Visual Perception Test, and the Bender-Gestalt Test, revealed no special profiles of strengths or weaknesses in children early-treated for PKU. Average school achievement was also near expected levels (Fishler et al., 1989).

It may be desirable for the teacher or other school personnel to provide a direct educational program to explain the child's need for a special diet to other children in the class, and perhaps to the parents of the non-PKU children. Young children can be thoughtless in dealing with a classmate whom they discover is "different" in some way. The teacher's simple explanation of the special diet should help the other children accept it.

As the child grows older, peer pressure to conform with dress standards and social behavior, including eating habits, increases the likelihood that the child will experiment with various foods that may contain excessive amounts of phe. For the adolescent female, remaining on the diet is especially important as she approaches childbearing age. Without restriction in phe-intake before and during pregnancy, a woman with PKU risks extensive damage to her unborn child. Directors of PKU clinics are recommending that females with PKU remain on a low phe diet throughout their school and childbearing years, as it is much more difficult to return to the diet after an unrestricted period (Holtzman et al., 1986). This represents a relatively recent change in policy. Previously, it was thought that the diet could be discontinued soon after the child entered school. Secondary school counselors and guidance personnel can be helpful in reinforcing the need for continued dietary restrictions during the adolescent years and into adulthood.

The Elementary School Student with PKU

By the time the child with PKU reaches school age, parents will have had several years' experience with dietary treatment. The child's medical experiences will be different from his or her peers due to the special diet, periodic visits to the PKU clinic, and frequent blood tests. As a result, it is important for the school to be sensitive not only to the child's diet but also to emotional and social needs. The child's emotional needs are best met by treating him or her as much like a non-PKU child as possible. However, children with special needs often require a little extra support from parents and teachers to feel accepted and "normal." Based on experience with children in the Collaborative Study of Children Treated for Phenylketonuria, teachers, counselors and administrators in preschool or elementary schools should take special note of the following:

- While children are curious about each other and are quick to note differences such as a special diet, they are also able to understand the concept of a "food allergy." Thus, no attempt should be made to hide the fact that the child with PKU has a different kind of lunch, nor should any lengthy explanation be required at this age.

- Since many schools utilize a "lunch supervisor," that individual should be acquainted with the basic dietary problems associated with PKU. The supervisor should also be aware of the need to avoid excessive attention to the child. Occasional indiscretions are not fatal, and as children with PKU grow older they must take more and more responsibility for their own dietary management. The teacher can assist the child in building the inner controls.

- Some school personnel have been known to overreact to a diagnosis of PKU. One school classified a child with PKU as "orthopedically handicapped" and imposed a limited, adaptive physical education program that was totally unwarranted. Unless the treatment has been initiated late, or the diet not maintained satisfactorily, the child with PKU is not different from other children in physical ability or general health. Similarly, regular school procedures should be followed when a child with PKU becomes ill at school. PKU is not associated with any sudden, dramatic episodes such as the insulin reaction experienced by diabetics, or the grand mal seizure of a child with epilepsy.

- The child with PKU who was diagnosed early and maintained on the special diet will most often have educational needs that are unaffected by PKU. The child with PKU needs to be treated as any normal child, with strengths and weaknesses, likes and dislikes, and a learning style unrelated to the PKU condition. Most early-diagnosed children with PKU whose diet has been well managed should be able to participate in the regular school program on an age-appropriate basis.

The Adolescent Student with PKU

By secondary school age, the adolescent with PKU should have assumed responsibility for much of his or her own dietary control. For example, he or she might consume some of the PKU medical food products before and after school, and select foods from the school luncheon menu, including salads, vegetables, fruits, and fruit juices (Rees and Trahms, 1986). As indicated earlier, school counselors and teachers should be aware of the recommendation by the Maternal PKU Collaborative Study that a restricted-phe diet be continued indefinitely. It is imperative that women maintain the diet throughout the entire childbearing years (Rohr, 1987).

At the junior or senior high school level, when the curriculum calls for nutrition or cooking classes, it is especially important for the teacher to be in close contact with the parents and the student. They will have, or know of, materials similar to that contained in the "Resources" section at the end of this chapter. These can be useful supplements to the regular school texts, thus enabling the student with PKU to be included. The need for students with PKU to monitor their diet can serve as a model, especially for children with other kinds of diet problems. Special low protein foods may be baked and served. Science fair projects can be designed by the students to illustrate the genetic and biochemical reactions involved in PKU (see references for teachers in Resources section).

Teachers and counselors in secondary schools can assist the Maternal PKU Collaborative Study in locating young women who were on the PKU diet as a child. This could be done by having the teacher, nurse, physical education or health instructor note on the health record which students they remember being on the "PKU diet" or a special diet in childhood. If appropriate, the young woman and/or her parents should be urged to call a PKU treatment center in order to obtain important information concerning the effect of PKU on pregnancy (Rohr, 1987; Acosta, 1991).

The Maternal PKU Collaborative Study is designed to locate young women with hyperphenylalaninemia (PKU), to inform them of the problems their babies will have if the PKU is not controlled before and during pregnancy, and to assist them in returning to a phe-restricted diet. Women wishing to return to the diet prior to considering pregnancy, or who are already pregnant, will be enrolled in the study. The pregnancy will be monitored to maintain the safe levels of phe and the other essential elements needed to have a much better chance of having healthy babies. The location of the nearest Maternal PKU Center can be obtained by contacting the appropriate regional Contributing Center of the Maternal PKU Collaborative Study (see list included in Resources section).

Research Programs

Phenylketonuria is an autosomally inherited metabolic disorder that has an incidence of one in every 10,000-15,000 newborn children. The condition is due to a defect in a liver enzyme, phenylalanine hydroxylase (PAH). Untreated babies with PKU exhibit severe mental retardation, behavioral problems, irritability, epilepsy, and other signs of brain impairment. Neonatal screening programs for PKU, which were initiated in the early 1960's, have been successful in diagnosing virtually all infants with PKU within a few weeks of birth. Treatment of genetically affected babies with a special diet containing restricted levels of phenylalanine, an amino acid that is essential for normal growth and development, has largely prevented or mitigated the development of severe intellectual and neurological handicaps that would otherwise occur in a majority of untreated cases.

Using recombinant DNA technology, a [National Institute of Child Health and Human Development]–supported investigator mapped the PAH locus on the long arm of chromosome 12 (12q22-24) and cloned the gene involved in PKU. Mutations in the human PAH gene producing PKU have now been identified in many patients from various ethnic groups.

Extensive population genetic studies have demonstrated that the majority of PKU mutations are restricted to a few major haplotypes. This led to the development of a simple, reliable, and sensitive DNA-based strategy for carrier screening and prenatal diagnosis, which cannot be accomplished with the current Guthrie filter paper blood test for PKU. Approximately 80-90% of all PKU mutations could be detected through the use of RFLP (restriction fragment length polymorphism), VNTR (variable number of tandem repeats), and STS (sequence tagged site) probes.

In related studies, researchers have examined the biochemical and clinical consequences of particular PKU mutations. This involves detailed structural and kinetic analysis on the PAH enzyme, including site-directed mutagenesis to alter specific aspects of enzyme function. This has aided in the diagnosis of specific types of PKU (i.e., genotypes), and the development of therapeutic strategies optimized for a particular genotype. More recently, a number of PKU alleles has been identified that lack any defect in the structural region of the PAH gene; this has prompted research into the regulatory aspects of PAH gene expression.

Current studies are laying the groundwork for gene therapy. Partial hepatectomy was performed in a mouse model for PKU. PAH-deficient hepatocytes were cultured and infected with a retroviral vector containing the PAH gene. The transfected cells regained the ability to convert phenylalanine to tyrosine in vitro. Experiments are now underway to transplant back these transfected cells into PAH-deficient mice to determine whether they can maintain high enough levels of liver PAH to prevent the occurrence of PKU-associated pathology.

Maternal PKU

In the past, virtually all phenylketonuric women of child-bearing age were mentally retarded and bore few, if any, children. Soon after Guthrie described a simple, rapid and economical method of testing for elevated levels of blood phenylalanine, newborn screening for PKU in the United States became an accepted standard of medical practice. Newborn screening followed by early dietary treatment with restricted levels of phenylalanine has resulted in normal physical and intellectual development among girls with PKU, many of whom have already reached, or are approaching, the child-bearing age. It has been known for several decades that elevated levels of maternal phenylalanine exert a teratogenic effect on the fetus. But it was not until 1980 when a landmark international survey was published, that the scientific significance and societal impact of maternal PKU became more obvious. The international survey demonstrated an association between blood phenylalanine levels during pregnancy and the prevalence of mental retardation, microcephaly, congenital heart disease, low birth weight in the offspring and spontaneous abortion. In addition to these observations, it has been projected that the incidence of new cases of PKU-related mental retardation will return to its former level after one generation, if women reproduce at a normal rate without dietary regulation of phenylalanine during pregnancy. Unless corrective measures are developed and applied, this epidemiologic projection will offset the demonstrated benefits of the neonatal screening for PKU.

In 1984, in response to this major public health problem, the MRDD Branch initiated a collaborative study designed to evaluate the efficacy of a phenylalanine-restricted diet during or before pregnancy in reducing the morbidity that is associated with maternal PKU. In order to enroll an adequate sample size for a meaningful analysis, the study was organized to include regional contributing centers which would coordinate the enrollment and follow-up of subjects. In addition, a data coordinating center was established which is responsible for the collection and analyses of data submitted by the contributing centers following a common protocol. About 130 centers are participating in the United States and 18 in all Canadian provinces. Last year, contributing clinics from Germany, Austria and Switzerland were added to the study to assure enrollment of sufficient number of women with PKU who are placed on a phenylalanine-restricted diet before, or shortly after, pregnancy.

The study has found that, based on a still limited number of subjects, babies born to mothers who were treated preconceptionally and have kept their phenylalanine levels between 2 and 6 mg/dL, appear to have improved reproductive outcome, based on weight, length, and head measurements at birth, compared to those whose mothers had higher levels during pregnancy. Definitive data are not yet available on postnatal growth and development or intellectual ability of the offspring of women with PKU. The children in this collaborative study are still too young for substantial evaluation of these parameters, especially for reliable intelligence testing or measurement of school achievement. Early developmental testing does suggest that metabolic control during pregnancy with a phenylalanine-restricted diet is important for psychosocial development, but confirmation of these results must await further evaluation of the offspring.

Glossary

Amino Acids: Organic compounds which combine to form proteins. An "essential" amino acid must be supplied by food; a "non-essential" amino acid can be produced within the body.

Enzyme: A chemical compound which changes one substance into another (i.e., a catalyst). The enzyme, phenylalanine hydroxylase, is the one that is defective in individuals with PKU—thus they are unable to convert the amino acid, phenylalanine, into other products.

"Equal": An artificial sweetener containing aspartame, which is 56% phenylalanine (phe) and thus must be totally avoided by persons with PKU.

Hyperphenylalaninemia: The term used to designate a number of conditions (one of which is classical PKU) in which the individual exhibits elevated levels of phenylalanine in the blood.

Maternal PKU: The problems associated with pregnancy where the mother-to-be has PKU.

Medical Foods: These are special formulas designed to provide the person with PKU with the needed protein, but with little or no phenylalanine. Some of these products and their manufacturers are:

- "Lofenalac" (Mead Johnson), "Analog XP" (Ross Laboratories), and "PKU I" (Mead Johnson) are commonly used with infants with PKU;

- "Maxamaid XP" (Ross Laboratories), "Phenyl-Free" (Mead Johnson), "PKU 2," "PKU 3" (Mead Johnson), and "PKU Aid" (Anglo-Dietetics Ltd.) provide school-aged children with the needed protein source.

- "Maxamum XP" (Ross Laboratories) and "PKU 3" (Mead Johnson) are utilized for pregnant PKU women.

"Nutra-Sweet": A sugar substitute found in many "diet" products such as soft drinks. It is made of aspartame which contains 56% phenylalanine and therefore, like "Equal" should not be used by persons with PKU.

Phenylketonuria: An inherited error of metabolism in which the individual cannot metabolize (or use) the essential amino acid, phenylalanine.

PKU: A common abbreviation for phenylketonuria.

Phenylalanine: The essential amino acid in all protein which a person with PKU cannot convert into useful products.

phe: A common abbreviation for phenylalanine.

Protein: Compounds made of amino acids that are essential for all living cells in the body.

Tyrosine: A non-essential amino acid present in all protein foods. In persons with PKU it becomes an essential amino acid because the enzyme necessary for its production from phenylalanine is defective.

Resources

For additional information or assistance beyond that presented in this text, the following sources are suggested:

Clinics for Treatment of PKU and Maternal PKU

A directory of the 115 PKU clinics in the United States is available in the publication:

Schuett, V.E. (1990) *National Survey of Treatment Programs for PKU and Selected Other Inherited Metabolic Diseases* (DHHS Pub. No. HRS-M-CH-89-5) which can be obtained from: National Center for Education in Maternal and Child Health, 38th and R Streets, NW, Washington, DC 20057.

The following regional contributing centers of the Maternal PKU Collaborative Study can also provide information and assistance concerning PKU and maternal PKU:

Northeast Region

Connecticut, Delaware, New Hampshire, Maine, Maryland, Massachusetts, New Jersey, New York, Pennsylvania, Rhode Island, Vermont, Virginia, West Virginia, District of Columbia.

Director: Harvey Levy, M.D.
Children's Hospital Medical Center
300 Longwood Avenue
Boston, Massachusetts 02115
Phone: (617) 735-6346

Midwest Region

Illinois, Indiana, Iowa, Kansas, Kentucky, Michigan, Minnesota, Missouri, Nebraska, North Dakota, Ohio, Oklahoma, South Dakota, Wisconsin.

Co-Directors: Reuben Matalon, M.D., Ph.D.
and Harvey Levy, M.D.
University of Illinois at Chicago
Department of Nutrition and Medical Dietetics
Mail Code 517,
College of Associate Health Professions
Chicago, Illinois 60612
Phone: (312) 996-0995

Southeast Region

Alabama, Arkansas, Florida, Georgia, Louisiana, Mississippi, North Carolina, South Carolina, Tennessee, Texas, Puerto Rico.

Director: Bobbye Rouse, M. D.
University of Texas Medical Branch
Department of Pediatrics
Galveston, Texas 77550
Phone: (409) 772-2356

Western Region

Alaska, Arizona, California, Colorado, Hawaii, Idaho, Montana, Nevada, New Mexico, Oregon, Utah, Washington, Wyoming.

Director: Richard Koch, M.D.
Co-Director: Julian Williams, M.D., Ph.D.
PKU Section, Children's Hospital of Los Angeles
4650 Sunset Boulevard
Los Angeles, California 90027
Phone: (213) 669-2152

All Provinces of Canada

Director: William B. Hanley, M.D.
The Hospital for Sick Children
555 University Avenue
Toronto, Ontario M5G 1X8, Canada
Phone: (416) 598-6356 or (416) 781-1805

Materials for Parents of Young Children with PKU

Parents' Guide to the Child with PKU. (1982, 66 pages: $8.00) Topics include understanding PKU, diet management, growth and development patterns, role of others in diet management, management of feeding and behavior problems, management of diet in special situations, future considerations. Ruth E. Pestle, Ph.D. Florida State University, Center for Family Study, 103 Sandels Bldg., Tallahassee, FL 32306-2033.

Understanding PKU. (1982, 12 pages: single copy free) Booklet created as a source of basic information concerning PKU. PKU Clinic, Children's Hospital Medical Center, 300 Longwood Avenue, Boston, MA 02115.

Living with PKU. (1990, 19 pages: single copy free) A booklet written by parents and staff, including discussion of what PKU is, the genetics and management; interviews with families; and helpful hints from experienced parents. Mead Johnson, phone (800) 222-9123.

A Babysitter's Guide to PKU. (1986, 8 pages: $2.50) An easy to understand pamphlet that helps parents discuss diet management of the child with the babysitter. Cristine M. Trahms, M.S., R.D., PKU Clinic, CDMRC WJ-10, University of Washington, Seattle, WA 98195.

Babysitters: My Child has PKU. (n.d., 9 pages: single copy free) Instructions for babysitter regarding diet. Emphasis placed on the fact that the child is like other children except for diet. Brief outline of diet with list of "free" foods. Karen M. Kinkus, R.D., Department of Pediatrics, Univ. of Louisville, Louisville, KY 40292.

The Child with PKU. (1986, 45 pages: $5.00) A booklet for parents; explains PKU, lists sources for information, supplies and assistance. PKU Section C 19, Child Development, Dept. of Pediatrics, University of Texas Medical Branch, Galveston, TX 77550.

Booklets and Videos Explaining PKU to Children and Youth

You and PKU. (1978, 50 pages: $5.00) A booklet for children ages 3 to 8 years old describing PKU and why they need to be on a special diet. Also includes suggestions for parents in teaching their child about PKU. Marketing Department, University of Wisconsin Press, 114 North Murray Street, Madison, WI 53715.

All About PKU. (1978, 18 pages: $1.50) A cartoon coloring book in which PKU and the diet are explained. This book is appropriate for 4-to 9-year-old children. (Also available in Spanish). Melanie M. Hunt, R.D., Metabolic Treatment Center, IDR 528, Children's Hospital Research Foundation, Elland and Bethesda Avenues, Cincinnati, OH 45229.

What is PKU? (n.d., 12 pages: single copy free) Children's coloring and reading book. PKU Section, Children's Hospital and Health Center, San Diego Regional Center for the Developmentally Disabled, 8001 Frost Street, San Diego, CA 92123.

Why Is Mary on a Diet? (n.d., 14 pages: single copy free) Simple explanation of the PKU diet for young children. Hazel M. Vespa, ACSW PKU Clinic, The Children's Memorial Hospital, 2300 Children's Plaza, Chicago, IL 60614.

Hidden from View: PKU and the Teenager. (n.d., 20 pages: $1.00; VHS videotape: $10.00) A booklet and video explaining PKU for teenagers. Questions answered include: What is PKU? How did I get PKU? How was I treated for PKU? Why should I think about PKU now? What can I do as a teen? Pediatric Neurology Metabolic Clinic, Box 54, C1054 Outpatient Building, University Hospital, Ann Arbor, MI 48109.

PKU and Teens: Planning Makes it Easier. (1987, 29 pages: single copy free) Designed to help teenagers with PKU learn more about PKU, its treatment and application of dietary needs to situations usually encountered by teenagers. Illinois Department of Public Health, Division of Family Health, Genetics Diseases Program, 535 West Jefferson Street, Springfield, IL 62761.

Teenagers and PKU. (1988, 18 minute VHS videotape, free on loan) Companion video to PKU and Teens booklet (above). Discusses issues teens face with respect to continuing the low phe diet; includes a segment on Maternal PKU (two weeks' notice required) Mead Johnson, phone (800) 222-9123.

Materials Concerning Maternal PKU

The Young Woman with PKU. (1986, 50 pages: $5.00) A thorough review of PKU and the required diet, with special emphasis on the problems associated with pregnancy in a woman who has PKU. PKU Treatment Center, Department of Pediatrics, University of Texas Medical Branch, C-19, Galveston, TX 77550.

Understanding Maternal PKU. (1990, 12 pages: single copy free) Booklet written to help women with PKU and their families understand Maternal PKU. Topics include basic information about Maternal PKU, description of PKU, genetics and treatment. PKU Clinic, Children's Hospital Medical Center, 300 Longwood Avenue, Boston, MA 02115.

Understanding Mild Hyperphenylalaninemia. (1986, 7 pages: single copy free) Description of the biochemistry, detection and genetics of mild hyperphenylalaninemia. PKU Clinic, Children's Hospital Medical Center, 300 Longwood Avenue, Boston, MA 02115.

Your Diet for Maternal PKU. (1987, 19 pages: single copy free) Discussion of the need for diet before conception and description of the low phe diet. (Also available in Spanish) PKU Clinic, Children's Hospital Medical Center, 300 Longwood Avenue, Boston, MA 02115.

PKU and Pregnancy. (1984, 28 pages: $3.00) A guide for women with phenylketonuria and other forms of hyperphenylalaninemia. Topics include the problem of PKU and pregnancy, preparing for pregnancy, the nature of the diet and meal planning. The Genetic Metabolic Disease Program, The Hospital for Sick Children, 555 University Ave., Toronto, Ontario M5G 1X8, CANADA

Maternal Hyperphenylalaninemia. (1984, 6 pages: single copy free) Booklet written for young women with PKU or hyperphenylalaninemia, their families and friends. PKU Clinic, St. Christopher's Hospital for Children, 2603 North 5th Street, Philadelphia, PA 19133.

Hidden from View: PKU and the Teenager (n.d., 12 minute VHS videotape: $10) A videocassette designed to draw attention to the concerns of PKU and pregnancy. Pediatric Neurology Metabolic Clinic, Box 54, C1045 Outpatient Building, University Hospital, Ann Arbor, MI 48109.

Women with PKU. (n.d., 18 pages; single copy free) Booklet written for young women with PKU, describing the California Maternal PKU project, and answering common questions about PKU and Maternal PKU. A list of all PKU clinics in California is also provided. California Maternal PKU Project, 2125 Berkeley Way, Annex 4, Room 300, Berkeley, CA 94704.

PKU, Pregnancy and You. (1987, 48 pages; single copy free) An attractively formatted 5 by 8 inch booklet for young women with PKU with extensive information concerning PKU, its genetic basis, as well as general pregnancy advice, sample diet menus, and answers to commonly asked questions. The list of PKU clinics in California is provided, together with the regional contributing centers of the Maternal PKU Collaborative Study. California Maternal PKU Project, 2125 Berkeley Way, Annex 4, Room 300. Berkeley, CA 94704.

References for Teachers and Other Professionals

A Teacher's Guide to PKU. (1985, 13 pages: $1.00) Resource book for preschool teachers and school staff; contains PKU basics, NutraSweet warning, suggestions of how teachers can help the child with PKU, questions and answers about PKU, classroom activities. Maria Nardella, M.A., R.D., Nutrition Consultant for Crippled Children's Service, Arizona Dept. of Health Services, 1740 West Adams (Room 208), Phoenix, AZ 85007.

Games that Teach. (1986, 8 pages: $2.50) For parents and teachers of preschool and kindergarten classes. Offers nutrition activities appropriate for a group of children including the child with phenylketonuria. Cristine M. Trahms, M.S., R.D., PKU Clinic, CDMRC WJ-10, University of Washington, Seattle, WA 98195.

PKU for Children: Learning to Measure. (1981, 24 pages: $3.00) "Lesson" format for parents and teachers. Goal of increased responsibility for self-management is approached through food preparation and accurate measuring. Cristine M. Trahms, M.S., R.D., PKU Clinic, CDMRC WJ-10, University of Washington, Seattle, WA 98195.

Low Protein Cookery for PKU. (1988, 569 pages: $13.75 plus $1.50 postage) Over 450 recipes plus helpful hints for managing the PKU diet. Marketing Department, University of Wisconsin Press, 114 North Murray Street, Madison, WI 53715.

Dental Health in Children with PKU. (1984, 28 pages: single copy free) Provides information for medical and dental professionals about the dental health needs of children with PKU. National Center for Education in Maternal and Child Health, 38th and R Streets, NW, Washington, DC 20057.

Screening and Treatment of PKU. (1985, slide/sound: 131 slides with a 38 minute audiotape: available for purchase: $283.80) Prepared by the staff at the Waisman Center of the University of Wisconsin, Madison, this is a comprehensive introduction to the condition. It includes an explanation of the metabolic basis for PKU, differences between treated and untreated cases, screening of newborns for PKU, and the dietary program needed to prevent damage due to excessive phenylalanine. Designed for parents and older children with PKU as well as professionals. Distribution Dept., Health Sciences Consortium, 201 Silver Cedar Court, Chapel Hill, NC 27514; phone (919) 942-8731.

References in the Professional Literature

Acosta, P.B. (1991) Phenylketonuria, impact of nutrition support on reproductive outcome. *Nutrition Today*, Jan-Feb: 43-47.

American Academy of Pediatrics (1965) Committee on the Handicapped Child: statement on treatment of phenylketonuria. *Pediatrics*, 35: 499.

American Academy of Pediatrics (1985) Committee on Genetics: Maternal Phenylketonuria. *Pediatrics*, 76 (2): 313-314.

Azen, C., Koch, R., and Friedman, E.G. (1991) Intellectual development in 12-year-old children treated for phenylketonuria. *American Journal of Diseases of Children*, 145: 35-39.

Fishler, K., Azen, C.G., Henderson, R., Friedman, E.G. and Koch, R. (1987) Psychoeducational findings among children treated for phenylketonuria. *American Journal of Mental Deficiency*, 92(1): 65-73.

Fishler, K., Azen, C.G., Friedman, E.G. and Koch, R. (1989) School achievement in treated PKU children. *Journal of Mental Deficiency Research*, 33: 493-498.

Heffernan, J. and Trahms, C. (1981) A model preschool for patients with phenylketonuria. *Journal of the American Dietetic Association*, 79: 306-308.

Holtzman, N.A., Kronmal, R.A., van Doorninck, W., Azen, C., and Koch, R. (1986) Effect of age at loss of dietary control on intellectual performance and behavior of children with phenylketonuria. *New England Journal of Medicine*, 314 (10): 593-598.

Hunt, M.M., Berry, H. and White, P.P. (1985) Phenylketonuria, adolescence and diet. *Journal of the American Dietetic Association*, 85: 1328-1334.

Koch, R., Azen, C., Friedman, E. and Williamson, M. (1984) Paired comparisons between early treated PKU children and their matched sibling controls on intelligence and school achievement test results at eight years of age. *Journal of Inherited Metabolic Diseases*, 7: 86-90.

Koch, R., Yusin, M. and Fishler, K. (1985) Successful adjustment to society by adults with phenylketonuria. *Journal of Inherited Metabolic Diseases*, 8: 209-211.

Koch, R. and Wenz, E. (1987) Phenylketonuria. *Annual Reviews in Nutrition*, 7: 117-138.

Koch, R., Hanley, W., Levy, H., Matalon, R., Rouse, B., de la Cruz, F., Azen, C., and Friedman, E. (1990) A preliminary report of the collaborative study of maternal phenylketonuria in the United States and Canada. *Journal of Inherited Metabolic Diseases*, 13: 641-650.

Lenke, R. and Levy, H. (1980) Maternal PKU and hyperphenyl-alaninemia. *New England Journal of Medicine*, 303: 1202-08.

Rees, J.M. and Trahms, C.M. (1987) The adolescent and phenylketonuria: promoting self-management. *Topics in Clinical Nutrition*, 2(3): 35-39.

Rohr, F. (1987) Maternal phenylketonuria: a new challenge in the dietary treatment of phenylketonuria. *Topics in Clinical Nutrition*, 2(3): 44-48.

Scriver, C.R. and Clow, C.L. (1980) Phenylketonuria: epitome of human biochemical genetics. *New England Journal of Medicine*, 303: 1336-42.

Trahms, C.M. (1986) Treatment of phenylketonuria. Long-term nutrition intervention model. *Topics in Clinical Nutrition*, 1: 62-72.

Williamson, M., Koch, R., Azen, C. and Chang, C. (1981) Correlates of intelligence test results in treated phenylketonuria children. *Pediatrics*, 68(2): 161-167.

Chapter 58

Wermer's Syndrome (FMEN1)

What is FMEN1?

Familial multiple endocrine neoplasia type 1 (FMEN1) is an inherited disorder that affects the endocrine glands. It is sometimes called familial multiple endocrine adenomatosis type 1 or Wermer's syndrome, after one of the first doctors to recognize it. FMEN1 is quite rare, occurring in about 3 to 20 persons out of 100,000. It affects both sexes equally and shows no geographical, racial, or ethnic preferences.

Endocrine glands are different from other organs in the body because they release hormones into the bloodstream. Hormones are powerful chemicals that travel through the blood, controlling and instructing the functions of various organs. Normally, the hormones released by endocrine glands are carefully balanced to meet the body's needs.

In patients with FMEN1, usually more than one group of endocrine glands, such as the parathyroid, the pancreas, and the pituitary become overactive at the same time. Most people who develop over activity of only one endocrine gland do not have FMEN1.

How Does FMEN1 Affect the Endocrine Glands?

The Parathyroid Glands

The parathyroids are the endocrine glands most often affected by FMEN1. The human body normally has four parathyroid glands,

NIH Pub. No. 96-3048, "Familial Multiple Endocrine Neoplasia Type I (Wermer's Syndrome," National Institute of Diabetes and Digestive and Kidney Diseases (NIDDK), at: www.niddk.nih.gov/fmen1/fmen1.html; October 1996.

which are located close to the thyroid gland in the front of the neck. The parathyroids release a chemical called parathyroid hormone, which helps maintain a normal supply of calcium in the blood, bones, and urine.

In FMEN1, all four parathyroid glands tend to be overactive. They release too much parathyroid hormone, leading to excess calcium in the blood. High blood calcium, known as hypercalcemia, can exist for many years before it is found by accident or by family screening. Unrecognized hypercalcemia can cause excess calcium to spill into the urine, leading to kidney stones or kidney damage.

Nearly everyone who inherits a susceptibility to FMEN1 will develop overactive parathyroid glands (hyperparathyroidism) by age 60, but the disorder can often be detected before age 20. Hyperparathyroidism may cause problems such as tiredness, weakness, muscle or bone pain, constipation, indigestion, kidney stones, or thinning of bones.

Treatment of Hyperparathyroidism. It is sometimes difficult to decide whether hyperparathyroidism in FMEN1 is severe enough to need treatment, especially in a person who has no symptoms. The usual treatment is an operation to remove the three largest parathyroid glands and all but a small part of the fourth. After parathyroid surgery, regular testing should continue, since the small piece of parathyroid tissue can grow back and cause recurrent hyperparathyroidism. People whose parathyroid glands have been completely removed by surgery must take daily supplements of calcium and vitamin D to prevent hypocalcemia (low blood calcium).

The Pancreas Gland

The pancreas gland, located behind the stomach, releases digestive juices into the intestines and key hormones into the bloodstream. Some hormones produced in the islet cells of the pancreas and their effects are:

- insulin—lowers blood sugar;
- glucagon—raises blood sugar;
- somatostatin—inhibits many cells.

In FMEN1, one or more tumors producing high amounts of gastrin tend to develop in the pancreas and small intestine. Gastrin is a hormone that normally circulates in the blood, causing the stomach to secrete enough acid needed for digestion. If exposed to too much gastrin, the stomach releases excess acid, leading to the formation of severe ulcers in the stomach and small intestine. Too much gastrin can also cause serious diarrhea.

About one in three patients with FMEN1 has gastrin-releasing tumors, called gastrinomas. (The illness associated with these tumors is sometimes called Zollinger-Ellison syndrome.) The ulcers caused by gastrinomas are much more dangerous than typical stomach or intestinal ulcers; left untreated, they can cause rupture of the stomach or intestine and even death.

Treatment of Gastrinomas. The gastrinomas associated with FMEN1 are difficult to cure by surgery, because it is difficult to find the multiple small gastrinomas in the pancreas and small intestine. In the past, the standard treatment for gastrinomas was the surgical removal of the entire stomach to prevent acid production. Recently, however, researchers have identified very powerful blockers of stomach acid release, called acid pump inhibitors. Taken by mouth, these have proven effective in controlling most cases of Zollinger-Ellison syndrome.

The Pituitary Gland

The pituitary is a small gland inside the head, behind the bridge of the nose. Though small, it produces many important hormones that regulate basic body functions. The major pituitary hormones and their effects are:

- prolactin—controls formation of breast milk, influences fertility, and influences bone strength;

- growth hormone—regulates body growth, especially during adolescence;

- adrenocorticotropin (ACTH)—stimulates the adrenal glands to produce cortisol;

- thyrotropin (TSH)—stimulates the thyroid gland to produce thyroid hormones;

- luteinizing hormone (LH)—stimulates the ovaries or testes to produce sex hormones that determine many features of "maleness" or "femaleness"; and

- follicle stimulating hormone (FSH)—regulates fertility in men through sperm production and in women through ovulation.

The pituitary gland becomes overactive in about one of six persons with FMEN1. This over activity can usually be traced to very small, benign tumors in the gland that release too much prolactin, called prolactinomas. High prolactin can cause excessive production of breast milk or it can interfere with fertility in women or with sex drive and fertility in men.

Treatment of Prolactinomas. Most prolactinomas are small, and treatment may not be needed. If treatment is needed, a very effective type of medicine known as a dopamine agonist can lower the production of prolactin and shrink the prolactinoma. Occasionally, prolactinomas do not respond well to this medication. In such cases, surgery, radiation, or both may be needed.

Rare Complications of FMEN1

Occasionally, a person who has FMEN1 develops islet tumors of the pancreas that secrete high levels of pancreatic hormones other than gastrin. Insulinomas, for example, produce too much insulin, causing serious low blood sugar, or hypoglycemia. Tumors that secrete too much glucagon or somatostatin can cause diabetes, and too much vasoactive intestinal peptide can cause watery diarrhea.

Other rare complications arise from pituitary tumors that release high amounts of ACTH, which in turn stimulates the adrenal glands to produce excess cortisol. Pituitary tumors that produce growth hormone cause excessive bone growth or disfigurement.

Another rare complication is an endocrine tumor inside the chest or in the stomach, known as a carcinoid. In general, surgery is the mainstay of treatment for all of these rare types of tumors, except for gastric carcinoids which usually require no treatment.

Are the Tumors Associated With FMEN1 Cancerous?

The overactive endocrine glands associated with FMEN1 may contain benign tumors, but usually they do not have any signs of cancer. Benign tumors can disrupt normal function by releasing hormones or by crowding nearby tissue. For example, a prolactinoma may become quite large in people with FMEN1. As it grows, the tumor can press against and damage the normal part of the pituitary gland or the nerves that carry vision from the eyes. Sometimes impaired vision is the first sign of a pituitary tumor in FMEN1.

Another type of benign tumor often seen in people with FMEN1 is a plum-sized, fatty tumor called a lipoma, which grows under the skin. Lipomas cause no health problems and can be removed by simple cosmetic surgery if desired. These tumors are also fairly common in the general population.

Benign tumors do not spread to or invade other parts of the body. Cancer cells, by contrast, break away from the primary tumor and spread, or metastasize, to other parts of the body through the bloodstream or lymphatic system.

The pancreatic islet cell tumors associated with FMEN1 tend to be numerous and small, but most are benign and do not release active hormones into the blood. A proportion of pancreatic islet cell tumors in FMEN1 are cancerous.

Treatment of Pancreatic Endocrine Cancer in FMEN1. Since the type of pancreatic endocrine cancer associated with FMEN1 can be difficult to recognize, difficult to treat, and very slow to progress, doctors have different views about the value of surgery in managing these tumors.

One approach is to "watch and wait," using medical, or nonsurgical treatments. According to this school of thought, pancreatic surgery has serious complications, so it should not be attempted unless it will cure a tumor that is secreting too much hormone.

Another school advocates early surgery, perhaps when a tumor grows to a certain size, to remove pancreatic endocrine cancers in FMEN1 before they spread and become dangerous. There is no clear evidence, however, that aggressive surgery to prevent pancreatic endocrine cancer from spreading actually leads to longer survival for patients with FMEN1.

Doctors agree that excessive release of certain hormones (such as gastrin) from pancreatic endocrine cancer in FMEN1 needs to be treated, and medications are often effective in blocking the effects of these hormones. Some tumors, such as insulin-producing tumors of the pancreas, are usually benign and single and are curable by pancreatic surgery. Such surgery needs to be considered carefully in each patient's case.

Is FMEN1 the Same in Everyone?

Although FMEN1 tends to follow certain patterns, it can affect a person's health in many different ways. Not only do the features of FMEN1 vary among members of the same family, but some families with FMEN1 tend to have a higher rate of prolactin-secreting pituitary tumors and a much lower frequency of gastrin-secreting pancreatic tumors.

In addition, the age at which FMEN1 can begin to cause endocrine gland over function can differ strikingly from one family member to another. One person may have only mild hyperparathyroidism beginning at age 50, while a relative may develop complications from tumors of the parathyroid, pancreas, and pituitary by age 20.

Can FMEN1 Be Cured?

There is no cure for FMEN1 itself, but most of the health problems caused by FMEN1 can be recognized at an early stage and controlled or treated before they become serious problems.

If you have been diagnosed with FMEN1, it is important to get periodic checkups because FMEN1 can affect different glands, and even after treatment, residual tissue can grow back. Careful monitoring enables your doctor to adjust your treatment as needed and to check for any new disturbances caused by FMEN1.

How Is FMEN1 Detected?

Each of us has millions of genes in each of our cells, which determine how our cells and bodies function. In people with FMEN1, there is a mutation, or mistake, in one gene. A carrier is a person who has the FMEN1 gene mutation. The FMEN1 gene mutation is transmitted directly to a child from a parent carrying the gene.

In the next few years, scientists hope to develop a simple test that will identify the abnormal FMEN1 gene. Such a test would be given once in a person's lifetime to find out whether he or she has inherited the FMEN1 gene.

In the meantime, though, screening of close relatives of persons with FMEN1, who are at high risk, generally involves testing for hyperparathyroidism, the most common and usually the earliest sign of FMEN1. Any doctor can screen for hyperparathyroidism by testing the blood for calcium and sometimes one or two other substances such as ionized calcium and parathyroid hormone. An abnormal result indicates that the person probably has FMEN1, but a normal finding cannot rule out the chance that he or she will develop hyperparathyroidism at a later time. Blood testing can usually show signs of early hyperparathyroidism many years before symptoms of hyperparathyroidism occur.

Why Screen for FMEN1?

FMEN1 is not an infectious or contagious disease, nor is it caused by environmental factors. Because FMEN1 is a genetic disorder inherited from one parent, and its transmission pattern is well understood, family members at high risk for the disorder can be easily identified.

Testing can detect the blood chemical problems caused by FMEN1 many years before these complications develop. Finding these hormonal imbalances early enables your doctor to begin preventive treatment, reducing the chances that FMEN1 will cause problems later.

Who Should Be Screened for FMEN1?

Close relatives of persons with FMEN1, such as parents, brothers, sisters, and children have a 50 percent risk of having inherited the FMEN1 gene, and they should be screened. Though the abnormal gene is present before birth, it tends to become evident at varying ages and in different organs. A "silent" carrier has the gene but has not yet shown any hormonal disturbance caused by the gene. Periodic testing may also be considered in people whose nearest affected relative is a grandparent, uncle, or aunt (that is, a second-degree relative), if there is reason to believe that the parent may be a silent FMEN1 gene-carrier.

When and How Often Should Screening Be Done?

Hyperparathyroidism, most often the first sign of FMEN1, can usually be detected by blood tests between the ages of 15 and 50. Periodic testing should begin around age 10 and be repeated every year. There is no age at which periodic testing should stop, since doctors cannot rule out the chance that a person has inherited the FMEN1 gene. However, a person with normal testing beyond age 50 is very unlikely to have inherited the FMEN1 gene.

Should a Person Who Has FMEN1 Avoid Having Children?

A person who has FMEN1 may have a hard time deciding whether to have a child. No one can make this decision for anyone else, but some of the important facts can be summarized as follows:

- A man or a woman with FMEN1 has a 50-50 risk with each pregnancy of having a child with FMEN1. At present, it is difficult to detect FMEN1 before birth or even before age 15.

- FMEN1 tends to fit a broad pattern within a given family, but the severity of the disorder varies widely from one family member to another. In particular, a parent's experience with FMEN1 cannot be used to predict the severity of FMEN1 in a child.

- FMEN1 is a problem that does not usually develop until adulthood. Treatment may require regular monitoring and considerable expense, but the disease usually does not prevent an active, productive adulthood.

- Prolactin-releasing tumors in a man or woman may inhibit fertility and make it difficult to conceive. Also, hyperparathyroidism in a woman during pregnancy may raise the risks of complications for mother and child.

Research in FMEN1

The National Institute of Diabetes and Digestive and Kidney Diseases (NIDDK) was established by Congress in 1950 as part of the National Institutes of Health (NIH), whose mission is to improve human health through biomedical research. The NIH is the research arm of the Public Health Service under the U.S. Department of Health and Human Services.

The NIDDK conducts and supports a variety of research in endocrine disorders, including FMEN1. Researchers have begun to locate the FMEN1 gene by showing that it is on chromosome 11. Researchers have also suggested that the FMEN1 gene contributes to common endocrine tumors outside of the familial setting.

Additional Information

After reading this chapter, you may think of questions that you would like answered. Some sources of additional information are medical textbooks, physicians, nurses, and genetic counselors. Genetic counseling can help couples through the decision-making process about family planning. Genetic counselors provide information but do not tell anyone what to do.

The following articles about FMEN1 can be found in medical libraries, some college and university libraries, and through interlibrary loan in most public libraries.

Metz, D. C., Jensen, R. T., Bale, A., Skarulis, M.C., Eastman, R.C., Nieman, L., Norton, J.A. Friedman, E., Larson, C., Amorosi, A., Brandi, M.L., Marx, S.J., "Multiple endocrine neoplasia type 1: Clinical features and management," in *The Parathyroids*, ed by Bilezekian, J.P., Levine, M.A., and Marcus R. Raven Press, 1994, 591–646.

Friedman, E., Larsson, C., Amorosi, A., Brandi, M.L., Bale, A., Metz, D., Jensen, R.T., Skarulis, M., Eastman, R.C., Nieman, L., Norton, J.A., Marx, S.J., "Multiple endocrine neoplasia type 1: Pathology, pathophysiology, and differential diagnosis," in Bilezekian et al, 647–680.

Other Resources

The following organizations might also be able to assist with certain types of information:

Office of Health Research Reports
National Institute of Diabetes and Digestive and Kidney Diseases
Building 31, Room 9A04
Bethesda, MD 20892

March of Dimes/Birth Defects Foundation
1275 Mamaroneck Avenue
White Plains, NY 10605
(914) 428-7100

Alliance for Genetic Support Groups
35 Wisconsin Circle, Suite 440
Chevy Chase, MD 20815
1-800-336-GENE or (301) 652-5553

—by Stephen J. Marx, M.D.
and Robert T. Jensen, M.D.

Index

Index

testes (testicles), continued
  formation 15
  hormones 272
    see also testosterone
  location *271*
  removal (castration, orchiectomy) 3
testicles *see* testes
testicular cancer
  steroid hormones 13
Testoderm 336
testosterone 16, 255, 325–26
  anabolic steroids 18–19
  hormone receptors 6
  skin patches 336
tests
  bilateral inferior petrosal sinus
    sampling 309–10
  Cushing's disease 219, 223–26
  diabetes 99, 106–7
  Diabetes Control and Complications
    Trial (DCCT) 76, 83–84, 91–93
  Diabetes Prevention Trial-Type 1
    75, 91–93
  endoscopic retrograde
    cholangiopancreatography
    (ERCP) 58
  galactose tolerance 450
  glucose tolerance 50, 99, 122–23,
    146, 189, 292
  glycosylated hemoglobin 107
  growth hormone deficiency 273–74
  Hashimoto's disease 408
  hemoglobin A1c test 81
  hormone levels 7
  hypothyroidism 396–97
  islet cell cancer 66
  pancreatitis 55
  percutaneous transhepatic cholang-
    iography (PTC) 58
  thyroid disorders 355–60
  water deprivation 309
  see also animal studies; blood tests;
    individual disorder diagnoses;
    urine tests
thirst, increased
  Cushing's syndrome 218
  insulin-dependent diabetes 75–76
  noninsulin-dependent diabetes mel-
    litus 97, 111

Thorner, Michael O. 334
Thryolar 337
thyroid cancer 352, 411–17
  follicular 413–14
  nodules (lumps) 419–22
    diagnosis 420–21
    treatment 421
  overview 346
  papillary 412–13
  well-differentiated 412–15
thyroid disorders 343–440
  additional information 347
  described 349–53
  research 25, 43, 353
  symptoms 355
  treatment 352, 370
  treatments 355–60
  see also Grave's disease;
    Hashimoto's disease; hyperthy-
    roidism; hypothyroidism; hyper-
    parathyroidism; thyroid cancer;
    thyroiditis
The Thyroid Foundation of America,
  Inc. 43, 347, 417
thyroid gland 3–4, 255
  described 349, 355, 371, 375, 397,
    405–6
  location *271*
  overview 343–47
  underactive 343, 399
  see also parathyroid glands
thyroid hormone deficiency 265, 343
thyroid hormones 12, 254, 349, 356,
  397
  see also triiodothyronine (T3); thy-
    roxine (T4)
thyroid nodules (lumps) 345–46, 419–
  22
"Thyroid Signpost" (Thyroid Society
  for Education and Research) 387
Thyroid Society for Education and
  Research 43, 353, 360, 369n, 372,
  376, 387, 398, 406, 422
thyroid stimulating hormone (TSH)
  254, 271, 300, 308, 313, 343–47,
  356, 375, 396, 416
thyroidectomy 359–60, 379, 389, 393–
  94, 401, 421

Environmentally Induced Disorders Sourcebook

Basic Information about Diseases and Syndromes Linked to Exposure to Pollutants and Other Substances in Outdoor and Indoor Environments Such As Lead, Asbestos, Formaldehyde, Mercury, Emissions, Noise, and More

Edited by Allan R. Cook. 620 pages. 1997. 0-7808-0083-4. $75.

Fitness & Exercise Sourcebook

Basic Information on Fitness and Exercise, Including Fitness Activities for Specific Age Groups, Exercise for People with Specific Medical Conditions, How to Begin a Fitness Program in Running, Walking, Swimming, Cycling, and Other Athletic Activities, and Recent Research in Fitness and Exercise

Edited by Dan R. Harris. 663 pages. 1996. 0-7808-0186-5. $75.

Food & Animal Borne Diseases Sourcebook

Basic Information about Diseases That Can Be Spread to Humans through the Ingestion of Contaminated Food or Water or by Contact with Infected Animals and Insects, Such As Botulism, E. Coli, Hepatitis A, Trichinosis, Lyme Disease, and Rabies, along with Information Regarding Prevention and Treatment Methods, and a Special Section for International Travelers Describing Diseases Such as Cholera, Malaria, Travelers' Diarrhea, and Yellow Fever, and Offering Recommendations for Avoiding Illness

Edited by Karen Bellenir and Peter D. Dresser. 535 pages. 1995. 0-7808-0033-8. $75.

"A comprehensive collection of authoritative information." — *Emergency Medical Services, Oct '95*

"Targeting general readers and providing them with a single, comprehensive source of information on selected topics, this book continues, with the excellent caliber of its predecessors, to catalog topical information on health matters of general interest. Readable and thorough, this valuable resource is highly recommended for all libraries."
— *Academic Library Book Review, Summer '96*

Gastrointestinal Diseases & Disorders Sourcebook

Basic Information about Gastroesophageal Reflux Disease (Heartburn), Ulcers, Diverticulosis, Irritable Bowel Syndrome, Crohn's Disease, Ulcerative Colitis, Diarrhea, Constipation, Lactose Intolerance, Hemorrhoids, Hepatitis, Cirrhosis and Other Digestive Problems, Featuring Statistics, Descriptions of Symptoms, and Current Treatment Methods of Interest for Persons Living with Upper and Lower Gastrointestinal Maladies

Edited by Linda M. Ross. 413 pages. 1996. 0-7808-0078-8. $75.

". . . very readable form. The successful editorial work that brought this material together into a useful and understandable reference makes accessible to all readers information that can help them more effectively understand and obtain help for digestive tract problems." — *Choice, Feb '97*

Genetic Disorders Sourcebook

Basic Information about Heritable Diseases and Disorders Such As Down Syndrome, PKU, Hemophilia, Von Willebrand Disease, Gaucher Disease, Tay-Sachs Disease, and Sickle-Cell Disease, along with Information about Genetic Screening, Gene Therapy, Home Care, and Including Source Listings for Further Help and Information on More Than 300 Disorders

Edited by Karen Bellenir. 642 pages. 1996. 0-7808-0034-6. $75.

". . . geared toward the lay public. It would be well placed in all public libraries and in those hospital and medical libraries in which access to genetic references is limited."
— *Doody's Health Sciences Book Review, Oct '96*

"Provides essential medical information to both the general public and those diagnosed with a serious or fatal genetic disease or disorder."
— *Choice, Jan '97*

Head Trauma Sourcebook

Basic Information for the Layperson about Open-Head and Closed-Head Injuries, Treatment Advances, Recovery, and Rehabilitation, along with Reports on Current Research Initiatives

Edited by Karen Bellenir. 414 pages. 1997. 0-7808-0208-X. $75.

Health Insurance Sourcebook

Basic Information about Managed Care Organizations, Traditional Fee-for-Service Insurance, Insurance Portability and Pre-Existing Conditions Clauses, Medicare, Medicaid, Social Security, and Military Health Care, along with Information about Insurance Fraud

Edited by Wendy Wilcox. 530 pages. 1997. 0-7808-0222-5. $75.

Continues next page

Immune System Disorders Sourcebook

Basic Information about Lupus, Multiple Sclerosis, Guillain-Barré Syndrome, Chronic Granulomatous Disease, and More, along with Statistical and Demographic Data and Reports on Current Research Initiatives

Edited by Allan R. Cook. 608 pages. 1997. 0-7808-0209-8. $75.

■

Kidney & Urinary Tract Diseases &Disorders Sourcebook

Basic Information about Kidney Stones, Urinary Incontinence, Bladder Disease, End-Stage Renal Disease, Dialysis, and More, along with Statistical and Demographic Data and Reports on Current Research Initiatives

Edited by Linda M. Ross. 602 pages. 1997. 0-7808-0079-6. $75.

■

Learning Disabilities Sourcebook

Basic Information about Disorders Such As Autism, Dyslexia, Hyperactivity, and Attention Deficit Disorder, along with Statistical and Demographic Data and Reports on Current Research Initiatives

Edited by Linda M. Ross. 600 pages. 1998. 0-7808-0210-1. $75.

■

Men's Health Concerns Sourcebook

Basic Information about Topics of Special Interest to Men, Including Prostate Enlargement, Impotence and Other Sexual Dysfunctions, Vasectomies, Condoms, Snoring, Sleep Apnea, Hair Loss, and More

Edited by Allan R. Cook. 600 pages. 1998. 0-7808-0212-8. $75.

■

Mental Health Disorders Sourcebook

Basic Information about Schizophrenia, Depression, Bipolar Disorder, Panic Disorder, Obsessive-Compulsive Disorder, Phobias and Other Anxiety Disorders, Paranoia and Other Personality Disorders, Eating Disorders, and Sleep Disorders, along with Information about Treatment and Therapies

Edited by Karen Bellenir. 548 pages. 1995. 0-7808-0040-0. $75.

"... provides information on a wide range of mental disorders, presented in nontechnical language."
— *Exceptional Child Education Resources, Spring '96*

"The text is well organized and adequately written for its target audience."
— *Choice, Jun '96*

"The great strengths of the book are its readability and its inclusion of places to find more information. Especially recommended." — *RQ, Winter '96*

"Recommended for public and academic libraries."
— *Reference Book Review, '96*

"... useful for public and academic libraries and consumer health collections."
— *Medical Reference Services Quarterly, Spring '97*

■

Ophthalmic Disorders Sourcebook

Basic Information about Glaucoma, Cataracts, Macular Degeneration, Strabismus, Refractive Disorders, and More, along with Statistical and Demographic Data and Reports on Current Research Initiatives

Edited by Linda M. Ross. 631 pages. 1996. 0-7808-0081-8. $75.

■

Oral Health Sourcebook

Basic Information about Diseases and Conditions Affecting Oral Health, Including Cavities, Gum Disease, Dry Mouth, Oral Cancers, Fever Blisters, Canker Sores, Oral Thrush, Bad Breath, Temporomandibular Disorders, and other Craniofacial Syndromes, along with Statistical Data on the Oral Health of Americans, Oral Hygiene, Emergency First Aid, Information on Treatment Procedures and Methods of Replacing Lost Teeth

Edited by Allan R. Cook. 560 pages. 1997. 0-7808-0082-6. $75.

■

Pain Sourcebook

Basic Information about Specific Forms of Acute and Chronic Pain, Including Headaches, Back Pain, Muscular Pain, Neuralgia, Surgical Pain, and Cancer Pain, along with Pain Relief Options Such As Analgesics, Narcotics, Nerve Blocks, Transcutaneous Nerve Stimulation, and Alternative Forms of Pain Control, Including Biofeedback, Imaging, Behavior Modification, and Relaxation Techniques

Edited by Allan R. Cook. 608 pages. 1997. 0-7808-0213-6. $75.

■

Pregnancy & Birth Sourcebook

Basic Information about Planning for Pregnancy, Fetal Growth and Development, Labor and Delivery, Postpartum and Perinatal Care, Pregnancy in Mothers with Special Concerns, and Disorders of Pregnancy, Including Genetic Counseling, Nutrition and Exercise, Obstetrical Tests, Pregnancy Discomfort, Multiple Births, Cesarean Sections, Medical Testing of Newborns, Breastfeeding, Gestational Diabetes, and Ectopic Pregnancy

Edited by Heather Aldred. 752 pages. 1997. 0-7808-0216-0. $75.